PHYSICAL DIAGNOSIS OF PAIN

AN ATLAS OF SIGNS
AND SYMPTOMS

3rd Edition

PHYSICAL DIAGNOSIS OF PAIN

AN ATLAS OF SIGNS AND SYMPTOMS

STEVEN D. WALDMAN, MD, JD

Chairman and Professor
Department of Medical Humanities and Bioethics
Clinical Professor of Anesthesiology
University of Missouri–Kansas City School of Medicine
Kansas City, Missouri

ELSEVIER

ELSEVIER

3251 Riverport Lane
St. Louis, Missouri 63043

PHYSICAL DIAGNOSIS OF PAIN: AN ATLAS OF SIGNS
AND SYMPTOMS, Third Edition

ISBN: 978-0-323-37748-5

Notices

Knowledge and best practice in this field are constantly changing. As new research and experience broaden
our understanding, changes in research methods, professional practices, or medical treatment may become
necessary.

Practitioners and researchers must always rely on their own experience and knowledge in evaluating and
using any information, methods, compounds, or experiments described herein. In using such information or
methods they should be mindful of their own safety and the safety of others, including parties for whom they
have a professional responsibility.

With respect to any drug or pharmaceutical products identified, readers are advised to check the most
current information provided (i) on procedures featured or (ii) by the manufacturer of each product to be
administered, to verify the recommended dose or formula, the method and duration of administration, and
contraindications. It is the responsibility of practitioners, relying on their own experience and knowledge of
their patients, to make diagnoses, to determine dosages and the best treatment for each individual patient,
and to take all appropriate safety precautions.

To the fullest extent of the law, neither the Publisher nor the authors, contributors, or editors assume any
liability for any injury and/or damage to persons or property as a matter of products liability, negligence or
otherwise, or from any use or operation of any methods, products, instructions, or ideas contained in the
material herein.

Library of Congress Cataloging-in-Publication Data
Waldman, Steven D., author.
  Physical diagnosis of pain : an atlas of signs and symptoms / Steven D. Waldman.—Third edition.
    p. ; cm.
  Includes index.
  ISBN 978-0-323-37748-5 (hardcover)
  I. Title.
  [DNLM: 1. Musculoskeletal Diseases—diagnosis—Atlases. 2. Pain—diagnosis—Atlases. 3. Physical
Examination—methods—Atlases. WE 17]
  RC925.7
  616.7′07540223—dc23

2015032343

Publishing Manager: Michael Houston
Content Development Manager: Margaret Nelson
Publishing Services Manager: Catherine Jackson
Senior Project Manager: Clay S. Broeker
Design Direction: Amy Buxton

Working together
to grow libraries in
developing countries

www.elsevier.com • www.bookaid.org

Printed in Canada

Last digit is the print number: 9 8 7 6 5 4 3 2 1

Every Long Journey Begins with a First Step
Confucius

*This book is dedicated to my children—
David Mayo, Corey, Jennifer, and Reid—
all of whom are sick of hearing me invoke the above quote …
but have nevertheless steadfastly followed its timeless wisdom
in their daily lives!*

Preface

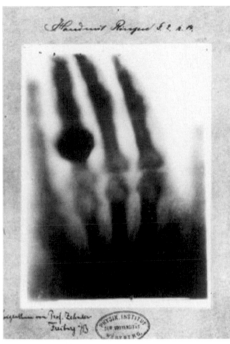

"I knew it was too good to be true ... some things never change!"
(From Kaplan EL, Mhoon D, Kaplan SP, Angelos P. Radiation-induced thyroid cancer: The Chicago experience. *Surgery* 146:979, 2009.)

While it's true that I hadn't quite finished medical school when Wilhelm Roentgen took an x-ray of his wife's hand, there is no doubt in my mind that this simple act forever changed the way medicine would be practiced. (Rumor has it he was actually trying to find a way to make her wedding ring disappear rather than diagnosis anything, as he was in love with his much younger and sexier x-ray tech!) Be that as it may, from that point on, physicians have constantly been looking for a way to make the diagnosis without actually examining the patient. X-ray gave way to fluoroscopy, which gave way to computerized tomography, which gave way to ultrasound, which gave way to magnetic resonance imaging, which has recently given way to PET scanning. Each modality's initial promise of an easier way to make the diagnosis always seemed to fall short of the mark. Yet hope springs eternal in the human breast, and many hope that rather than medical imaging, it will be the human genome that finally releases the medical profession from actually having to examine the patient!

In our perennial search for a less up close and personal way to come up with what's wrong with the patient, we must constantly be reminded that "some things never change" ... and one of those things is the amazing clinical utility of the properly taken history and properly performed physical examination. Yes, we actually have to touch the patient. Yes, we actually have to exert some effort. However, can you think of anything that has a higher yield for the patient and physician alike? I certainly can't.

In reviewing the Prefaces for the first and second editions of this text, I was struck by the spot-on accuracy of the musing of the great baseball player Yogi Berra when he said, "It's like déjà vu all over again!" Put another way, when all else fails ... EXAMINE THE PATIENT!

Steven D. Waldman
Summer 2015

Contents

Section 6: The Chest Wall, Thorax, and Thoracic Spine

Section 7: The Lumbar Spine

Section 8: The Abdominal Wall and Pelvis

Section 9: The Hip

Section 10: The Knee

Section 11: The Ankle and Foot

Video Contents

SECTION 1

The Cervical Spine

1 Functional Anatomy of the Bony Cervical Spine

THE VERTEBRAE OF THE CERVICAL SPINE

To fully understand the functional anatomy of the cervical spine and the role its unique characteristics play in the evolution of the myriad painful conditions that have the cervical spine as their nidus, one must first recognize that unlike the thoracic and lumbar spine, whose functional units are quite similar, the cervical spine must be thought of as being composed of two distinct and dissimilar functional units. The first type of functional unit consists of the atlanto-occipital unit and the atlantoaxial units (Figs. 1-1 and 1-2). While these units help to provide structural static support for the head, they are uniquely adapted to their

primary function of facilitating focused movement of the head to allow the optimal functioning of the eyes, ears, nose, and throat. The uppermost two functional units are susceptible to trauma and the inflammatory arthritides as well as to the degenerative changes that occur as a result of the aging process.

The second type of functional unit that makes up the cervical spine is very similar to the functional units of the thoracic and lumbar spine and serves primarily as a structural support for the head and secondarily functions to aid in the positioning of the sense organs located in the head (Fig. 1-3, *A-C*). Disruption of this second type of functional unit, which comprises the lower five cervical vertebrae and

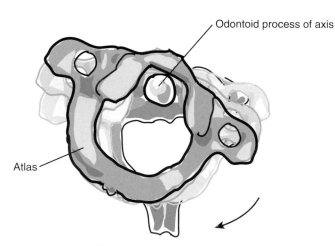

• **Figure 1-1** Atlanto-occipital unit.

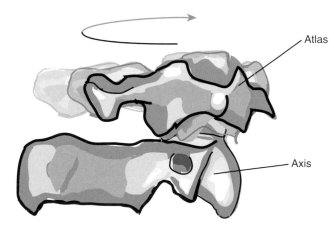

• **Figure 1-2** Atlantoaxial unit.

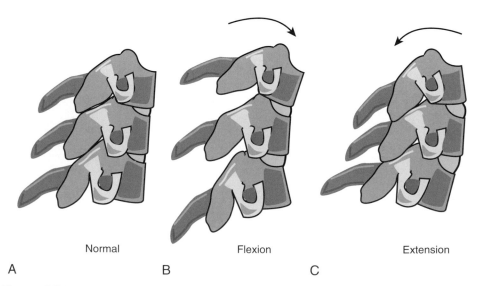

• **Figure 1-3** Functional units of the cervical spine in normal **(A)**, flexed **(B)**, and extended **(C)** positions.

their corresponding intervertebral discs, is responsible for the majority of painful conditions encountered in clinical practice (see Chapter 15).

THE MOBILITY OF THE CERVICAL SPINE

The cervical spine has the greatest range of motion of the entire spinal column and allows movement in all planes. Its greatest movement occurs from the atlanto-occipital joint to the third cervical vertebra. Movement of the cervical spine occurs as a synchronized effort of the entire cervical spine and its associated musculature, with the upper two cervical segments providing the greatest contribution to rotation, flexion, extension, and lateral bending. During flexion of the cervical spine, the spinal canal is lengthened, the intervertebral foramina become larger, and the anterior portion of the intervertebral disc becomes compressed (Fig. 1-3, B). During extension of the cervical spine, the spinal canal becomes shortened, the intervertebral foramina become smaller, and the posterior portion of the anterior disc becomes compressed (Fig. 1-3, C). With lateral bending or rotation, the contralateral intervertebral foramina become larger, while the ipsilateral intervertebral foramina become smaller. In health, none of these changes in size results in

functional disability or pain; however, in disease, these movements may result in nerve impingement with its attendant pain and functional disability.

THE CERVICAL VERTEBRAL CANAL

The bony cervical vertebral canal serves as a protective conduit for the spinal cord and as an exit point of the cervical nerve roots. Owing to the bulging of the cervical neuromeres as well as the other fibers that must traverse the cervical vertebral canal to reach the lower portions of the body, the cervical spinal cord occupies a significantly greater proportion of the space available in the spinal canal relative to the space occupied by the thoracic and lumbar spinal cord. This decreased space results in less shock-absorbing effect of the spinal fluid during trauma and also results in compression of the cervical spinal cord with attendant myelopathy when bone or intervertebral disc compromises the spinal canal (Fig. 1-4). Such encroachment of the cervical cord by degenerative changes or disc herniation can occur over a period of time, and the resultant loss of neurologic function due to myelopathy can be subtle; as a result, a delay in diagnosis is not uncommon.

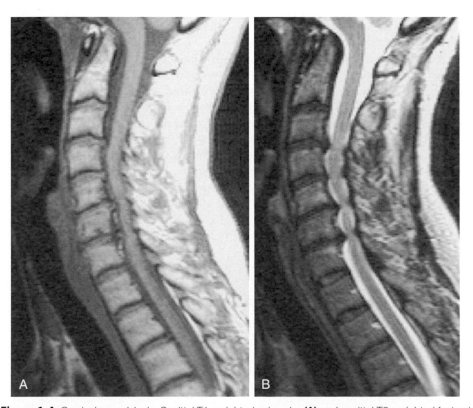

• **Figure 1-4** Cervical spondylosis. Sagittal T1-weighted spin echo **(A)** and sagittal T2-weighted fast spin echo **(B)** magnetic resonance images of the cervical spine demonstrate disc degeneration at essentially every cervical level, in addition to loss of disc space height and, in **B,** diminished signal intensity. Severe central canal stenosis is related to both anterior disc herniation with osteophytes and posterior ligamentous hypertrophy at most of the cervical levels. A focal area of high signal intensity within the cord at the C5-C6 level reflects posttraumatic myelomalacia. (From Resnick D, Kransdorf MJ, editors: *Bone and joint imaging*, ed 3, Philadelphia, 2005, Saunders, p 147.)

The cervical vertebral canal is funnel-shaped, with its largest diameter at the atlantoaxial space and progressing to its narrowest point at the C5-C6 interspace. It is not surprising that this narrow point serves as the nidus of many painful conditions of the cervical spine. The shape of the cervical vertebral canal in humans is triangular but is subject to much anatomic variability among patients. Those patients with a more trifoil shape generally are more susceptible to cervical radiculopathy in the face of any pathologic process that narrows the cervical vertebral canal or negatively affects the normal range of motion of the cervical spine.

THE CERVICAL NERVES AND THEIR RELATION TO THE CERVICAL VERTEBRAE

The cervical nerve roots are each composed of fibers from a dorsal root that carries primarily sensory information and a ventral root that carries primarily motor information. As the dorsal and ventral contributions to the cervical nerve roots move away from the cervical spinal cord, they coalesce into a single anatomic structure that becomes the individual cervical nerve roots. As these coalescing nerve fibers pass through the intervertebral foramen, they give off small branches, with the anterior portion of the nerve providing innervation to the anterior pseudo-joint of Luschka and the annulus of the disc and the posterior portion of the nerve providing innervation to the zygapophyseal joints of each adjacent vertebra between which the nerve root is exiting. These nerve fibers are thought to carry pain impulses from these anatomic structures, and this notion of the intervertebral disc and zygapophyseal joint as distinct pain generators diverges from the more conventional view of the compressed spinal nerve root as the sole source of pain emanating from the cervical spine. As the nerve fibers exit the intervertebral foramen, they fully coalesce into a single nerve root and travel forward and downward into the protective gutter made up of the transverse process of the vertebral body to provide innervation to the head, neck, and upper extremities (Fig. 1-5).

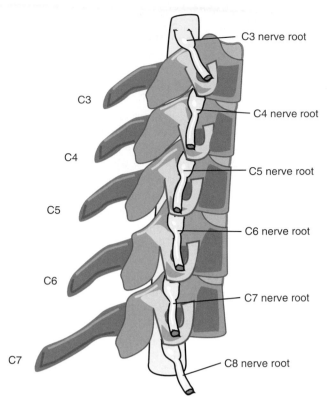

•**Figure 1-5** Position of cervical nerves relative to cervical vertebrae.

IMPLICATIONS FOR THE CLINICIAN

The bony cervical spine is a truly amazing anatomic structure in terms of both its structure and its function. The two uppermost segments of the cervical spine are vitally important to a human's day-to-day safety and survival, but with the exception of cervicogenic and tension-type headaches, they are not the source of the majority of painful conditions involving the cervical spine that are commonly encountered in clinical practice. However, the lower five segments provide ample opportunity for the evolution of myriad common painful complaints, most notably cervical radiculopathy and cervicalgia, including cervical facet syndrome.

2 Functional Anatomy of the Cervical Intervertebral Disc

The cervical intervertebral disc has two major functions: (1) to serve as the major shock-absorbing structure of the cervical spine and (2) to facilitate the synchronized movement of the cervical spine while at the same time helping to prevent impingement of the neural structures and vasculature that traverse the cervical spine. Both the shock-absorbing function and the movement and protective function of the cervical intervertebral disc are a function of the disc's structure as well as the laws of physics that affect it.

To understand how the cervical intervertebral disc functions in health and becomes dysfunctional in disease, it is useful to think of the disc as a closed, fluid-filled container. The outside of the container is made up of a top and a bottom called the endplates, which are composed of relatively inflexible hyaline cartilage. The sides of the cervical intervertebral disc are made up of a woven crisscrossing matrix of fibroelastic fibers that tightly attaches to the top and bottom endplates. This woven matrix of fibers is called the annulus, and it completely surrounds the sides of the disc (Fig. 2-1). The interlaced structure of the annulus results in an enclosing mesh that is extremely strong yet at the same time very flexible, which facilitates the compression of the disc during the wide range of motion of the cervical spine (Fig. 2-2).

Inside this container of the top and bottom endplates and surrounding annulus is water that contains a mucopolysaccharide gel-like substance called the nucleus pulposus (see Fig. 2-1). The nucleus is incompressible and transmits any pressure placed on one portion of the disc to the surrounding nucleus. In health, the water-filled gel creates a positive intradiscal pressure that forces the adjacent vertebrae apart and helps to protect the spinal cord and exiting nerve roots. When the cervical spine moves, the incompressible nature of the nucleus propulsus maintains a constant intradiscal pressure, while some fibers of the disc relax and others contract.

As the cervical intervertebral disc ages, it becomes less vascular and loses its ability to absorb water into the disc. This results in a degradation of the disc's shock-absorbing and motion-facilitating functions. This problem is made worse by degeneration of the annulus, which allows portions of the disc wall to bulge, distorting the ability of the nucleus pulposus to evenly distribute the forces placed on it through the entire disc. This exacerbates the disc dysfunction and can contribute to further disc deterioration, which can ultimately lead to actual complete disruption of the annulus and extrusion of the nucleus as well as render the disc more susceptible to damage from even minor trauma (Fig. 2-3; also see Chapter 3). The deterioration of the disc is responsible for many of the painful conditions that emanate from the cervical spine that are encountered in clinical practice (see Chapter 15).

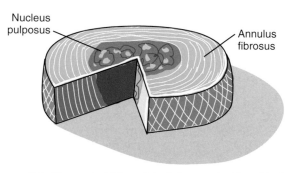

•**Figure 2-1** The cervical intervertebral disc can be thought of as a closed, fluid-filled container.

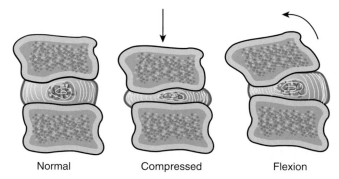

•**Figure 2-2** The cervical intervertebral disc is a strong yet flexible structure, shown here in the range of motion of the cervical spine.

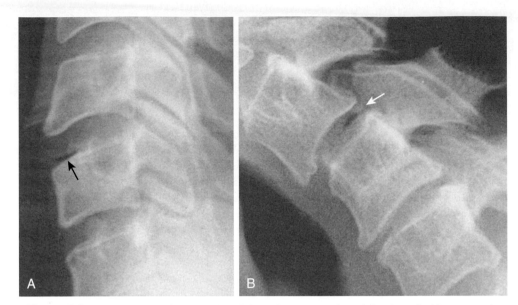

•**Figure 2-3** Posttraumatic discovertebral injury: lucent annular cleft sign. **A,** Hyperextension injury. Lateral radiograph shows a linear collection of gas within the annular fibers of the intervertebral disc adjacent to the vertebral endplate. The lucent cleft sign *(arrow),* often seen after hyperextension injuries, is believed to represent traumatic avulsion of the annulus fibrosus from its attachment to the anterior cartilaginous endplate. **B,** Hyperflexion injury. Observe the gas density within the posterior portion of the C4-C5 disc *(arrow)* on this lateral radiograph obtained in flexion. This patient was recently involved in a rear-end impact motor vehicle collision and had severe neck pain. (From Taylor JAM, Hughes TH, Resnick D: *Skeletal imaging: atlas of the spine and extremities,* ed 2, St. Louis, 2010, WB Saunders.)

3 Nomenclature of the Diseased Cervical Disc

Much confusion surrounds the nomenclature that is used to describe the diseased cervical disc. Such confusion exists in part because of the use of a system of nomenclature that was devised before the advent of computed tomography and magnetic resonance imaging and in part because of the focus by radiologists and clinicians alike on the impingement of the intervertebral disc on neural structures as the sole source of pain emanating from the spine. This second viewpoint ignores the disc and facet joint as an independent source of spine pain and leads to misdiagnosis, treatment plans with little chance of success, and needless suffering for the patient. By standardizing the nomenclature of the diseased cervical disc, the radiologist and clinician can do much to avoid these pitfalls when caring for the patient with spinal pain. The following classification system will allow the radiologist and clinician to communicate with each other in the same language. It also takes into account the fact that the intervertebral disc may be the sole source of spinal pain and that certain findings on magnetic resonance imaging should point the clinician toward a discogenic source of pain and an early consideration of discography as a diagnostic maneuver prior to surgical interventions. More than 90% of clinically significant disc abnormalities of the cervical spine occur at C5-C6 or C6-C7.

THE NORMAL DISC

As was discussed in Chapter 2, the normal disc consists of the central gel-like nucleus pulposus, which is surrounded concentrically by a dense fibroelastic ring called the annulus. The top and bottom of the disc are made up of cartilaginous endplates that are adjacent to the vertebral body. The laws of physics (primarily Pascal's law) allow the disc to maintain an adequate intradiscal pressure to push the adjacent vertebrae apart. On magnetic resonance imaging, the normal cervical disc appears symmetrical with low signal intensity on T1-weighted images and high signal intensity throughout the disc on T2-weighted images. In health, the margins of the cervical disc do not extend beyond the margins of the adjacent vertebral bodies (Fig. 3-1).

THE DEGENERATED DISC

As the disc ages, both the nucleus and the annulus undergo structural and biochemical changes that affect both the disc's appearance on magnetic resonance imaging and the disc's ability to function properly. Although this degenerative process is a normal part of aging, it can be accelerated by trauma to the cervical spine, infection, and smoking. If the degenerative process is severe enough, many but not all patients will experience clinical symptoms.

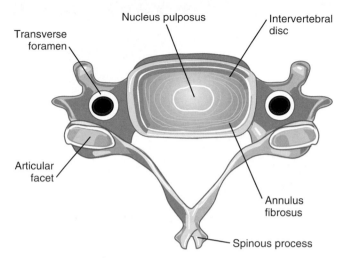

• **Figure 3-1** Normal cervical disc.

As the degenerative process occurs, the nucleus pulposus begins to lose its ability to maintain an adequate level of hydration as well as its ability to maintain a proper mixture of proteoglycans necessary to keep the gel-like consistency of the nuclear material. Degenerative clefts develop within the nuclear matrix, and portions of the nucleus become replaced with collagen, which leads to a further degradation of the shock-absorbing abilities and flexibility of the disc. As this process continues, the disc's ability to maintain an adequate intradiscal pressure to push the adjacent vertebrae apart begins to break down, leading to a further deterioration of function with the onset of clinical symptoms.

In addition to degenerative changes affecting the nucleus pulposus, the degenerative process affects the annulus as well (Fig. 3-2). As the annulus ages, the complex interwoven mesh of fibroelastic fibers begins to break down, with small tears within the mesh occurring. As these tears occur, the exposed collagen fibers stimulate the ingrowth of richly innervated granulation tissue that can account for discogenic pain. These tears can be easily demonstrated in magnetic resonance imaging as linear structures of high signal intensity on T2-weighted images that correlate with positive results when provocative discography is performed on the affected disc. When identified as the source of pain on discography, these annular tears can be treated with intradiscal electrothermal annuloplasty with good results (Fig. 3-3).

THE DIFFUSELY BULGING DISC

As the degenerative process continues, further breakdown and tearing of the annular fibers and continued loss of hydration of the nucleus propulsus lead to a loss of intradiscal pressure with resultant disc space narrowing, which can

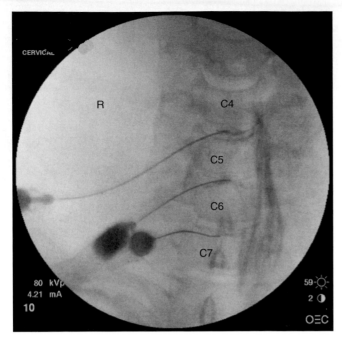

• **Figure 3-2** Contrast within the epidural space suggesting complete disruption of the disc annulus. *R*, Right. (From Waldman SD: *Atlas of interventional pain management*, ed 2, Philadelphia, 2004, Saunders, p 554.)

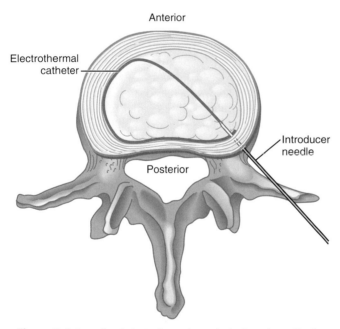

• **Figure 3-3** Intradiscal electrothermal annuloplasty: schematic view. (From Waldman SD: *Atlas of interventional pain management*, ed 2, Philadelphia, 2004, Saunders, p 554.)

lead to an exacerbation of clinical symptoms. As the disc space gradually narrows owing to decreased intradiscal pressure, the anterior and posterior longitudinal ligaments grow less taut and allow the discs to bulge beyond the margins of the vertebral body (Fig. 3-4, *A, B*). This causes impingement of bone or disc on nerve and spinal cord, adding impingement-induced pain to the pain emanating

from the disc annulus itself (Fig. 3-5). These findings are clearly demonstrated on magnetic resonance imaging and should alert the clinician to the possibility of multifactorial sources of the patient's pain and functional disability.

THE FOCAL DISC PROTRUSION

As the disc annulus and nucleus propulsus continue to degenerate, the ability of the annulus to completely contain and compress the nucleus propulsus is lost and with it the incompressible nature of the nucleus propulsus. This leads to focal areas of annular wall weakness, which allow the nucleus propulsus to protrude into the spinal canal or against pain-sensitive structures (Fig. 3-4, *C*). Such protrusions are focal in nature and are easily seen on both T1- and T2-weighted magnetic resonance images (Fig. 3-6). These focal disc protrusions may be either relatively asymptomatic if the focal bulge does not impinge on any pain-sensitive structures or highly symptomatic, presenting clinically as pure discogenic pain or as radicular pain if the focal protrusion extends into a neural foramen or the spinal canal.

THE FOCAL DISC EXTRUSION

Focal disc extrusion is frequently symptomatic because the disc material often migrates cranially or caudally, resulting in impingement of exiting nerve roots and the creation of an intense inflammatory reaction as the nuclear material irritates the nerve root. This chemical irritation is thought to be responsible for the intense pain that is experienced by many patients with focal disc extrusion and may be seen on magnetic resonance imaging as high-intensity signals on T2-weighted images (Fig. 3-7). Although more pronounced than a focal disc protrusion, focal disc extrusion is similar in that the extruded disc material remains contiguous with the parent disc material (Fig. 3-4, *D*).

THE SEQUESTERED DISC

When a portion of the nuclear material detaches itself from its parent disc material and migrates, the disc fragment is called a sequestered disc (Fig. 3-4, *E*). Sequestered disc fragments frequently migrate in a cranial or caudal direction and become impacted beneath a nerve root or between the posterior longitudinal ligament and the bony spine. Sequestered disc fragments can cause significant clinical symptoms and pain and often require surgical intervention. Sequestered disc fragments will often enhance on contrast-enhanced T1-weighted images and demonstrate a peripheral rim of high-intensity signal due to the inflammatory reaction the nuclear material elicits on T2-weighted images. Failure to identify and remove sequestered disc fragments often leads to a poor surgical result. Magnetic resonance imaging of the cervical spine, cervical myelography with contrast-enhanced computed tomography, and discography will help the clinician to further delineate the type of disc herniation the patient is suffering from and aid in formulation of a treatment plan (Fig. 3-8).

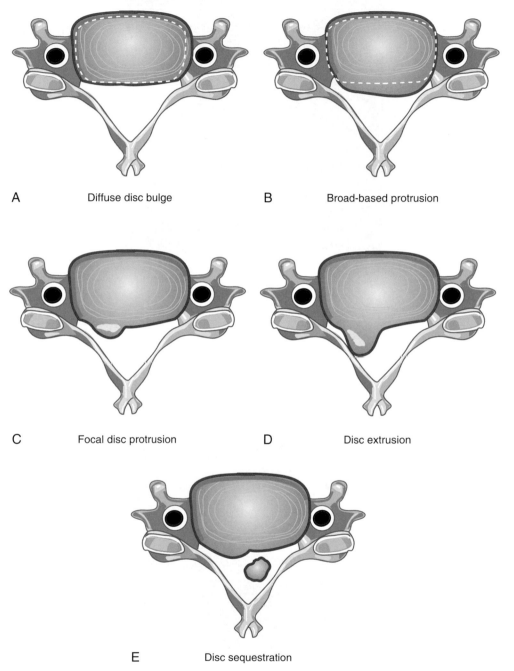

A   Diffuse disc bulge   B   Broad-based protrusion

C   Focal disc protrusion   D   Disc extrusion

E   Disc sequestration

• **Figure 3-4** Various types of cervical disc degeneration.

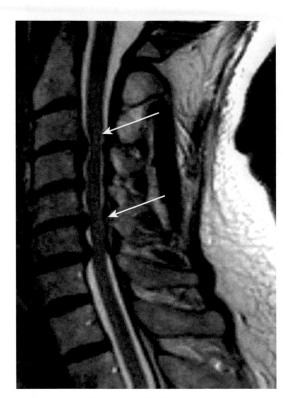

•**Figure 3-5** Sagittal T2-weighted MRI scan showing significant cervical degenerative disk disease with broad-based disk bulging at C3-4, C5-6, and C6-7. Cord signal changes are evident at C3-4 and C5-6 *(arrows)*. (From Jandial R, Garfin SR, Ames CP: *Best evidence for spine surgery: 20 cardinal cases*, Philadelphia, 2012, Saunders/Elsevier, p 152, fig 13-2.)

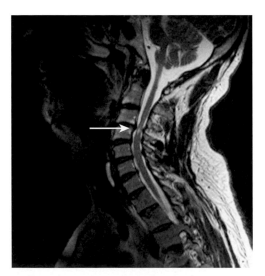

•**Figure 3-6** T2-weighted, sagittal MRI image in a patient with C3-4 disc protrusion, causing compressive intramedullary signal change in the cervical spinal cord *(arrow)*. (From Davis W, Allouni AK, Mankad K, et al: Modern spinal instrumentation. Part 1: normal spinal implants, *Clin Radiol* 68(1):65, 2013, fig 1a.)

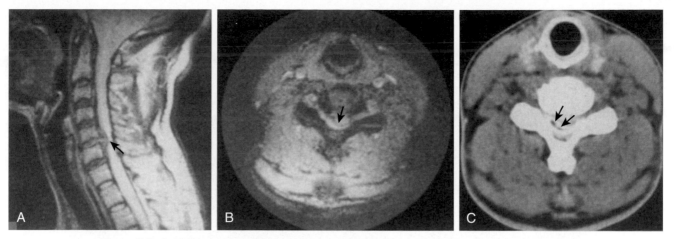

•**Figure 3-7 A,** Midline sagittal magnetic resonance (MR) image, showing extrusion of disk material into spinal canal at fifth cervical interspace *(arrow)*. Disk material extends both above and below level of interspace. (Repetition time [TR] = 1,500 ms; echo time [TE] = 60 ms.) **B,** Axial MR image, confirming large disk extrusion in midline and extending to the left. Note considerable compression of spinal cord and subarachnoid space *(arrow)*. Image is "noisy" because of small slice thickness and small field of view required when imaging the cervical spine. (TR = 400 ms; TE = 20 ms; flip angle = 10 degrees.) **C,** Post-myelographic computed tomogram, showing better detail of large disk protrusion. Note substantial compression of spinal cord *(arrows)* within dural sac. (From Miller GM, Forbes GS, Onofrio BM: Magnetic resonance imaging of the spine, *Mayo Clin Proc* 64(8):986–1004, 1989, fig 3.)

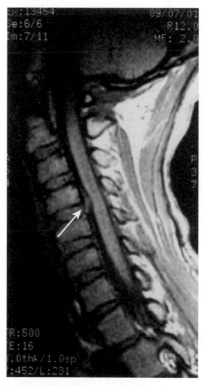

•**Figure 3-8** Magnetic resonance imaging of the cervical spine depicting a sequestered disc *(white arrow)* at C4-5 causing moderate cervical cord compression. (From Fung GPG, Chan KY: Cervical myelopathy in an adolescent with hallervorden-spatz disease, *Pediatr Neurol* 29(4):337–340, 2003, fig 2.)

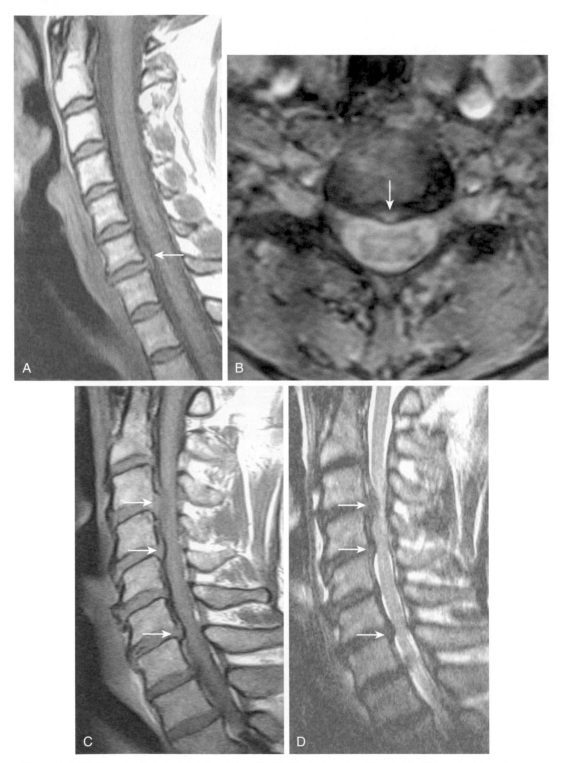

• **Figure 3-9** MR images of cervical disk herniation. Sagittal fast spin-echo, T1-weighted **(A)** and axial gradient-echo **(B)** images show a small central disk herniation *(arrows)*. In the cervical spine, herniations can be quite subtle. Sagittal fast spin-echo, T1-weighted **(C)** and T2-weighted **(D)** images of multiple disk herniations *(arrows)* in the same patient. (From Haaga J, Lanzieri C, Gilkeson R, editors: *CT and MR imaging of the whole body*, ed 4, Philadelphia, 2002, Mosby.)

4 Painful Conditions Emanating from the Cervical Spine

The initial general physical examination of the cervical spine and cervical dermatomes guides the clinician in narrowing his or her differential diagnosis and helps suggest which specialized physical examination maneuvers and laboratory and radiographic testing will aid in confirming the cause of the patient's neck and upper extremity pain and dysfunction. For the clinician to make best use of the initial information gleaned from the general physical examination of the cervical spine and cervical dermatomes, a grouping of the common causes of pain and dysfunction emanating from the cervical spine is exceedingly helpful. Although no classification of cervical spine pain and dysfunction can be all inclusive or all exclusive, owing to the frequently overlapping and multifactorial nature of cervical spine pathology, Table 4-1 should help to improve the diagnostic accuracy of the clinician confronted with the patient complaining of neck or upper extremity pain and dysfunction and help him or her to avoid overlooking less common diagnoses. Although the list is by no means comprehensive, it does aid the clinician in organizing the potential sources of pathology that presents as pain and dysfunction emanating from the cervical spine. It should be noted that the most commonly missed categories of neck and upper extremity pain and the categories that most often result in misadventures in diagnosis and treatment are the last three categories in the table. The knowledge of this potential pitfall should help the clinician to keep these sometimes overlooked causes of neck and upper extremity pain and dysfunction in the differential diagnosis.

TABLE 4-1 Overview of Causes of Neck and Upper Extremity Pain

Localized Bony, Disc Space, or Joint Space Pathology	Primary Shoulder Pathology	Systemic Disease	Sympathetically Mediated Pain	Referred from Other Body Areas
Vertebral fracture	Bursitis	Rheumatoid arthritis	Causalgia	Thyroiditis
Primary bone tumor	Tendinitis	Collagen vascular	Reflex sympathetic	Eagle's syndrome
Facet joint disease	Rotator cuff tear	disease	dystrophy	Hyoid syndrome
Localized or generalized	Impingement syndromes	Reiter syndrome	Shoulder/hand	Malignancy of the
degenerative arthritis	Adhesive capsulitis	Gout	syndrome	retropharyngeal
Osteophyte formation	Joint instability	Other crystal	Dressler syndrome	space
Disc space infection	Muscle strain	arthropathies	Intrathoracic tumors	Brachial
Herniated cervical disc	Muscle sprain	Charcot's neuropathic	Fibromyalgia	plexopathy
Degenerative disc	Periarticular infection not	arthritis	Myofascial pain	
disease	involving joint space	Multiple sclerosis	syndromes such as	
Whiplash injuries	Entrapment neuropathies	Ischemic pain secondary	scapulocostal	
Primary spinal cord	Ankylosing spondylitis	to peripheral vascular	syndrome	
pathology	Subdiaphragmatic pathology	insufficiency	Parsonage-Turner	
Osteomyelitis	such as subcapsular	Thoracic outlet	syndrome (idiopathic	
Epidural abscess	hematoma of the spleen	syndrome	brachial neuritis)	
Epidural hematoma	with positive Kerr sign	Pneumothorax		

Physical examination of the cervical spine should begin with a visual inspection of the anterior, lateral, and posterior cervical spine. The clinician should note the presence or absence of the normal cervical lordotic curve (Figs. 5-1 and 5-2). Loss or straightening of the cervical lordotic curve is often indicative of spasm of the cervical paraspinal musculature caused by pain. This finding can be confirmed on lateral radiographic imaging of the spine. The clinician then notes any abnormality in head or neck position suggestive of a central neurologic process such as spasmodic torticollis. The clinician then looks for any skin lesions, including vesicular lesions suggestive of acute herpes zoster, as well as any abnormal mass that might be suggestive of primary or metastatic tumor (Fig. 5-3).

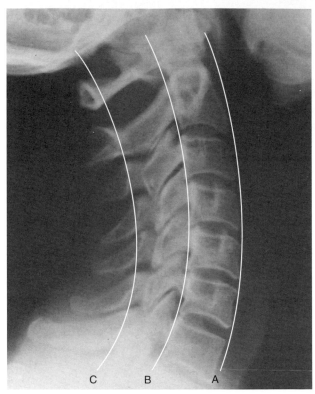

• **Figure 5-2** Plain lateral radiograph of a normal cervical spine. Lines joining the anterior part of the vertebral body **(A),** the posterior aspect of the vertebral body **(B),** and the anterior border of the laminae **(C)** should describe a smooth arc. (From Klippel JH, Dieppe PA: *Rheumatology*, ed 2, London, 1998, Mosby, p 5.5.)

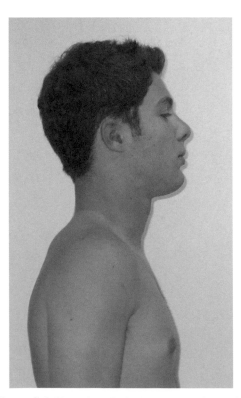

• **Figure 5-1** Normal cervical spine on visual inspection.

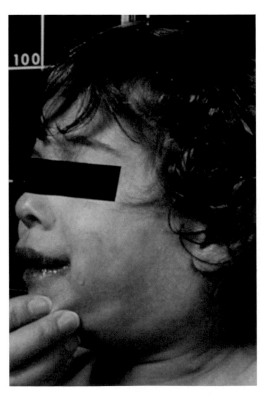

• **Figure 5-3** Cervical adenopathy in a patient with neck pain and fever. (From Scuccimarri R: Kawasaki disease, *Pediatr Clin North Am* 59(2):425–445.)

6 Palpation of the Cervical Spine

Palpation of the cervical spine is carried out primarily to identify abnormalities of the soft tissues. Careful palpation of the anterior cervical region is performed to identify abnormalities of the thyroid, including thyroiditis, deep lesions such as thyroglossal duct cysts, primary or metastatic tumors, and carotidynia (Figs. 6-1 and 6-2). The lateral cervical region is also palpated to identify spasm of the sternocleidomastoid muscles and occult abnormal mass (Fig. 6-3). The posterior cervical spine is palpated to identify any obvious bony abnormality that might be suggestive of severe degenerative disease or primary or metastatic tumor. The clinician should always be on the lookout for abnormal mass of the paraspinous musculature, including sarcoma. Spasm of the posterior cervical paraspinous musculature is a common finding following trauma (Fig. 6-4). A careful palpation of the posterior cervical paraspinous musculature will allow the clinician to identify myofascial trigger points that suggest fibromyalgia. Palpation of these trigger points should elicit a positive "jump" sign, which is pathognomonic for fibromyalgia (Fig. 6-5). Diffuse muscle tenderness should suggest the possibility of collagen vascular disease such as polymyositis or lupus, and this finding should cue the clinician to order appropriate laboratory testing to confirm the diagnosis.

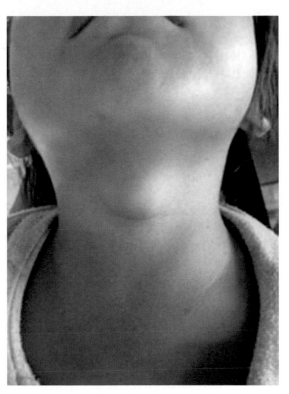

• **Figure 6-2** Thyroglossal duct cyst. (From Marom T, Dagan D, Weiser G, et al. Pediatric otolaryngology in a field hospital in the Philippines, *Int J Pediatr Otorhinolaryngol* 78(5):807–811, 2014, fig 5a.)

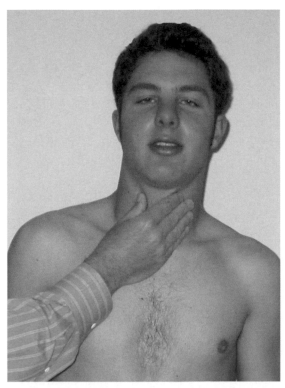

• **Figure 6-1** Palpation of the anterior cervical spine.

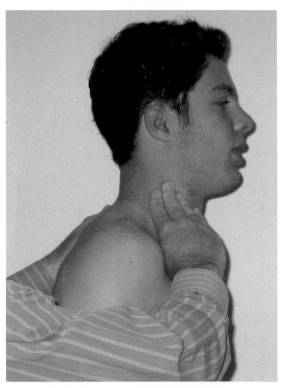

• **Figure 6-3** Palpation of the lateral cervical spine.

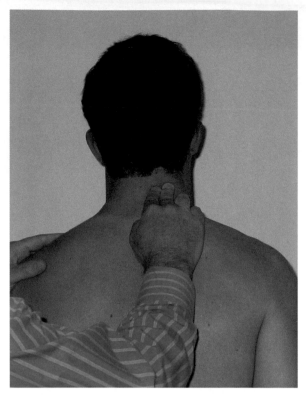

• **Figure 6-4** Palpation of the posterior cervical spine.

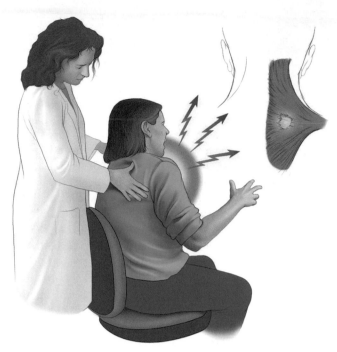

• **Figure 6-5** Palpation of a trigger point will result in a positive "jump" sign. (From Waldman SD: *Atlas of common pain syndromes*, Philadelphia, 2002, Saunders, p 53.)

7 Physical Examination of the Cervical Spine Range of Motion

As was mentioned in Chapter 1, the cervical spine has a wide and varied range of motion due to the unique nature of the upper two segments, namely, the atlanto-occipital and atlantoaxial joints. In fact, the majority of movement of the cervical spine occurs in the upper three segments. In health, movement of the cervical spine requires synchronized movement of all the elements of the spine. In disease, problems at one level can cause functional disability at other levels.

FLEXION AND EXTENSION

To assess the range of motion of the cervical spine, the clinician has the patient place his or her spine in neutral position (Fig. 7-1). The patient is then asked to flex his or her cervical spine forward while the clinician observes for any limitation in range of motion or a lack of a smooth, synchronized flexion that is indicative of pain or spinal segment dysfunction. In general, patients with normal flexion of the cervical spine should be able to smoothly and easily touch the chin to the chest. The patient is then asked to return the cervical spine to neutral position and then to extend the cervical spine while the clinician observes for any limitation in range of motion or a lack of a smooth, synchronized extension that might be indicative of pain or spinal segment dysfunction (Fig. 7-2, *A* and *B*). With both of these maneuvers, the clinician should be sure that movement occurs only at the level of the cervical spine and that the patient is not using

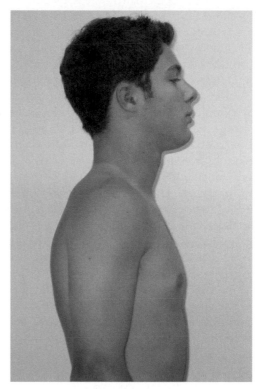

• **Figure 7-1** Neutral position.

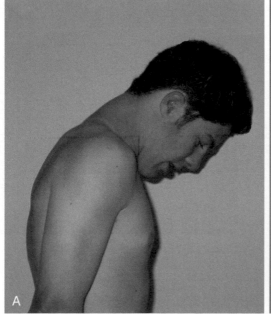
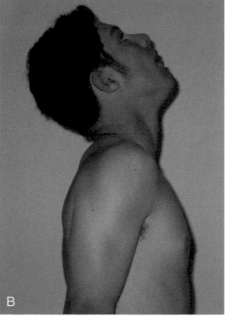

• **Figure 7-2 A,** Flexed position. **B,** Extended position.

the thoracic spine to compensate for a limitation of range of motion of the cervical segments.

ROTATION AND LATERAL BENDING

To assess the range of motion of rotation of the cervical spine, the clinician has the patient place his or her spine in neutral position. The patient is then asked to fully rotate his or her cervical spine in both the left and right directions while the clinician observes for any limitation in range of motion or a lack of a smooth, synchronized rotation that might be indicative of pain or spinal segment dysfunction (Fig. 7-3). The patient is then asked to return the cervical spine to neutral position and then to laterally bend the cervical spine while the clinician observes for any limitation in range of motion or a lack of a smooth, synchronized lateral bending that might be indicative of pain or spinal segment dysfunction (Fig. 7-4). With both of these maneuvers, the clinician should be sure that movement occurs only at the level of the cervical spine and that the patient is not using the thoracic spine to compensate for a limitation of range of motion of the cervical segments. It should be remembered that the clinician should use care when performing these maneuvers in any patient with symptoms suggestive of cervical myelopathy, cervical radiculopathy, or carotid or vertebral artery insufficiency to avoid precipitating an acute neurologic event. Care should also be exercised when performing these maneuvers in patients suffering from rheumatoid arthritis, as occult erosion of the odontoid process can render the upper cervical spine extremely susceptible to instability (Fig. 7-5).

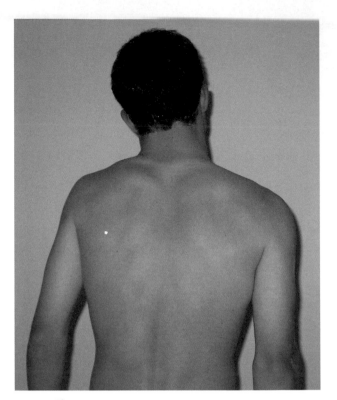

• **Figure 7-4** Lateral bending of the cervical spine.

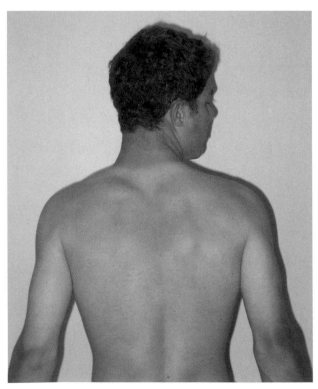

• **Figure 7-3** Rotation of the cervical spine.

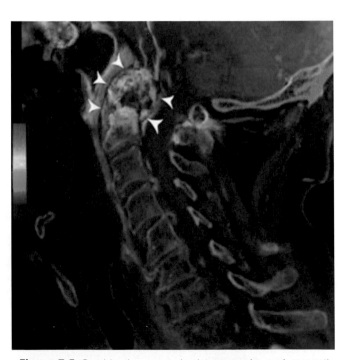

• **Figure 7-5** Combined computerized tomography and magnetic resonance imaging of the odontoid process demonstrating significant bony erosions and synovitis in a patient presenting with difficulty walking and urinary and fecal incontinence. (From de Parisot A, Ltaief-Boudrigua A, Villani A-P, et al: Spontaneous odontoid fracture on a tophus responsible for spinal cord compression: a case report, *Joint Bone Spine* 80(5):550–551, 2013, fig 2.)

In humans, the innervation of the skin, muscles, and deep structures is determined embryologically at an early stage of fetal development, and there is amazingly little inter-subject variability. Each segment of the spinal cord and its corresponding spinal nerves have a consistent segmental relationship that allows the clinician to ascertain the probable spinal level of dysfunction based on the pattern of pain, muscle weakness, and deep tendon reflex changes.

Figure 8-1 is a dermatomal chart that the clinician will find useful in determining the specific spinal level that subserves a patient's pain. In general, the cervical spinal segments move down the upper extremity from cephalad to caudad on the lateral border of the upper extremity and from caudad to cephalad on the medial border.

In general, in humans, the more proximal the muscle, the more cephalad is the spinal segment, with the ventral muscles innervated by higher spinal segments than the corresponding dorsal muscles. It should be remembered that pain perceived in the region of a given muscle or joint might not be coming from the muscle or joint but simply be referred by problems at the same cervical spinal segment that innervated the muscles.

Furthermore, the clinician needs to be aware that the relatively consistent pattern of dermatomal and myotomal distribution breaks down when the pain is perceived in the deep structures of the upper extremity, such as the joints and tendinous insertions. With pain in these regions, the clinician should refer to the sclerotomal chart in Figure 8-2. This is particularly important if a neurodestructive procedure at the spinal cord level is being considered, as the sclerotomal level of the nerves subserving the pain might be several segments higher or lower than the dermatomal or myotomal levels the clinician would expect.

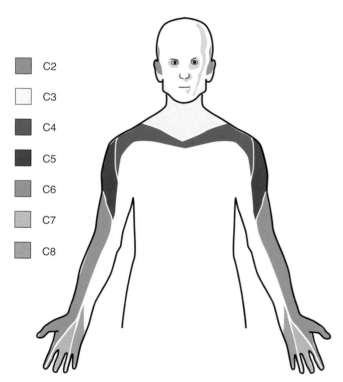

C2
C3
C4
C5
C6
C7
C8

• **Figure 8-1** Cervical dermatomal chart.

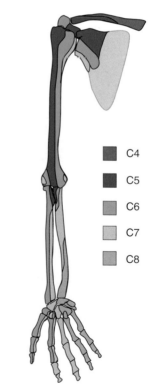

C4
C5
C6
C7
C8

• **Figure 8-2** Cervical sclerotomal chart.

The concept of diagnosing a problem at a specific neurologic level via physical examination has its basis in the fact that pathology at the cervical spinal cord or cervical nerve root level manifests itself in a relatively consistent manner by dysfunction, numbness, and pain of the upper extremity, which occurs in a dermatomal distribution. Although not foolproof, a careful physical examination of the upper extremity with an eye to the neurologic level affected can frequently guide the clinician in designing a more targeted workup and treatment plan (Video 9-1). By overlapping the information gleaned from physical examination with the neuroanatomic information gained from magnetic resonance imaging and the neurophysiologic information from electromyography, a highly accurate diagnosis can be made as to which level of the cervical spine is responsible for the patient's symptoms.

Testing for the C5 dermatome is best carried out by a careful sensory evaluation of the lateral aspect of the more cephalad portion of the upper extremity (Fig. 9-1). Decreased sensation in this anatomic region can be ascribed

to proximal lesions of the spinal cord, such as a syrinx; more distal lesions of the C5 nerve root, such as impingement by a herniated disc; or a lesion of the more peripheral axillary nerve. For this reason, correlation with manual muscle testing and evaluation of the deep tendon reflex combined with radiographic and electromyographic testing can help to determine the exact site of pathology.

Testing for the C5 myotome is best carried out by manual muscle testing of the deltoid muscle. The deltoid muscle is primarily innervated by the C5 nerve with a small contribution in most patients from the C6 nerve. Because in most patients abduction of the deltoid is a C5 function, the muscle should be tested as follows. The patient is placed in the standing position with the affected extremity resting against the patient's side. The patient is asked to flex the elbow to 90 degrees and then asked to forcefully abduct the affected extremity at the shoulder (Fig. 9-2). If the manual muscle testing is normal, the examiner should not be able to resist abduction nor to force the arm back toward the patient's side. If the patient has primary shoulder pathology

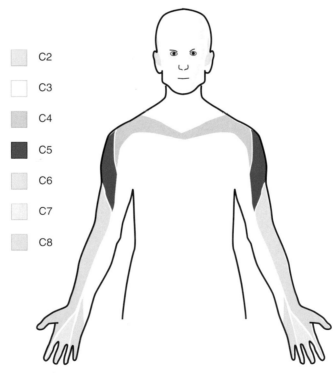

C2
C3
C4
C5
C6
C7
C8

• **Figure 9-1** Sensory distribution of the C5 dermatome.

C5

Motor

Sensory

Deltoid

Biceps

Reflex

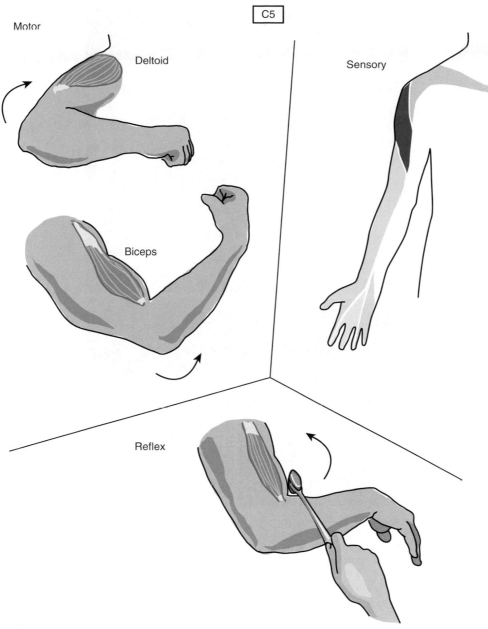

• **Figure 9-2** C5 myotome integrity testing.

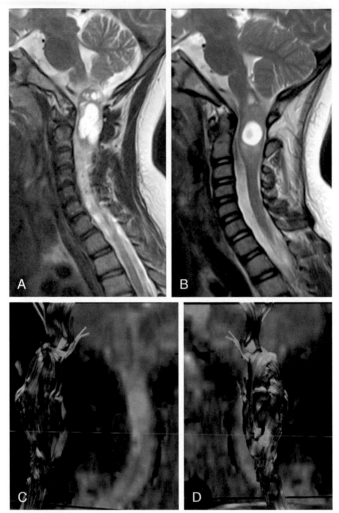

• **Figure 9-3** Pilocytic astrocytoma in an 18-year-old male patient with slowly progressive symptoms of cervical myelopathy. **A,** Sagittal T2 weighted image (WI) shows a moderate-sized intramedullary space-occupying lesion within the uppermost part of the cervical cord spanning the C1-C2 levels. This lesion has a mostly cystic septated well-defined component causing expansion of the cervical cord at that region. **B,** Sagittal post contrast T1 WI shows an associated small solid intensely enhancing component along the superior left aspect of this cystic lesion. **C** and **D,** Magnetic resonance tractography of the cord particularly emphasizing that such lesion is splaying apart the projectional fibers of the cord. The overall pattern as such confirms that this is a low-grade neoplastic lesion with no infiltration of destruction. (From El Maati AAA, Chalabi N: Diffusion tensor tractography as a supplementary tool to conventional MRI for evaluating patients with myelopathy, *Egyptian J Radiol Nuclear Med* 45(4):1223–1231, 2014, fig 1.)

that precludes this test, the clinician may test the strength of flexion of the biceps, which is also primarily innervated by C5.

The biceps deep tendon reflex is mediated via the C5 spinal segment. To test the biceps reflex, the patient is asked to relax and lay the affected extremity against the clinician's arm. The clinician then strikes the biceps tendon at the elbow with a neurologic hammer and grades the response (see Fig. 9-2). A diminished or absent reflex might point to compromise of the C5 segment, whereas a hyperactive response might suggest an upper motor neuron lesion, such as cervical myelopathy (Fig. 9-3).

The concept of diagnosing a problem at a specific neurologic level via physical examination has its basis in the fact that pathology at the cervical spinal cord or cervical nerve root level manifests itself in a relatively consistent manner by dysfunction, numbness, and pain of the upper extremity, which occurs in a dermatomal distribution. Although not foolproof, a careful physical examination of the upper extremity with an eye to the neurologic level affected can frequently guide the clinician in designing a more targeted workup and treatment plan (Video 10-1). By overlapping the information gleaned from physical examination with the neuroanatomic information gained from magnetic resonance imaging and the neurophysiologic information from electromyography, a highly accurate diagnosis can be made as to which level of the cervical spine is responsible for the patient's symptomatology.

Testing for the C6 dermatome is best carried out by a careful sensory evaluation of the lateral aspect of the more distal portion of the upper extremity (Fig. 10-1). Decreased sensation in this anatomic region can be ascribed to proximal lesions of the spinal cord, such as a syrinx; more distal lesions of the C6 nerve root, such as impingement by a herniated disc; or a lesion of the more peripheral portion of the nerve (Fig. 10-2). For this reason, correlation with

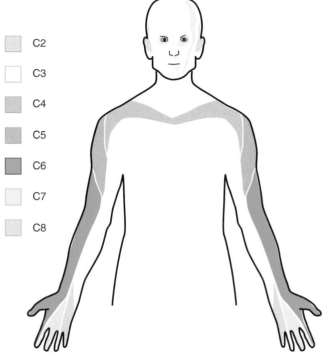

C2
C3
C4
C5
C6
C7
C8

• **Figure 10-1** Sensory distribution of the C6 dermatome.

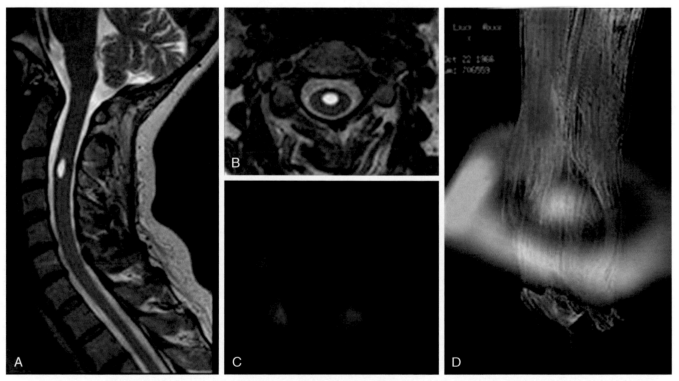

A   B   C   D

• **Figure 10-2** Focal syrinx of the cervical spinal cord in patient with cervical myelopathy. Sagittal **(A)** and axial **(B)** T2-weighted images demonstrate a focal syrinx in the central spinal cord at the C3 level. **C,** Axial color-coded fractional anisotropy map demonstrates no fiber tracts running through the lesion. **D,** Tractography shows displacement of the fiber tracts around the syrinx. Identical tractography findings are seen with spinal cord ependymomas. In contradistinction spinal cord astrocytoma tractography would show infiltrated or attenuated fibers traversing the lesion. (From Lerner A, Mogensen MA, Kim PE, et al: Clinical applications of diffusion tensor imaging, *World Neurosurg* 82(1–2):96–109, 2014, Fig. 3.)

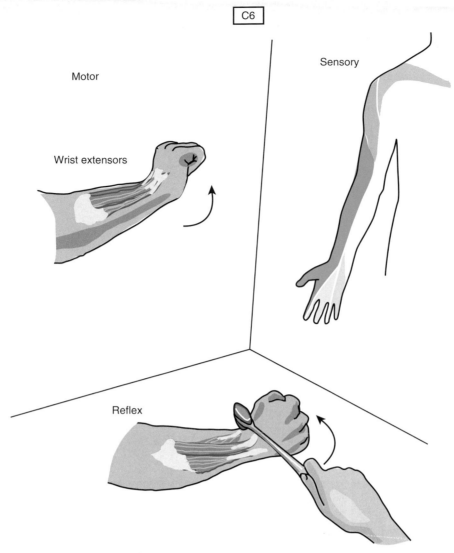

• **Figure 10-3** C6 myotome integrity testing.

manual muscle testing and evaluation of the deep tendon reflex combined with radiographic and electromyographic testing can help to determine the exact site of pathology.

Testing for the C6 myotome is best carried out by manual muscle testing of the radial wrist extensors. The radial wrist extensors are primarily innervated by the C6 nerve. Because extension on the radial of the wrist is a C6 function, with C7 providing innervation for the ulnar wrist extensor, C6 integrity should be tested as follows. The patient is placed in the sitting position with the fingers slightly flexed to avoid any extensor activity of the muscles of finger extension. The patient is then asked to extend the wrist in a radial direction while the clinician applies resistance (Fig. 10-3). If the manual muscle testing

for the C6 myotome is normal, the examiner should not be able to resist the radial wrist extension. If the C6 myotome is compromised and the C7 myotome is intact, then the clinician will observe ulnar wrist deviation on extension.

The brachioradialis deep tendon reflex is mediated via the C6 spinal segment. To test the brachioradialis reflex, the patient is asked to relax and lay the affected extremity against the clinician's arm. The clinician then strikes the brachioradialis tendon with a neurologic hammer and grades the response (see Fig. 10-3). A diminished or absent reflex might point to compromise of the C6 segment, whereas a hyperactive response might suggest an upper motor neuron lesion, such as cervical myelopathy.

The concept of diagnosing a problem at a specific neurologic level via physical examination has its basis in the fact that pathology at the cervical spinal cord or cervical nerve root level manifests itself in a relatively consistent manner by dysfunction, numbness, and pain of the upper extremity, which occurs in a dermatomal distribution. Although not foolproof, a careful physical examination of the upper extremity with an eye to the neurologic level affected can frequently guide the clinician in designing a more targeted workup and treatment plan (Video 11-1). By overlapping the information gleaned from physical examination with the neuroanatomic information gained from magnetic resonance imaging and the neurophysiologic information gleaned from electromyography, a highly accurate diagnosis can be made as to which level of the cervical spine is responsible for the patient's symptomatology.

Testing for the C7 dermatome is best carried out by a careful sensory evaluation of the middle finger of the hand of the affected upper extremity (Fig. 11-1). The clinician should be aware that there is some interpatient variability in the sensory innervation of the middle finger, with some patients having contribution of either C6 or C8. Decreased sensation in this anatomic region can be ascribed to proximal lesions of the spinal cord, such as a syrinx; more distal lesions of the C7 nerve root, such as impingement by a herniated disc; or a lesion of the more peripheral portion of the nerve (Fig. 11-2). For this reason, correlation with

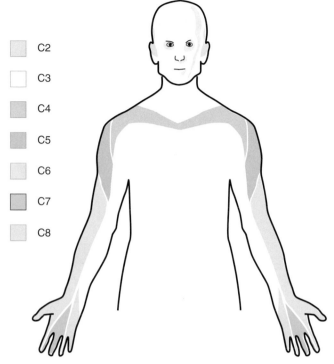

C2
C3
C4
C5
C6
C7
C8

• **Figure 11-1** Sensory distribution of the C7 dermatome.

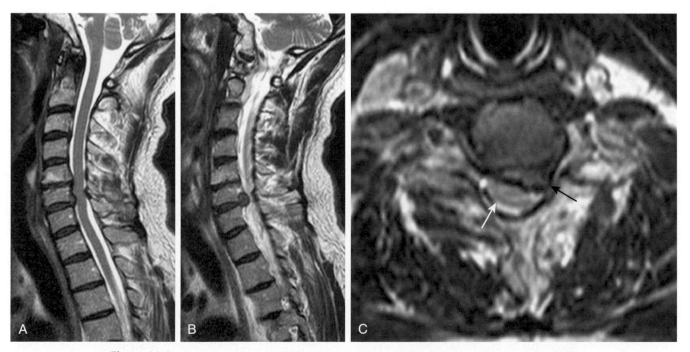

• **Figure 11-2** Magnetic resonance (MR) images of a patient with left-sided radicular symptoms. **A,** The midline sagittal T2W MR image shows disc degeneration at C5-C6 with disc space narrowing. There is less marked disc narrowing at C6-C7, but there is also a posterior disc herniation, which is much more prominent on the parasagittal T2W MR image **(B). C,** The axial T2W MR image demonstrates a large paracentral disc herniation *(black arrow)* that is compressing the cervical cord *(white arrow)*.

C7

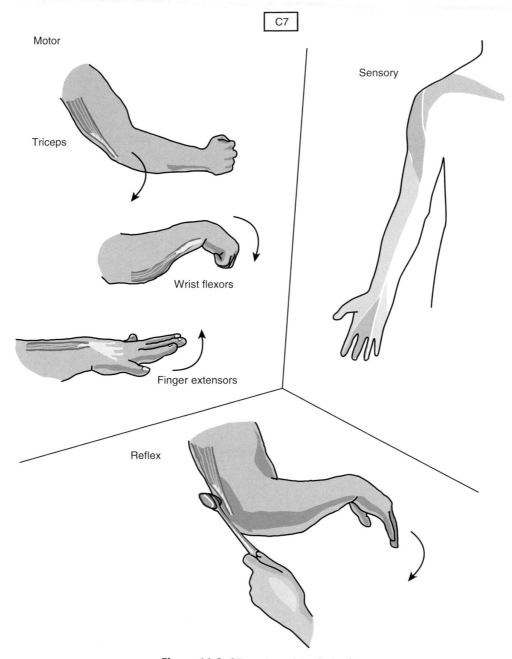

Motor

Triceps

Wrist flexors

Finger extensors

Sensory

Reflex

• **Figure 11-3** C7 myotome integrity testing.

manual muscle testing and evaluation of the deep tendon reflex combined with radiographic and electromyographic testing can help to determine the exact site of pathology.

Testing for the C7 myotome is best carried out by manual muscle testing of the flexor carpi radialis. The wrist extensors are primarily innervated by the C7 nerve, with the flexor carpi ulnaris usually innervated by C8. C7 myotome integrity should be tested as follows. The patient is placed in the sitting position with the fingers in extension to eliminate any finger flexor activity of the muscles of finger flexion. The patient is then asked to flex the wrist in a radial direction while the clinician applies resistance (Fig. 11-3). If the manual muscle testing for the C7 myotome is

normal, the examiner should not be able to resist the radial wrist flexion. If the C7 myotome is compromised and the C8 myotome is intact, then the clinician will observe ulnar wrist deviation on flexion.

The triceps deep tendon reflex is mediated via the C7 spinal segment. To test the triceps reflex, the patient is asked to relax and lay the affected extremity against the clinician's arm. The clinician then strikes the distal triceps tendon with a neurologic hammer and grades the response (see Fig. 11-3). A diminished or absent reflex might point to compromise of the C7 segment, whereas a hyperactive response might suggest an upper motor neuron lesion, such as cervical myelopathy.

The concept of diagnosing a problem at a specific neurologic level via physical examination has its basis in the fact that pathology at the cervical spinal cord or cervical nerve root level manifests itself in a relatively consistent manner by dysfunction, numbness, and pain of the upper extremity, which occurs in a dermatomal distribution. Although not foolproof, a careful physical examination of the upper extremity with an eye to the neurologic level affected can frequently guide the clinician in designing a more targeted workup and treatment plan (Video 12-1). By overlapping the information gleaned from physical examination with the neuroanatomic information gained from magnetic resonance imaging and the neurophysiologic information gleaned from electromyography, a highly accurate diagnosis can be made as to which level of the cervical spine is responsible for the patient's symptomatology.

Testing for the C8 dermatome is best carried out by a careful sensory evaluation of the ulnar aspect of the little finger of the hand of the affected upper extremity (Fig. 12-1). The clinician should be aware that there is some interpatient variability in the sensory innervation of the little finger, with most patients having sensory innervation from the ulnar nerve, which is made up of predominantly C8 fibers. Decreased sensation in this anatomic region can

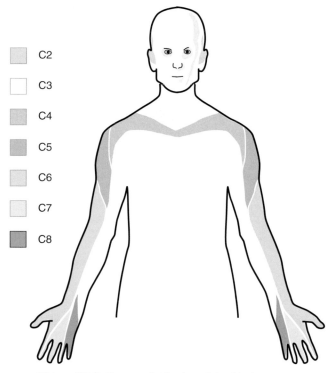

• **Figure 12-1** Sensory distribution of the C8 dermatome.

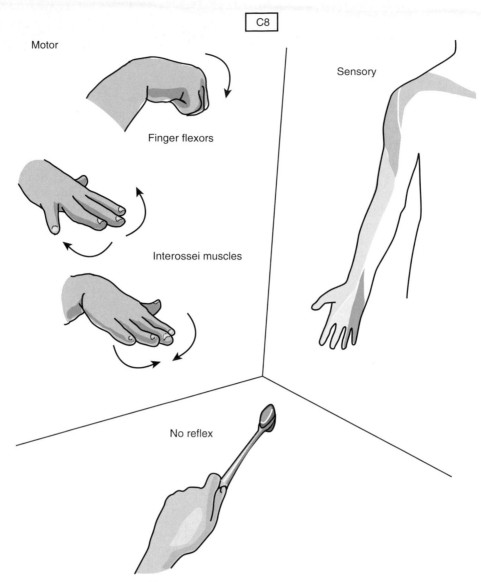

C8

Motor

Finger flexors

Interossei muscles

No reflex

Sensory

• **Figure 12-2** C8 myotome integrity testing.

be ascribed to proximal lesions of the spinal cord, such as a syrinx; more distal lesions of the C8 nerve root, such as impingement by a herniated disc; or a lesion of the more peripheral portion of the nerve. For this reason, correlation with manual muscle testing and evaluation of the deep tendon reflex combined with radiographic and electromyographic testing can help to determine the exact site of pathology.

Testing for the C8 myotome is best carried out by manual muscle testing of the flexor digitorum sublimus of the ring finger. The finger flexors are primarily innervated by the C8 nerve, with the flexor digitorum sublimus predominantly innervated by C8. The C8 myotome integrity should be tested as follows. The patient is placed in the sitting position with the middle, index, and little fingers stabilized in extension. The patient is then asked to flex the ring finger while the clinician applies resistance (Fig. 12-2).

There is no deep tendon reflex that is mediated predominantly by the C8 spinal segment.

13 The Spurling Test for Cervical Radiculopathy Secondary to Herniated Disc or Cervical Spondylosis

The Spurling test for cervical radiculopathy secondary to herniated disc or cervical spondylosis is performed by having the patient assume the standing position. The examiner stands behind the patient and examines the cervical spine for any abnormality. The examiner then has the patient extend the neck while tilting the head to the affected side (Fig. 13-1). Patients who suffer from cervical radiculopathy will experience a marked increase in pain secondary to compression of the nerve root as the neural foramen narrows with the maneuver (Video 13-1).

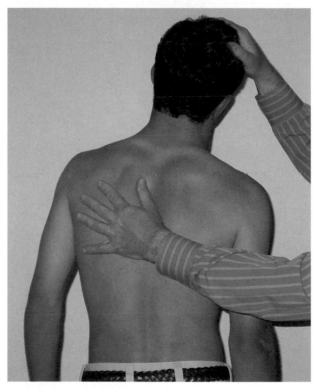

• **Figure 13-1** The Spurling test for cervical radiculopathy.

14 The Axial Loading Test for Cervical Discogenic Disease

The axial loading test for cervical discogenic disease is performed by having the patient assume the standing position. The examiner stands behind the patient and examines the cervical spine for any abnormality. The examiner then has the patient place the neck in neutral position while the examiner applies a steady downward pressure on the top of the patient's head, thereby loading the axial spine (Fig. 14-1). Patients who suffer from cervical discogenic disease will experience a marked increase in neck and upper extremity radicular pain secondary to compression of the nerve root as the cervical discs are compressed.

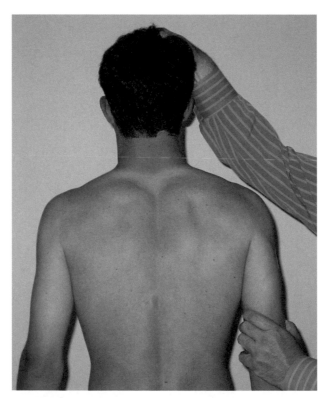

• **Figure 14-1** The axial loading test for cervical discogenic disease.

15 The Hoffmann Test for Cervical Myelopathy

The Hoffmann test or reflex can help the clinician identify patients who suffer from cervical myelopathy. The basis of the test is compression of the long tract fibers of the spinal cord. To perform the Hoffmann test, the examiner places the patient in a comfortable, relaxed position, and the patient's hand is cradled gently in the examiner's hand. The examiner then flicks the nail of the patient's middle finger and observes the hand for reflex flexion of the thumb and index finger (Fig. 15-1).

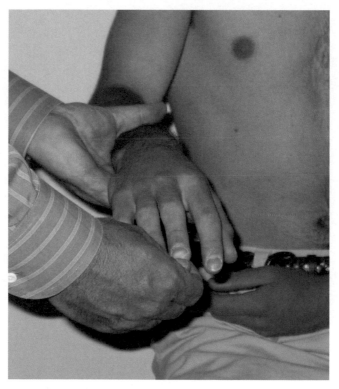

• **Figure 15-1** The Hoffmann test for cervical myelopathy.

The Sharp Purser test can help the clinician identify patients who suffer from instability of the atlantoaxial joint. This condition is most commonly seen in patients suffering from rheumatoid arthritis (Fig. 16-1). The basis of the test is identification of the loss of the functional integrity of the relationship with the odontoid process with the ring formed by the anterior arch and the transverse ligament of the atlas (Fig. 16-2). When this functional integrity is lost, atlas (C1 vertebra) will translate forward relative to axis (C2 vertebra). To perform the Sharp Purser test, the examiner places the

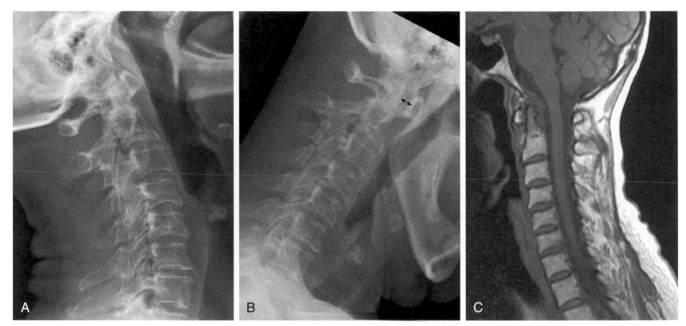

• **Figure 16-1 A,** Lateral radiograph of the cervical spine in extension shows normal C1-C2 alignment. **B,** On cervical flexion, however, there is widening of the predental space due to C1-C2 instability *(double-headed arrow).* **C,** The sagittal T1W magnetic resonance image shows erosion of the dorsal aspect of the odontoid peg.

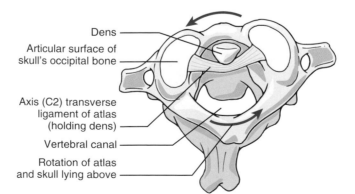

Dens
Articular surface of skull's occipital bone
Axis (C2) transverse ligament of atlas (holding dens)
Vertebral canal
Rotation of atlas and skull lying above

• **Figure 16-2** The anatomy of atlas and axis demonstrating the relationship of the odontoid process to the anterior arch and transverse ligament of atlas (C1 vertebra) with the odontoid process (dens) of axis (C2 vertebra). (From Waldman SD, Campbell, RSD: *Imaging of pain,* Philadelphia, 2010, Saunders/Elsevier, p 66, fig 24-1.)

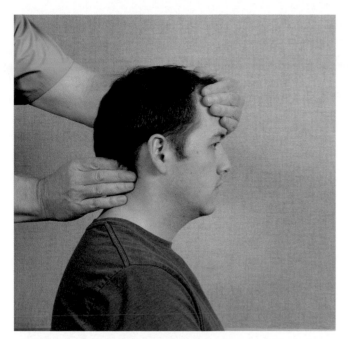

• **Figure 16-3** The Sharp Purser test for atlantoaxial joint instability, step 1. The examiner places the patient in a comfortable, relaxed sitting position, and the patient's forehead is cradled gently in the examiner's hand. The examiner then places his or her thumb and index finger of the contralateral hand on the tip of axis (C2).

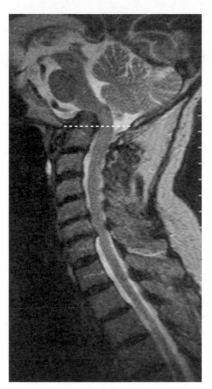

• **Figure 16-5** Sagittal T2W magnetic resonance image of a patient with chronic rheumatoid arthritis with cranial settling. The odontoid peg projects through the foramen magnum *(dotted line),* and there is impingement of the brainstem. (From Waldman SD, Campbell, RSD: *Imaging of pain,* Philadelphia, 2010, Saunders/Elsevier, p 66, fig 24-3.)

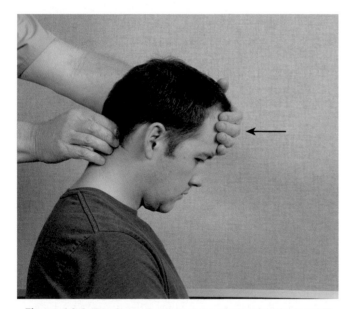

• **Figure 16-4** The Sharp Purser test for atlantoaxial joint instability, step 2. The patient is asked to slowly nod, which will flex the patient's cervical spine forward while the examiner simultaneously firmly presses on the patient's forehead in a controlled manner.

patient in a comfortable, relaxed sitting position, and the patient's forehead is cradled gently in the examiner's hand. The examiner then places his or her thumb and index finger of the contralateral hand on the tip of axis (C2) (Fig. 16-3). The patient is then asked to slowly nod, which will flex the patient's cervical spine forward while the examiner simultaneously firmly presses on the patient's forehead in a controlled manner (Fig. 16-4). If the test is positive, the examiner will perceive a sliding motion of the patient's head in relationship to axis (C2). The patient may also perceive a clunk or click in the roof of the mouth as atlas translates forward in relationship to axis. It should be noted that this test should be used with extreme caution in patients suffering from long-standing rheumatoid arthritis or in the presence of trauma to avoid serious neurological sequella (Fig. 16-5).

SECTION 2

The Shoulder

17 Functional Anatomy of the Shoulder Joint

The shoulder is a unique joint for a variety of reasons. Unlike the knee and the hip, with their inherent primary stability that results from their solid bony architecture, the shoulder is a relatively unstable joint that is held together by a complex combination of ligaments, tendons, muscles, and unique soft tissues, most notably the labrum and rotator cuff. What the shoulder lacks in stability, it more than makes up for in its extensive range of motion. Although not a true weight-bearing joint like the hip or knee, the shoulder joint is subjected to extreme mechanical forces owing to its extensive range of motion. Common activities such as lifting objects overhead or throwing can magnify these mechanical load factors and make the joint susceptible to repetitive motion injuries.

To make the most of the information that is gleaned from the physical examination of the shoulder, one must fully understand the functional anatomy of the shoulder. To fully understand the functional anatomy of the shoulder, one must recognize that the shoulder joint cannot be thought of as a single joint like the knee but must be thought of as four separate joints working in concert to function as one (Figs. 17-1 and 17-2). These four joints are as follows:
- The sternoclavicular joint
- The acromioclavicular joint
- The glenohumeral joint
- The scapulothoracic joint

The glenohumeral joint is responsible for the main functional mobility of the shoulder joint, and each of the other joints works synergistically with its counterparts to allow for the extensive and extremely varied range of motion of the shoulder joint. This unique range of motion is further enhanced by the unusual physical characteristics of the humeral head and the glenoid fossa. Whereas the articular surfaces of most joints are well matched in terms of their complementary shape with one another, such as the acetabulum and the femoral head, the large, rounded humeral head is amazingly mismatched to the much smaller and shallower, ovoid-shaped glenoid fossa (Fig. 17-3). This mismatch allows for the unique range of motion of the shoulder joint, but it also contributes to the relative instability of the joint and is in large part responsible for the shoulder joint's propensity for injury. As a result, the shoulder joint is the most commonly dislocated large joint in the body.

The unique nature of the shoulder joint has been the subject of medical commentary since early recorded medical history, with Hippocrates discussing the diagnosis and treatment of shoulder dislocation some 300 years B.C., and the recent advances of magnetic resonance imaging,

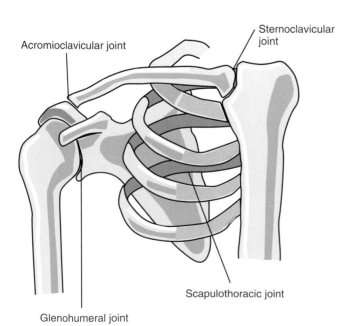

• **Figure 17-1** Four joints constituting the shoulder.

Acromioclavicular joint

Sternoclavicular joint

Scapulothoracic joint

Glenohumeral joint

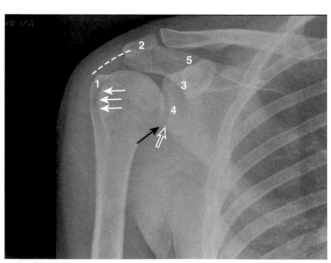

• **Figure 17-2** Anterior-posterior radiograph of the shoulder. *1,* greater tuberosity; *2,* acromion; *3,* coracoid process; *4,* glenoid (anterior rim); *5,* scapula spine; *white solid arrows,* lesser tuberosity; *black solid arrow,* acromioclavicular joint; *white open arrow,* glenohumeral joint; *dashed line,* subdeltoid fat plane (outline of subacromial bursa). (From Waldman SD, Campbell, RSD: *Imaging of pain,* Philadelphia, 2010, Saunders/Elsevier, p 218, fig 85-1.)

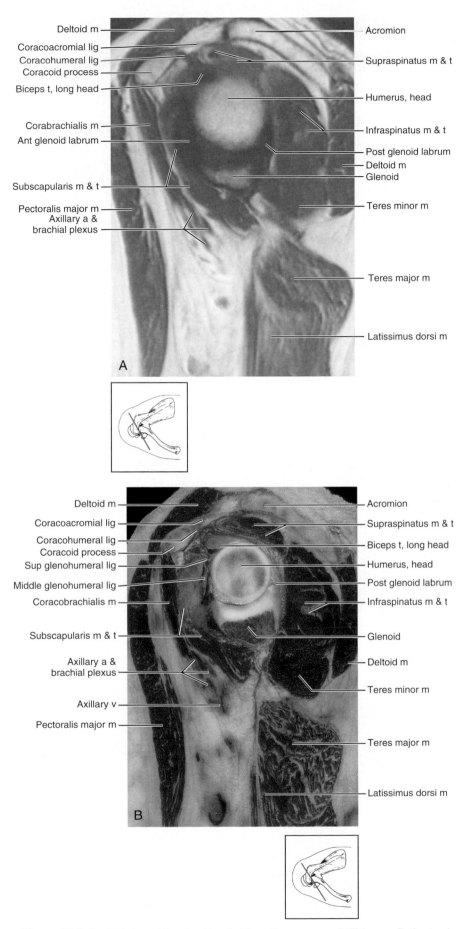

• **Figure 17-3** Sagittal view of the shoulder. **A,** Magnetic resonance (MR) image. **B,** Anatomic image. (From Kang HS, Ahn JM, Resnick D: *MRI of the extremities*, ed 2, Philadelphia, Saunders, 2002, pp 32–33.)

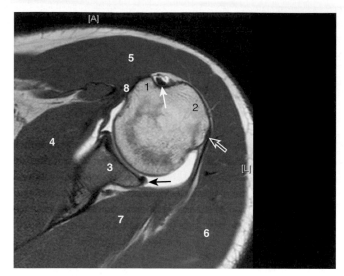

• **Figure 17-4** Axial T1-weighted magnetic resonance arthrogram image of the shoulder. *1,* lesser tuberosity; *2,* greater tuberosity; *3,* glenoid; *4,* subscapularis muscle; *5,* anterior deltoid muscle; *6,* posterior deltoid muscle; *7,* teres minor muscle; *8,* subscapularis tendon; *white arrow,* long head of biceps tendon; *open white arrow,* teres minor tendon; *black arrow,* glenoid labrum. (From Waldman SD, Campbell, RSD: *Imaging of pain,* Philadelphia, 2010, Saunders/Elsevier, p 218, fig 85-3.)

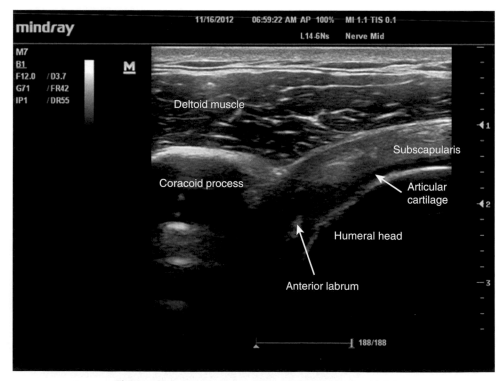

• **Figure 17-5** Ultrasound anatomy of the glenohumeral joint.

arthroscopy, and dynamic sonography have provided a clearer understanding of the shoulder joint in health and disease. This information has allowed the clinician to fine-tune his or her physical examination skills by correlating the patient's physical findings with magnetic resonance imaging and arthroscopy findings (Figs. 17-4 and 17-5). The information provided in the following chapters draws heavily on this recently gained knowledge and should aid the clinician in the care of the patient suffering from shoulder pain or dysfunction.

18   Visual Inspection of the Shoulder

The starting point in the physical examination of the shoulder is the visual inspection of the joint and surrounding structures. Asking the patient whether he or she is having any problem putting on undergarments or shirts can provide the examiner with useful clues as to the presence and etiology of shoulder dysfunction. For example, the inability to fasten or unfasten a bra might suggest anterior shoulder instability, adhesive capsulitis, or some other problem.

The visual inspection of the shoulder must be carried out with the patient undressed to avoid missing physical signs that might be masked by clothing. The anterior, lateral, and posterior aspects of the shoulder should be observed for muscle wasting, swelling, erythema, or ecchymosis that is suggestive of acute and chronic shoulder pathology, including traumatic rupture of tendons or chronic rotator cuff tear. Careful inspection of the acromioclavicular (AC) joints for asymmetry that suggests AC joint separation should be carried out next. The examiner should then evaluate the position of the shoulders relative to the neck and thorax to identify protective "splinting" or overprotraction of the joint that might be indicative of a painful or unstable joint (Fig. 18-1). Special attention should be paid to any evidence of scapular winging that might be suggestive of weakness of the serratus anterior muscle or compromise of the long thoracic nerve of Bell.

Positive findings during the initial visual inspection of the shoulder should help guide the examiner in his or her additional physical examination as well as provide a guide as to the ordering of specialized plain radiographic views and magnetic resonance imaging to further ascertain the etiology of the patient's shoulder pain and dysfunction.

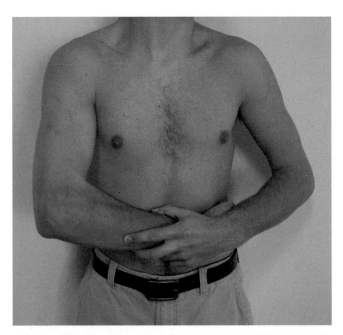

• **Figure 18-1** Visual inspection of the shoulder should include evaluation of the position of the shoulders relative to the neck and thorax.

Careful palpation of the shoulder joint and surrounding structures should be the next step after visual inspection of the shoulder in examining the patient who presents with shoulder pain and dysfunction.

Palpation of the shoulder must be carried out with the patient undressed to avoid missing physical signs, such as increased temperature, that may be masked by clothing. The anterior, lateral, and posterior aspects of the shoulder as well as the axilla should be palpated for abnormal mass, swelling, increased temperature, joint effusion, and bone spurs.

Targeted palpation of the bursae of the shoulder with particular attention to the subacromial and subdeltoid bursae will allow the examiner to identify inflamed and painful bursae that could serve as either a primary or a contributing cause of the patient's shoulder pain and dysfunction (Fig. 19-1 and Fig. 19-2). Targeted palpation of the tendon of the long head of the biceps as well as palpation of the tendinous insertions of the rotator cuff will assist the examiner in identifying tendinitis that might also be contributing to the patient's shoulder pain and dysfunction. The examiner should also assess the shoulder for the presence of joint instability and crepitus that are suggestive of tendinitis, adhesive capsulitis, or arthritis. The examiner should also examine the neck and the intrascapular and subscapular regions for the presence of myofascial trigger points as characterized by a positive "jump" sign that might be responsible for referred pain to the shoulder.

Positive findings during the palpation of the shoulder should help guide the examiner in his or her additional physical examination as well as provide a guide to the ordering of specialized plain radiographic views, ultrasound, and magnetic resonance imaging to further ascertain the etiology of the patient's shoulder pain and dysfunction (see Fig. 19-2).

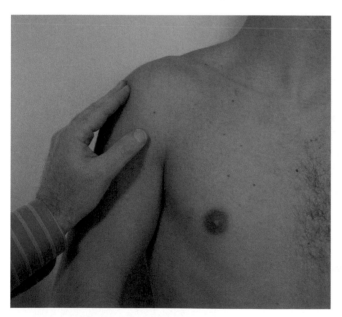

• **Figure 19-1** Palpation of the shoulder.

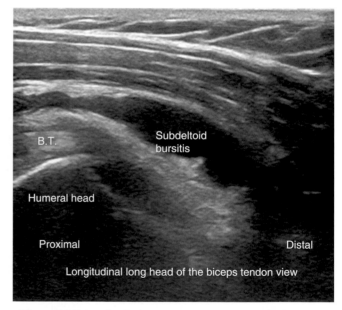

• **Figure 19-2** Longitudinal ultrasound image demonstrating subdeltoid bursitis. *B.T.,* Biceps tendon.

To adequately assess external rotation of the shoulder and identify subtle pathology, evaluation must be carried out with the arm first fully adducted and then abducted to at least 90 degrees. With the patient in the sitting position and the arms fully adducted, ask the patient to slowly externally rotate both arms (Fig. 20-1). The arms should move back rather than up as they reach the full extent of external rotation. Observe the patient for asymmetry of motion or apprehension that is suggestive of primary shoulder pathology.

Next, ask the patient to slowly abduct the arms to 90 degrees. Then have the patient slowly externally rotate the arm as far as it will go (Fig. 20-2). The normal shoulder should allow external rotation of the arm to at least parallel to the floor. Ascertain any limitation of the range of motion or pain on range of motion that would suggest primary shoulder pathology.

If either test is positive, physical examination for specific pathologic processes of the shoulder should then be carried out, such as the Neer impingement test or apprehension test for anterior and posterior instability, as well as obtaining plain radiographs, ultrasound, and magnetic resonance imaging of the affected joints and surrounding soft tissue to further clarify the pathology that is responsible for the patient's shoulder pain and dysfunction.

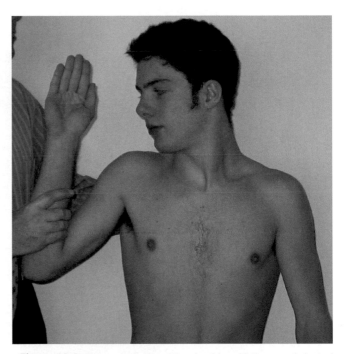

• **Figure 20-2** External rotation of the shoulder with the arm abducted to 90 degrees.

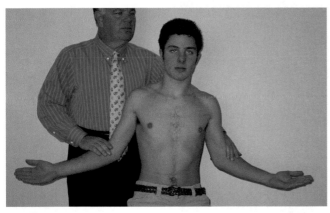

• **Figure 20-1** External rotation of the shoulder with the arms fully adducted.

To adequately assess internal rotation of the shoulder, ask the patient to fully adduct the arm with the palm facing toward the back. Then have the patient reach behind the back and, using the fully extended thumb, touch the uppermost spinal process that he or she can reach (Fig. 21-1). After noting the level that the patient was able to reach, have the patient repeat this maneuver with the contralateral arm, and note any asymmetry of movement or apprehension that is suggestive of primary shoulder pathology.

If this test is positive, physical examination for specific pathologic processes of the shoulder should then be carried out, such as the Neer impingement test or apprehension test for anterior and posterior instability. The examiner should also obtain plain radiographs, ultrasound, and magnetic resonance imaging of the affected joints and surrounding soft tissue to further clarify the pathology that is responsible for the patient's shoulder pain and dysfunction.

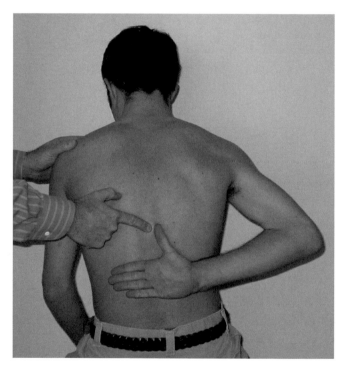

• **Figure 21-1** Internal rotation of the shoulder.

Evaluation of shoulder adduction using the crossed-arm maneuver is useful in identifying problems in the posterior shoulder, including adhesive capsulitis, bursitis, and tendinopathy. To perform this maneuver, place the patient in the seated position and have the patient slowly bring the arm across the chest, observing for any hesitancy or unevenness in movement that might be suggestive of pain (Fig. 22-1). The maneuver is then repeated with the contralateral arm, and the ranges of motion are compared. The patient with a normal shoulder or a minimal amount of primary shoulder pathology should be able to grasp the contralateral triceps without difficulty.

If this test is positive, physical examination for specific pathologic processes of the shoulder should then be carried out, such as the Neer impingement test or apprehension test for anterior and posterior instability. The examiner should also obtain plain radiographs, ultrasound, and magnetic resonance imaging of the affected joints and surrounding soft tissue to further clarify the pathology that is responsible for the patient's shoulder pain and dysfunction.

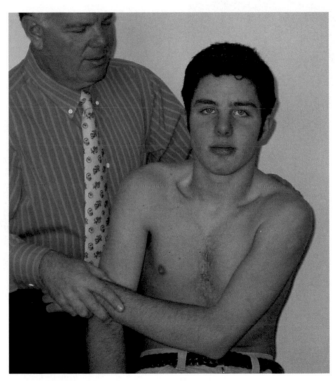

• **Figure 22-1** Crossed-arm adduction of the shoulder.

23 Abduction of the Shoulder

Evaluation of shoulder abduction is useful in identifying primary shoulder pathology, including tendinopathy, bursitis, and impingement syndromes. To evaluate shoulder abduction, have the patient stand, and ask the patient to fully extend the arms as far as they will go behind the back, observing for any asymmetry, apprehension, or limitation of motion (Fig. 23-1). Then ask the patient to fully abduct each shoulder, again observing for any asymmetry or limitation of motion (Fig. 23-2).

If this test is positive, physical examination for specific pathologic processes of the shoulder should then be carried out, such as the Neer impingement test or apprehension test for anterior and posterior instability. The examiner should also obtain plain radiographs, ultrasound, and magnetic resonance imaging of the affected joints and surrounding soft tissue to further clarify the pathology that is responsible for the patient's shoulder pain and dysfunction.

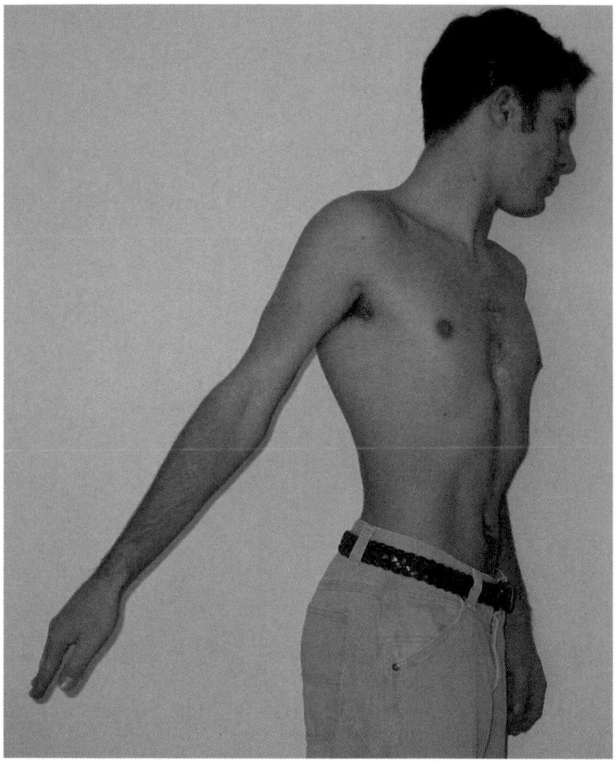

• **Figure 23-1** Begin assessment of shoulder abduction by asking the patient to fully extend the arms as far as they will go behind the back.

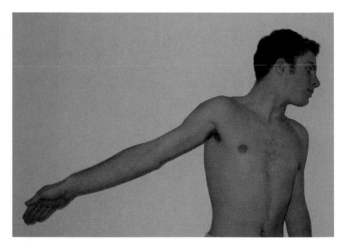

• **Figure 23-2** Continue assessment by asking the patient to fully abduct each shoulder.

As was previously indicated, it is the initial general physical examination of the shoulder that guides the clinician in narrowing his or her differential diagnosis and helps to suggest which specialized physical examination maneuvers and laboratory and radiographic testing will aid in confirming the cause of the patient's shoulder pain and dysfunction. For the clinician to make best use of the initial information gleaned from the general physical examination of the shoulder, a grouping of the common causes of shoulder pain and dysfunction is exceedingly helpful. Although no classification of shoulder pain and dysfunction can be all-inclusive or all-exclusive owing to the frequently overlapping and multifactorial nature of shoulder pathology, Table 24-1 should help to improve the diagnostic accuracy and help the clinician to avoid overlooking less common diagnoses.

The list in Table 24-1 is by no means comprehensive, but it does aid the clinician in organizing the potential sources of pathology that present as shoulder pain and dysfunction. It should be noted that the most commonly missed categories of shoulder pain and the categories that most often result in misadventures in diagnosis and treatment are the last three categories. The knowledge of this potential pitfall should help clinicians keep these sometimes overlooked causes of shoulder pain and dysfunction in their differential diagnosis. Table 24-2 provides a graphic correlation of the signs and symptoms of some of the more common causes of shoulder pain and dysfunction; it should aid the clinician in narrowing the differential diagnosis and ordering appropriate diagnostic testing to help confirm the diagnosis and guide treatment.

TABLE 24-1 Causes of Shoulder Pain

Localized Bony or Joint Space Pathology	Periarticular Pathology	Systemic Disease	Sympathetically Mediated Pain	Referred from Other Body Areas
Fracture	Bursitis	Rheumatoid arthritis	Causalgia	Brachial plexopathy
Primary bone tumor	Tendinitis	Collagen vascular disease	Reflex sympathetic dystrophy	Cervical radiculopathy
Primary synovial tissue tumor	Rotator cuff tear	Reiter syndrome	Shoulder-hand syndrome	Cervical spondylosis
Joint instability	Impingement syndromes	Gout	Dressler syndrome	Fibromyalgia
Localized arthritis	Adhesive capsulitis	Other crystal arthropathies	Postmyocardial infarction adhesive capsulitis of the shoulder	Myofascial pain syndromes such as scapulocostal syndrome
Osteophyte formation	Joint instability	Charcot's neuropathic arthritis		Parsonage-Turner syndrome (idiopathic brachial neuritis)
Joint space infection	Muscle strain			Thoracic outlet syndrome
Hemarthrosis	Periarticular infection not involving joint space			Entrapment neuropathies
Villonodular synovitis	Muscle sprain			Intrathoracic tumors
Intraarticular foreign body				Pneumothorax
				Subdiaphragmatic pathology such as subcapsular hematoma of the spleen with Kerr sign

TABLE 24-2 Differential Diagnosis of Shoulder Pain

Diagnosis	Age	Type of Onset	Location of Pain	Night Pain	Active Range of Motion	Passive Range of Motion	Impingement Signs	Radiation of Pain	Paresthesia	Weakness	Instability	Radiographic Changes	Special Features
Rotator cuff tendinitis	Any	Acute or chronic	Deltoid region	+	↓↓ Guarding	Normal	+++	−	−	Only due to pain	Look for	In chronic cases	Painful arc of abduction
Rotator cuff tears (chronic)	Older than 40 years	Often chronic	Deltoid region	++	↓↓	Normal (may later ↓)	++	−	−	++	−	+	Wasting of cuff muscles
Bicipital tendinitis	Any	Overuse	Anterior	−	↓ Guarding	Normal	+	Occasionally into biceps	−	Only due to pain	Look for	None	Special examination tests
Calcific tendinitis	30-60 years	Acute	Point of shoulder	++	↓↓ Guarding	Normal except for pain	+++	−	−	Only due to pain	−	++	Tenderness ++
Capsulitis ("frozen shoulder")	Older than 40 years	Insidious	Deep in shoulder	++	↓↓	↓↓	+	−	−	−	−	−	Global range of motion ↓
Acromioclavicular joint	Any	Acute or chronic	Over joint	Lying on side	↓ Full elevation	Normal	−	−	−	−	−	In chronic cases	Local tenderness
Osteoarthrosis of glenohumeral joint	Older than 40 years usually	Insidious	Deep in shoulder	++	↓↓	↓↓	−	−	−	May have mild + with acute episodes	−	+++	Crepitus
Glenohumeral instability	25 years	Episodic	Anterior or posterior	−	Only apprehension	Only apprehension	Possible	−	+ With acute episodes	+++	Often	Stress tests	
Cervical spondylosis	Older than 40 years	Insidious	Suprascapular	Often	Normal	Normal	−	++	+++	+	−	In cervical spine	Pain with neck movement
Thoracic outlet syndrome	Any	Usually with activity	Neck, shoulder, arm	−	Normal	Normal	−	++	++	++	−	−	Special examination tests
Sympathetically mediated pain	Any	With contact	Neck, shoulder, arm diffuse	Often	↓ Guarding	↓ Guarding	Possible	Ill-defined	−	With disuse	−	+ Bone scan, articular changes, and demineralization	Vasomotor and sudomotor changes

Modified from Dalton SE: The shoulder. In Klippel JH, Dieppe PA, editors: *Rheumatology*, ed 2, London, 1998, Mosby, p 76.

The father of modern medicine, Hippocrates, was no stranger to the problems of shoulder joint instability, as evidenced by his description of how to reduce an anterior shoulder dislocation in a treatise on medicine written around 300 B.C. While the knowledge of shoulder instability advanced in tandem with the other great advances in medicine, including anatomic dissection, asepsis for surgery, anesthesia, and radiography, it was not until the advent of magnetic resonance imaging (MRI), dynamic ultrasound, and arthroscopy that the construct of shoulder dislocation à la Bankhart as a primary model of shoulder instability gave way to a new, more comprehensive construct that embraced a continuum of dysfunction that ranged from subluxation to frank shoulder dislocation.

This new, refined construct allows the clinician to identify more subtle physical findings that point to the cause of shoulder pain and dysfunction and allow for a more comprehensive range of conservative treatment short of open or laparoscopic surgical procedures. To understand this new construct, the clinician might find the following definitions of subluxation and dislocation useful. Subluxation is defined as an abnormal movement of the humeral head relative to the glenoid. It is often transient in nature, making its recognition by the patient and unsuspecting clinician more difficult than the more obvious shoulder dislocation. Dislocation, with its complete lack of contact between the surfaces of the humeral head and glenoid fossa, is more dramatic and often (especially in the acute setting) does not resolve itself spontaneously, forcing the patient to seek urgent medical attention.

For the purposes of diagnosis of shoulder instability syndromes, the clinician will find it useful to categorize the abnormalities of shoulder instability that are identified during physical examination on the basis of the following:

- Acuity, such as acute or chronic
- Direction of instability, such as anterior, posterior, superior, or inferior
- The degree of instability, such as subluxation versus complete dislocation
- The pathogenesis of the instability, if known, such as MRI-proven labral tear

It should be noted that an individual patient may suffer from more than one type of shoulder instability and that the same shoulder might undergo anterior dislocation and also be subject to posterior, inferior, or superior subluxation or dislocation if different forces are placed on it.

The classifying of shoulder instability as acute or chronic is based on the chronology of the instability, with acute shoulder instability arbitrarily defined in those patients who seek medical attention within 25 hours after a shoulder

problem occurs. Chronic shoulder instability is arbitrarily defined in those patients who seek medical attention for a shoulder problem that has existed longer than 25 hours. Many patients with chronic shoulder instability have recurrent shoulder dislocations with attenuated pain and, because of the decreased amount of pain, often delay seeking medical attention. At first glance, it might seem unlikely that a person would delay seeking treatment for a shoulder dislocation, but it is in fact not uncommon for the diagnosis of posterior shoulder dislocation to be delayed for a period of days, especially if other shoulder pathology is present.

Shoulder instability can be further classified as to the direction in which the humeral head moves relative to the glenoid fossa. The most common direction of shoulder instability is anterior, with more than 90% of all shoulder dislocations occurring in this direction. Anterior subluxation may be identified on physical examination by performing the anterior drawer test (see Chapter 26), the apprehension test (see Chapter 28), and the Jobe relocation test (see Chapter 29). Anterior dislocations can be divided on the basis of where the humeral head dislocates and becomes fixed in order of frequency as follows:

- Subcoracoid (Fig. 25-1)
- Subglenoid (Fig. 25-2)
- Subclavicular (Fig. 25-3)
- Intrathoracic

Posterior subluxation may be diagnosed on physical examination with the posterior drawer test and the jerk test (see Chapter 31). True posterior shoulder dislocations are much less common than anterior shoulder dislocations and often are missed on initial evaluation in spite of a history of trauma to the outstretched arm. Such delay in diagnosis often results in the subsequent development of severe secondary osteoarthritis of the affected joint. Posterior dislocations of the shoulder can be divided on the basis of where the humeral head dislocates and becomes fixed in order of frequency as follows:

- Subacromial (Fig. 25-4)
- Subglenoid (Fig. 25-5)
- Subspinous (Fig. 25-6)

Superior and inferior subluxation of the shoulder are less common than anterior or posterior subluxation but are by no means uncommon. True superior or inferior dislocations are extremely rare, however, and are invariably associated with significant trauma such as falls from a great height or acceleration or deceleration injuries (Figs. 25-7 and 25-8). Concomitant fractures of the glenoid rim, acromion, clavicle, and humerus are also commonly associated with posterior shoulder dislocations, further confusing the diagnosis.

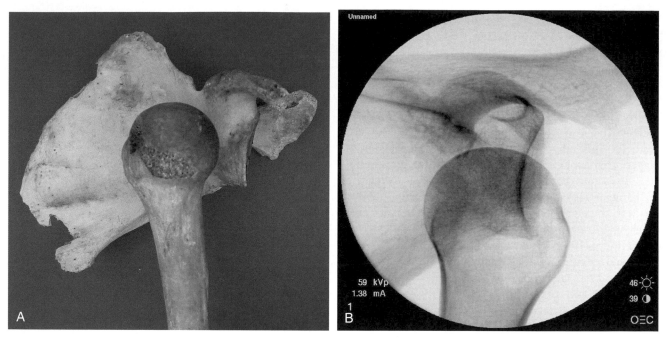

• **Figure 25-1 A** and **B,** Anterior dislocations of the shoulder: subcoracoid.

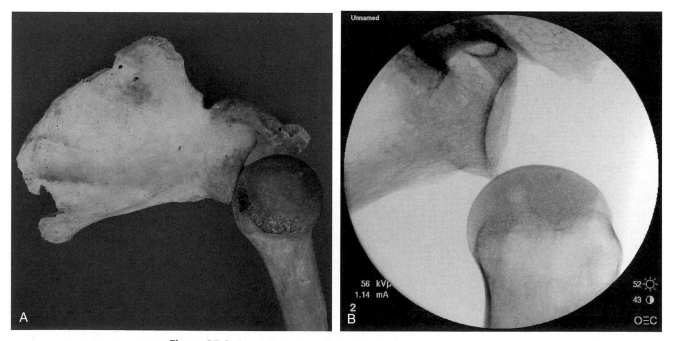

• **Figure 25-2 A** and **B,** Anterior dislocations of the shoulder: subglenoid.

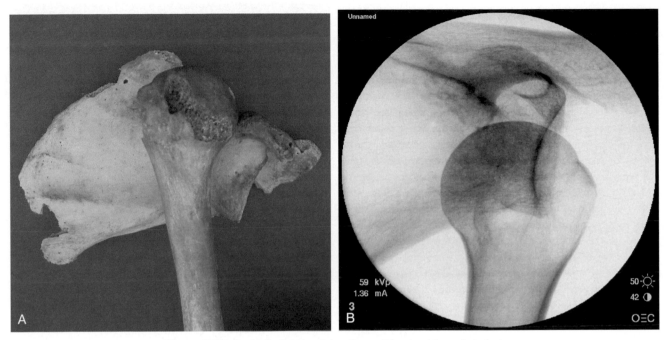

• **Figure 25-3 A** and **B,** Anterior dislocations of the shoulder: subclavicular.

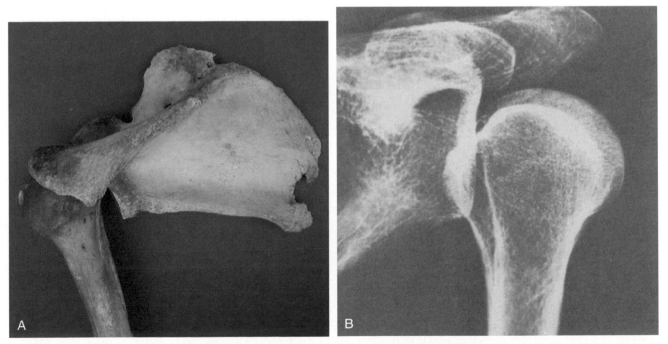

• **Figure 25-4 A** and **B,** Posterior dislocations of the shoulder: subacromial. (**B** from Resnick D: *Diagnosis of bone and joint disorders,* ed 4, Philadelphia, 2002, Saunders, p 2793.)

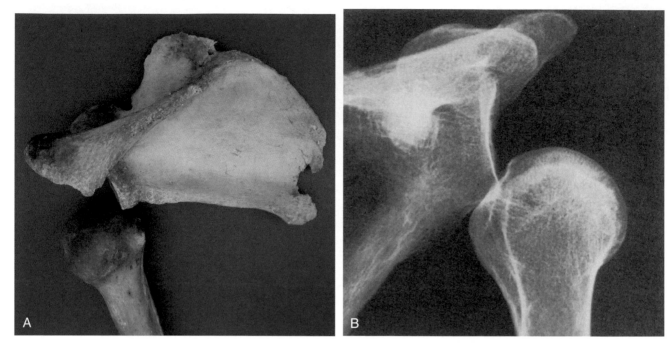

• **Figure 25-5 A** and **B,** Posterior dislocations of the shoulder: subglenoid. (**B** from Resnick D: *Diagnosis of bone and joint disorders,* Philadelphia, 2002, Saunders, p 2793.)

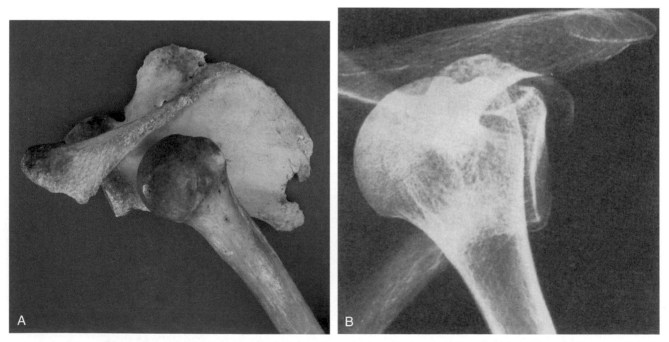

• **Figure 25-6 A** and **B,** Posterior dislocations of the shoulder: subspinous. (**B** from Resnick D: *Diagnosis of bone and joint disorders,* Philadelphia, 2002, Saunders, p 2793.)

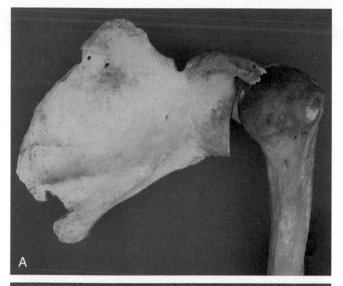

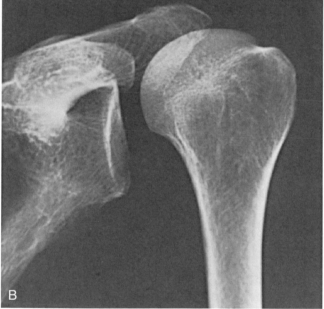

• **Figure 25-7 A** and **B,** True superior dislocation of the shoulder. (**B** from Resnick D, Kang HS: *Internal derangements of joints: emphasis on MR imaging,* Philadelphia, 1997, Saunders, p 239.)

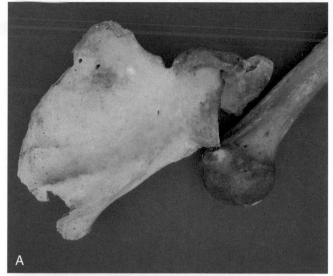

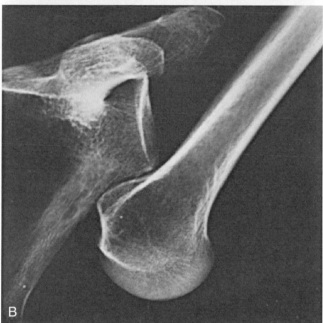

• **Figure 25-8 A** and **B,** True inferior dislocation of the shoulder. (**B** from Resnick D, Kang HS: *Internal derangements of joints: emphasis on MR imaging,* Philadelphia, 1997, Saunders, p 239.)

Careful physical examination should identify the shoulder instability in the majority of patients. The astute clinician should recognize that it is possible for shoulder instability to be multidirectional, and treatment should be aimed at reducing the instability in the plane in which it occurs. Specialized radiographic views, dynamic ultrasound, computed views with 3-dimensional reconstructions, and MRI will help to clarify many of the structural lesions that are responsible for shoulder instability (Fig. 25-9). Arthroscopy with active visualization of the shoulder during actual movement of the affected joint might also be required for the clinician to fully appreciate the functional abnormalities that are contributing to the patient's shoulder pain and dysfunction.

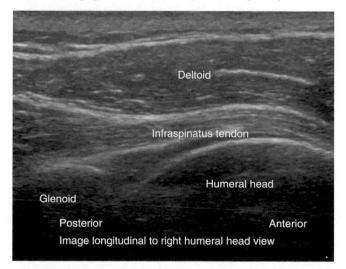

• **Figure 25-9** Longitudinal ultrasound image of patient with rotator cuff tear and resultant high riding humeral head.

The anterior drawer test is useful in identifying anterior shoulder instability, especially after trauma to the shoulder. With the patient in the seated position, the examiner stabilizes the patient's clavicle and scapula with one hand and identifies the humeral head with the other. Anterior force is then gradually applied to the humeral head (Fig. 26-1). The normal shoulder will allow slight anterior translation of the humeral head with a firm, definite, and relatively painless endpoint. If there is a sudden slippage, pain, or apprehension, the examiner should suspect anterior joint instability (Video 26-1).

Anterior stability with resultant anterior shoulder dislocation should be relatively straightforward to diagnose on physical examination because of the obvious gross shoulder deformity associated with anterior dislocation (Fig. 26-2). This is not the case with posterior dislocations, which are often missed during initial evaluation following shoulder trauma.

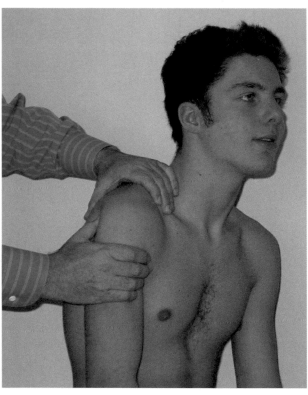

• **Figure 26-1** The anterior drawer test.

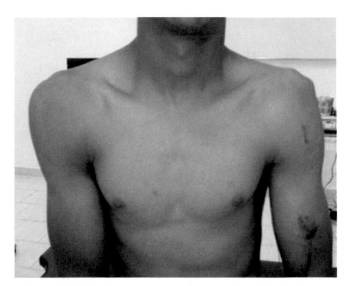

• **Figure 26-2** Typical appearance of a dislocation of the left shoulder. (From Lahrach K, Bennani A, Marzouki A, et al: Luxation antérieure de l'épaule associée à une fracture de la diaphyse humérale homolatérale (à propos d'un cas), *Journal de Traumatologie du Sport* 27(1):20–22, 2010.)

27 The Shift and Load Test for Shoulder Instability

With the patient in the sitting position with the affected arm positioned with 0 degrees abduction, the examiner places one hand along the edge of the scapula to stabilize it. With the opposite hand, the examiner grasps the head of the humerus and gently pushes the head into the glenoid fossa. The examiner then applies firm anterior and posterior pressure on the head of the humerus to assess the degree of anterior and posterior translation (Fig. 27-1). Subluxation of the humeral head in either direction indicates shoulder instability, and evaluation of the condition of the glenoid fossa, humeral head, and the supporting structures of the shoulder including the labrum with plain radiography, shoulder arthrography, computed tomography, sonography, and magnetic resonance imaging is indicated (Fig. 27-2).

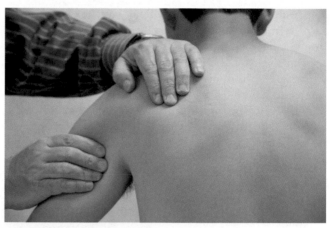

• **Figure 27-1** The shift and load test for shoulder instability.

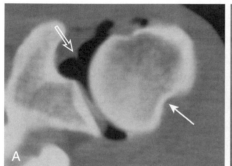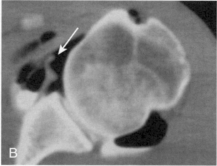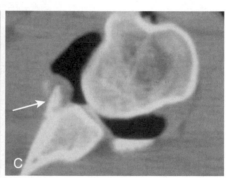

• **Figure 27-2** Glenohumeral joint instability: computed tomography (CT)—capsular, ligamentous, and labral abnormalities. Three transaxial CT arthrographic images obtained at the level of the superior aspect of the joint (level 1) **(A),** the midglenoid level (level 3) **(B),** and the inferior glenoid level (level 4) **(C)** show a number of abnormalities indicative of previous anterior glenohumeral joint dislocation. In **A,** observe a Hill-Sachs lesion *(arrow)*, irregularity of the superior glenohumeral ligament *(open arrow)*, and nonvisualization of the superoanterior portion of the labrum. In **B,** findings include avulsion of the anterior portion of the labrum at the site of attachment of the middle glenohumeral ligament *(arrow)* and a redundant anterior capsule. In **C,** observe a fracture *(arrow)* of the anterior surface of the glenoid rim. (From Resnick D, Kransdorf MJ, editors: *Bone and joint imaging*, ed 3, Philadelphia, 2005, Saunders, p 930.)

28 The Apprehension Test for Anterior Shoulder Instability

The apprehension test is useful in helping the clinician identify anterior shoulder instability and other painful conditions of the anterior shoulder. The test is performed by placing the patient in the sitting position and asking the patient to position his or her arm as if to throw a baseball. The examiner then *slowly* and *gradually* pulls the patient's hand backward to force the shoulder into ever-increasing extension and external rotation (Fig. 28-1). If there is anterior shoulder instability, the patient will actively drop the arm to the side to avoid subluxation or dislocation. If the patient is suffering from pathology of the anterior shoulder, such as tendinitis or bursitis, the patient will actively resist further backward movement of the arm to avoid pain. It is important that the examiner avoid any sudden or excessive application of backward pressure to the arm, if anterior stability is suspected, to avoid inadvertently dislocating the patient's shoulder.

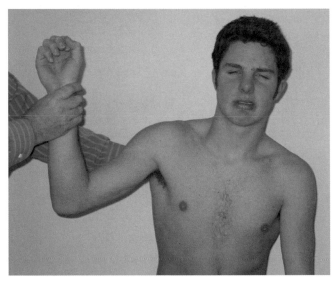

• **Figure 28-1** Apprehension test for anterior shoulder instability.

The Jobe relocation test for anterior shoulder instability is useful in helping the clinician to confirm the clinical suspicion of anterior shoulder instability following a positive apprehension test. The test is performed by placing the patient in the sitting position and applying firm posterior pressure to the anterior shoulder. The patient is then asked to place his or her arm in the baseball-throwing position, and the clinician then repeats the apprehension test for anterior shoulder instability by asking the patient to position his or her arm as if to throw a baseball (see Fig. 29-1). The examiner then *slowly* and *gradually* pulls the patient's hand backward to force the shoulder into ever-increasing extension and external rotation while continuing to apply firm posterior pressure on the anterior

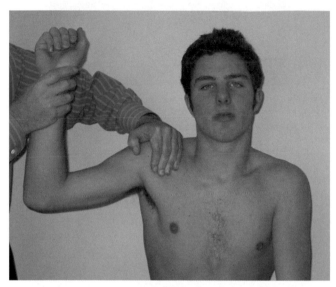

• **Figure 29-1** Jobe relocation test for anterior shoulder instability.

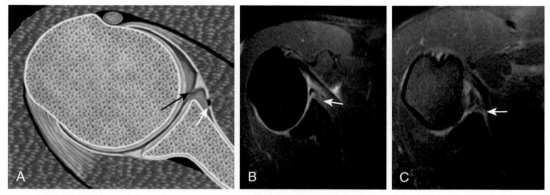

• **Figure 29-2** Bankart lesion, magnetic resonance (MR) imaging. Color diagram in the axial plane **(A)** reveals a tear and detachment of the anterior labrum *(black arrow),* with corresponding tear of the scapular periosteum *(white arrow).* Axial indirect MR arthrogram images **(B, C)** reveal a tear and detachment *(white arrow)* of the anterior inferior labrum. Also note some associated bone loss along the subjacent bony glenoid but no bone Bankart fragment. In **C,** note the displaced labral fragment. (From Zlatkin MB, Sanders TG: Magnetic resonance imaging of the glenoid labrum, *Radiol Clin North Am* 51(2): 279–297, 2013.)

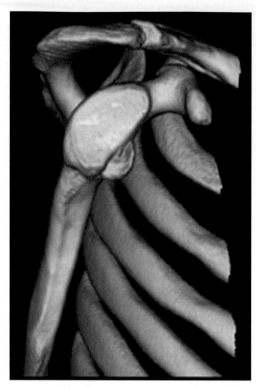

• **Figure 29-3** Three-dimensional computed tomography with humerus digitally subtracted of right shoulder. Bony Bankart lesion visible off anterior-inferior glenoid. (From Harris JD, Romeo AA: Arthroscopic management of the contact athlete with instability, *Clin Sports Med* 32(4):709–730, 2013.)

shoulder (Fig. 29-1). If the presence of this posterior force delays the point at which the patient demonstrates a positive apprehension sign, there is a very high probability of anterior shoulder instability, and magnetic resonance imaging of the shoulder is indicated. Many clinicians believe that a positive relocation test following a positive apprehension test is pathognomonic for a Bankart lesion, which is a disruption of the bony attachment of the anterior labrum to the rim of the glenoid (Figs. 29-2 and 29-3).

30 The Andrews Anterior Apprehension Test for Anterior Shoulder Instability

The Andrews anterior apprehension test for anterior shoulder instability is a useful technique to help confirm the physical findings suggesting anterior instability of the shoulder seen on the anterior apprehension test and Jobe relocation test. It is especially useful when evaluating the patient with shoulder pain who is unable to fully relax because of fear of pain or inadvertent shoulder dislocation during shoulder examination. To perform the Andrews anterior apprehension test for anterior shoulder instability, the patient is placed in the prone position and encouraged to relax. The patient is reassured by the examiner that he or she will be gentle and that by relaxing, the patient can avoid any needless discomfort. The patient's affected arm is then gently abducted and externally rotated while gentle pressure is placed on the posterior shoulder with the examiner's opposite hand (Fig. 30-1). The patient's shoulder is assessed for abnormal anterior movement as well as sudden apprehension due to pain. Care must be taken not to accidentally dislocate the patient's shoulder during this maneuver.

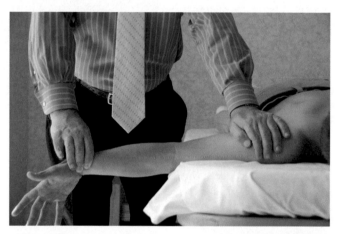

• **Figure 30-1** The Andrews anterior apprehension test for anterior shoulder instability.

The posterior drawer test is useful in identifying posterior shoulder instability, especially after trauma to the shoulder. With the patient in the seated position, the examiner stabilizes the patient's clavicle and scapula with one hand and identifies the humeral head with the other. Posterior force is then gradually applied to the humeral head (Fig. 31-1). The normal shoulder will allow slight posterior translation of the humeral head with a firm, definite, and relatively painless endpoint. If there is a sudden slippage, pain, or apprehension, the examiner should suspect posterior joint instability (Video 31-1).

In contradistinction to anterior instability with resultant anterior shoulder dislocation, which is easy to diagnose because of its obvious shoulder deformity, posterior dislocations are often missed even by experienced clinicians because of the less obvious shoulder deformity being limited to a subtle flattening of the anterior shoulder and slight posterior prominence associated with limited external rotation and forward elevation of the shoulder. Magnetic resonance and/or ultrasound imaging will help clarify the clinical diagnosis (Fig. 31-2).

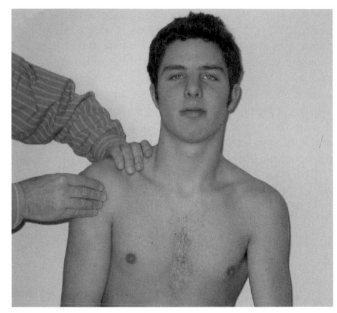

• **Figure 31-1** Posterior drawer test for posterior shoulder instability.

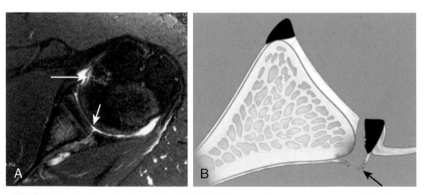

• **Figure 31-2** Posterior shoulder instability. Axial T2 FS magnetic resonance image **(A)** and corresponding diagram **(B).** Note the torn and detached posterior labrum with disruption of the scapular periosteum posteriorly consistent with a reverse Bankart lesion (*white arrow* in **A,** *black arrow* in **B**). Note the reverse Hill-Sachs lesion anteromedially in **A** (*longer white arrow*). (From Zlatkin MB, Sanders TG: Magnetic resonance imaging of the glenoid labrum. *Radiol Clin North Am* 51(2):279–297, 2013.)

32 The Jerk Test for Posterior Shoulder Instability

The jerk test is useful in identifying posterior shoulder instability and, when combined with the posterior drawer test, will increase the clinical accuracy of the diagnosis of the commonly misdiagnosed shoulder pathology. The jerk test is performed with the patient in the sitting position. The patient is asked to fully internally rotate the arm and then flex the arm at the elbow to 90 degrees. The examiner then exerts steady, even posterior force to the arm at the elbow, and the arm is then slowly moved across the body (Fig. 32-1). A sudden jerk may be felt as the humeral head slides off the back of the glenoid. This jerk may again be appreciated when the arm is then moved back to its original position of full rotation and 90-degree flexion as the head of the humerus slides back into the glenoid fossa. If this test is positive, further evaluation with plain radiographs, arthrography, computed tomography, and magnetic resonance imaging is indicated (Fig. 32-2).

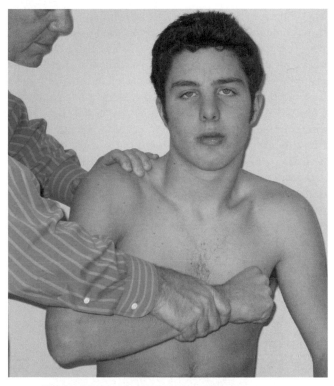

• **Figure 32-1** Jerk test for posterior shoulder instability.

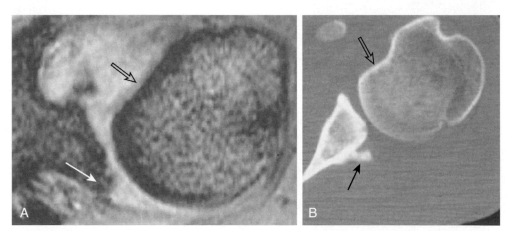

• **Figure 32-2** Posterior glenohumeral joint instability. **A,** Transaxial SPGR (TR/TE, 45/15; flip angle, 20 degrees) magnetic resonance image shows posterior subluxation of the humeral head, irregularity of the posterior glenoid rim *(solid arrow),* and a trough fracture *(open arrow)* involving the anterior surface of the humeral head. **B,** Transaxial computed tomography scan at a slightly lower level in the same patient confirms posterior displacement of the humeral head, a fracture of the posterior glenoid region *(solid arrow),* and a trough fracture of the humeral head *(open arrow).* (Courtesy of M. Schweitzer, MD, Philadelphia, PA; in Resnick D, Kransdorf MJ, editors: *Bone and joint imaging,* ed 3, Philadelphia, 2005, Saunders, p 932.)

33 The Posterior Clunk Test for Posterior Shoulder Instability

The posterior clunk test is useful in helping identify posterior shoulder instability and is often used in combination with the posterior drawer test and jerk test to confirm the suspicion of posterior shoulder instability. To perform the posterior clunk test, the patient is placed in the sitting position and the affected shoulder is internally rotated and then abducted to 90 degrees with the elbow flexed (Fig. 33-1). The examiner then places gentle posterior pressure on the elbow while the affected extremity is moved toward the patient's contralateral shoulder (Fig. 33-2). A clunk is appreciated by both patient and examiner as the humeral head subluxes posteriorly. The patient may also experience pain as the humeral head subluxes. Care must be taken not to apply too much posterior pressure to the elbow when performing this test or the shoulder may inadvertently be dislocated posteriorly (Fig. 33-3).

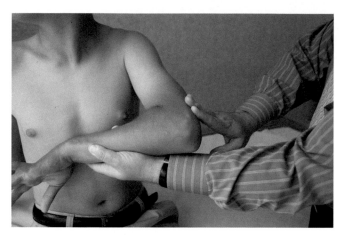

• **Figure 33-2** Clunk test maneuver.

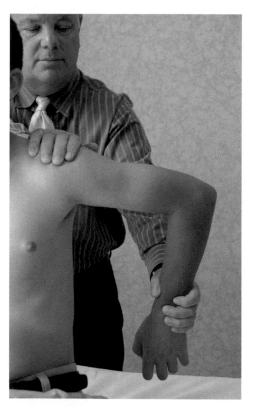

• **Figure 33-1** Initial positioning for the posterior clunk test.

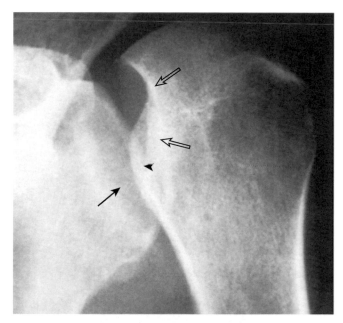

• **Figure 33-3** Glenohumeral joint: posterior dislocation. Findings on the anteroposterior radiograph include distortion of the normal elliptic radiodense region created by the overlying humeral head and glenoid fossa *(arrowhead)*, a "vacant" glenoid cavity *(solid arrow)*, loss of parallelism between the articular surfaces of the glenoid cavity and humeral head, internal rotation of the humerus, and an impaction fracture *(open arrows)*. (From Resnick D, Kransdorf MJ, editors: *Bone and joint imaging*, ed 3, Philadelphia, 2005, Saunders, p 833.)

34 The Sulcus Sign Test for Inferior Glenohumeral Instability

A positive sulcus sign is highly suggestive of inferior glenohumeral instability. To perform the sulcus sign test, the patient is placed in the sitting position with the affected upper extremity relaxed. The examiner then exerts firm inferior traction on the affected upper extremity while observing for the appearance of a dimple, or sulcus, between the acromion and humeral head (Fig. 34-1). More than 2 cm of inferior subluxation is highly suggestive of inferior glenohumeral instability, especially if the sulcus sign remains present as the affected extremity is abducted from 0 to 45 degrees.

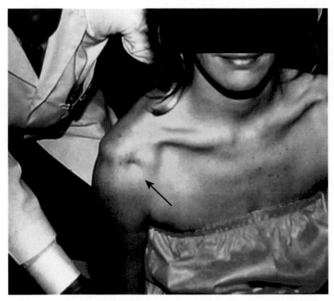

• **Figure 34-1** The positive sulcus sign. (Courtesy of Dr. Tom R. Norris of the San Francisco Shoulder, Elbow, and Hand Clinic.)

A positive crank test is highly suggestive of injury to the labrum of the glenohumeral joint (Fig. 35-1). To perform the crank test, the patient is placed in the sitting position with the affected upper extremity abducted and the elbow flexed 90 degrees (Fig. 35-2). The examiner then exerts firm pressure against the elbow to push the humeral head firmly into the glenohumeral joint (see Fig. 35-2). The humerus is then internally and externally rotated like a "crank" (Fig. 35-3). The test is positive if the rotation of the humerus elicits pain and/or a painful catching or clicking sensation.

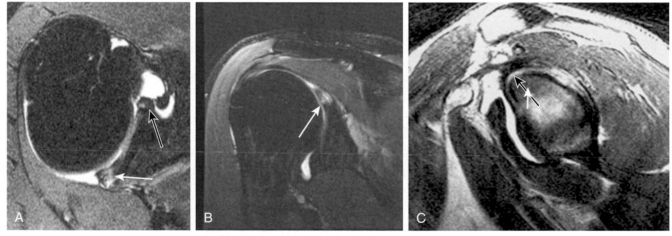

• **Figure 35-1** Axial **(A)**, coronal **(B)**, and sagittal **(C)** magnetic resonance arthrogram images demonstrating tearing of both the anterior superior *(black arrows)* and posterior superior labrum *(white arrows)* with posterior predominance. Some posterior inferior extension is best seen on the sagittal views. (From Zlatkin MB, Sanders TG: Magnetic resonance imaging of the glenoid labrum, *Radiol Clin North Am* 51(2):279–297, 2013, fig 15.)

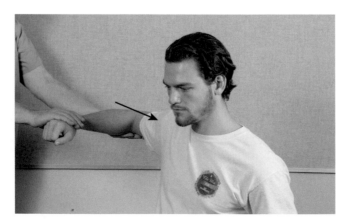

• **Figure 35-2** To perform the crank test, the patient is placed in the sitting position with the affected upper extremity abducted and the elbow flexed 90 degrees. The examiner then exerts firm pressure against the elbow to push the humeral head firmly into the glenohumeral joint.

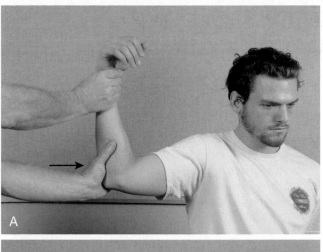

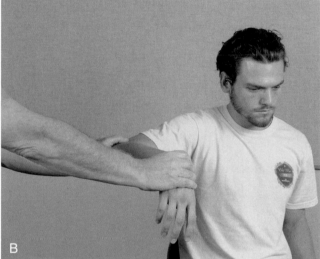

• **Figure 35-3 A** and **B,** The humerus is then internally and externally rotated like a "crank."

36 An Overview of Shoulder Impingement Syndromes

Just as with the pathology of shoulder instability, the understanding of shoulder impingement syndromes has been greatly enhanced by information obtained from magnetic resonance imaging (MRI) and direct arthroscopic visualization of the shoulder joint in health and disease. Unfortunately, as can be seen from Table 36-1, rather than simplifying the classification system for shoulder impingement, this new knowledge served to confirm what many clinicians had long suspected: that rather than being a disease that results from a single or unified pathology, shoulder impingement syndrome is in fact a clinical manifestation of myriad pathologic states.

Fortunately, in spite of the large number of things that can cause shoulder impingement syndrome, what these pathologic states have in common is constriction of the space bounded by the coracohumeral arch above and the humeral head and greater and lesser tuberosities of the humerus below (Figs. 36-1 to 36-3). Through this space pass the tendons of the rotator cuff, the coracohumeral ligament, and, with forward flexion of the humerus, the long tendon of the biceps (Fig. 36-4). In health, the movement of these structures underneath the coracohumeral arch is facilitated by lubrication from the subacromial and subdeltoid bursae, although inflammation, infection, or calcification of these bursae can in fact cause a shoulder impingement syndrome by themselves.

In spite of the multiple potential causes of shoulder impingement syndrome, in most patients, its clinical

TABLE 36-1	Factors Potentially Increasing Rotator Cuff Impingement
Structural Factors	**Functional Factors**
Acromioclavicular joint	Scapula
Congenital abnormality	Abnormal position
Degenerative spurs	Thoracic kyphosis
Nonsurgical foreign body in joint space	Acromioclavicular separation
Pins, wires, or sutures projecting into joint space	Abnormal motion
Acromion	Paralysis (e.g., of trapezius)
Unfused (bipartite acromion)	Fascioscapulohumeral muscular dystrophy
Abnormal shape (flat or overhanging)	Restriction of motion at the scapulothoracic joint
Degenerative spur	Loss of normal humeral head depression mechanism
Nonunion of fracture	Rotator cuff weakness (e.g., suprascapular nerve palsy or
Malunion of fracture	C5-C6 radiculopathy)
Coracoid	Rotator cuff tear (partial or full thickness)
Congenital abnormality	Constitutional or posttraumatic rotator cuff laxity
Posttraumatic change in shape or location	Rupture of long head of biceps
Postsurgical change in shape or location	Tightness of posterior shoulder capsule forcing the humeral
Bursa	head to rise up against the acromion during shoulder
Primary inflammatory bursitis (e.g., rheumatoid arthritis)	flexion
Chronic thickening from previous injury, inflammation, or	Capsular laxity
injection	
Nonsurgical foreign bodies in bursal space	
Pins, wires, or sutures projecting into the bursal space	
Rotator cuff	
Thickening related to chronic calcium deposits	
Thickening from retraction of partial-thickness tears	
Flaps and other irregularities of upper surface due to	
partial or complete tearing	
Postoperative or posttraumatic scarring	
Humerus	
Congenital abnormalities or fracture malunions producing	
relative or absolute prominence of the greater tuberosity	
Abnormally inferior position of humeral head prosthesis	
producing relative prominence of the greater tuberosity	

Modified from O'Brien SJ, Amoczky SP, Warren RF, et al: Developmental anatomy of the shoulder and anatomy of the glenohumeral joint. In Rockford CA Jr, Matsen FA III, editors: *The shoulder,* Philadelphia, 1990, Saunders, p 627.

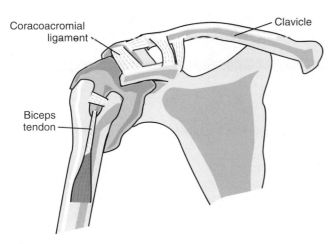

• **Figure 36-1** Anatomic depiction of the shoulder impingement syndrome.

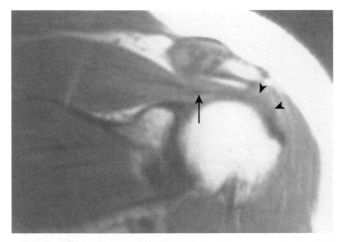

• **Figure 36-2** Acromioclavicular (AC) joint impingement: short-TE oblique coronal image. Callus and osteophyte at the AC joint may be more extensive than represented on plain radiographs and commonly cause shoulder impingement *(arrow)*. The portion of the tendon involved in the impingement process is thickened, with increased signal intensity and indistinct margins *(arrowheads)*. (From Stark DD, Bradley WG: *Magnetic resonance imaging,* ed 3, St. Louis, 1999, Mosby, p 706.)

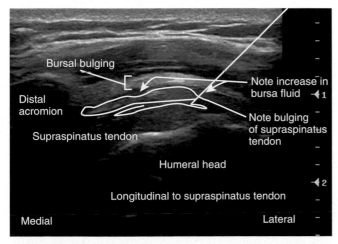

• **Figure 36-3** Longitudinal ultrasound image demonstrating changes consistent with subacromial impingement syndrome.

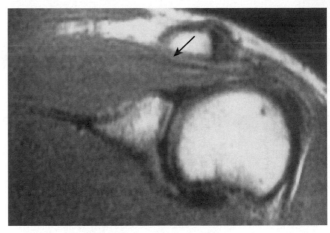

• **Figure 36-4** Hypertrophy of the supraspinatus muscle. Impingement symptoms may accompany severe hypertrophy of the supraspinatus muscle in the presence of a normal bony arch. Contour changes of the superior margin of the supraspinatus muscle from a normal AC joint may be seen in this process *(arrow)*. (From Stark DD, Bradley WG: *Magnetic resonance imaging,* ed 3, St. Louis, 1999, Mosby, p 707.)

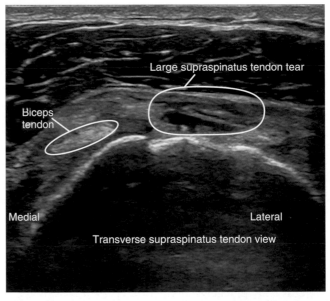

• **Figure 36-5** Transverse ultrasound image demonstrating tear of the supraspinatus tendon.

presentation is classic and easily distinguished from other causes of shoulder pain and dysfunction on physical examination. It must be emphasized, however, that other pathologic conditions of the shoulder frequently coexist with shoulder impingement syndrome, most notably anterior joint instability and rotator cuff tendinitis, and these coexistent pathologic conditions might confuse the clinical diagnosis (Fig. 36-5).

Shoulder impingement syndrome most often presents as ill-defined shoulder pain that is worse after overhead activities or overuse of the shoulder. People in occupations that

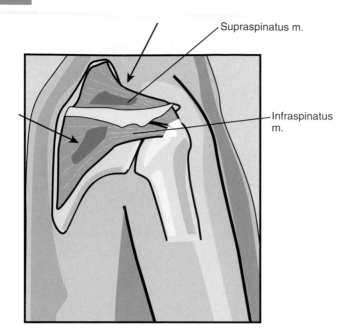

Supraspinatus m.

Infraspinatus m.

• **Figure 36-6** Atrophy of the supraspinatus and infraspinatus muscles in shoulder impingement syndrome.

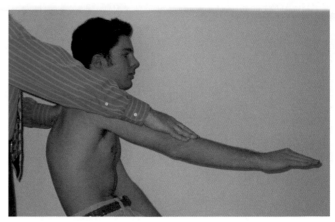

• **Figure 36-7** Manual muscle testing for shoulder impingement syndrome.

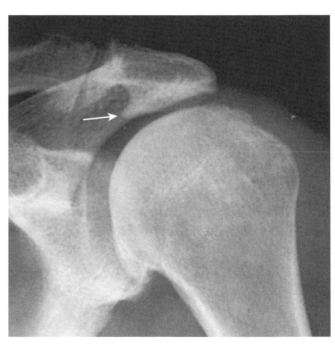

• **Figure 36-8** Shoulder impingement syndrome: routine radiographic abnormalities. A frontal radiograph of the shoulder shows a large enthesophyte *(arrow)* with osteophytes at the acromioclavicular joint and in the inferior portion of the humeral head. (From Resnick D, Kang HS: *Internal derangements of joints: emphasis on MR imaging,* Philadelphia, 1997, Saunders, p 185.)

require repetitive overhead activity, such as fruit pickers, carpenters, painters, and drywall hangers, are particularly susceptible to the development of shoulder impingement syndrome. Swimming, throwing, and tennis playing have also been implicated in the development of this painful condition.

If the pathologic process that is responsible for the shoulder impingement continues, the ill-defined pain will frequently localize to the anterior and lateral shoulder. The patient will often present to the clinician with the complaint of being unable to lie on the affected side at night. The pain is often worse at night, and the patient will begin to notice the inability to perform simple overhead tasks, such as putting dishes away or changing a light bulb.

On physical examination, the anterior and lateral shoulder may be acutely tender to palpation, and there may be crepitus and apprehension when the patient actively raises the arm above 60 degrees. Chronically, inspection of the shoulder may reveal atrophy of the muscles of the rotator cuff, most commonly the supraspinatus and infraspinatus muscles (Fig. 36-6). There may also be rather marked limitation of range of motion on elevation of the upper extremity. The shoulder may "catch" as the patient raises his or her arm. Manual muscle testing may reveal weakness of the muscles of the rotator cuff, in particular the supraspinatus (Fig. 36-7).

Specialized physical examination tests for shoulder impingement include the Neer and Hawkins tests for shoulder impingement (see Figs. 37-1 and 38-1). As was mentioned previously, because anterior instability of the glenohumeral joint is thought to be the most common contributing factor to the development of shoulder impingement syndrome, specific physical examination tests

including the anterior drawer sign, the apprehension test, and the relocation test should be performed on any patient who is suspected of suffering from shoulder impingement syndrome.

Plain radiographs including axillary views of the shoulder will often demonstrate significant osteophyte formation arising from the anteroinferior portion of the acromion (Fig. 36-8). If the clinical presentation and physical examination suggest shoulder impingement syndrome, magnetic resonance and ultrasound images of the shoulder joint and surrounding soft tissues should also be obtained, with

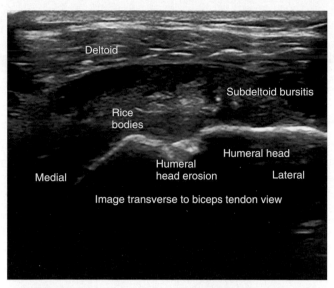

• **Figure 36-9** Transverse ultrasound image demonstrating subdeltoid bursitis with significant erosion of the humeral head. Note the Rice bodies within the subdeltoid bursa.

special attention to the acromion, the rotator cuff, the long tendon of the biceps, and the subacromial and subdeltoid bursae (Fig. 36-9). Computed tomographic scanning with 3-dimensional reconstruction of the coracohumeral arch may also be of value. It should be noted that the purpose of this testing is to try to identify the structural abnormality that is responsible for the evolution of the shoulder impingement syndrome with an eye to finding pathologic processes that are amenable to physical therapy, injection with corticosteroid, or surgical correction.

37 The Neer Test for Shoulder Impingement Syndromes

In the Neer test for shoulder impingement syndromes, the patient is asked to assume a sitting position. While applying firm forward pressure on the patient's scapula, the examiner actively raises the patient's arm to an overhead position, paying particular attention to any pain or apprehension that occurs when the arm moves above 60 degrees of elevation as structures are impinged by the humerus against the acromioclavicular arch (Fig. 37-1 and Video 37-1).

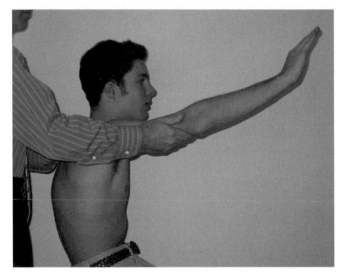

• **Figure 37-1** Neer test for shoulder impingement syndrome.

38 The Hawkins Test for Shoulder Impingement Syndromes

The Hawkins test for shoulder impingement is thought to identify patients whose shoulder impingement syndrome is caused by impingement of the supraspinatus tendon against the coracoacromial ligament. In the Hawkins test for shoulder impingement syndromes, the patient is placed in the sitting position and is then asked to place his or her arm in the throwing position. The examiner then flexes the arm forward approximately 30 degrees and firmly internally rotates the humerus (Fig. 38-1). Reproducible pain during internal rotation is considered a positive test and is highly suggestive of impingement of the supraspinatus tendon against the coracoacromial ligament.

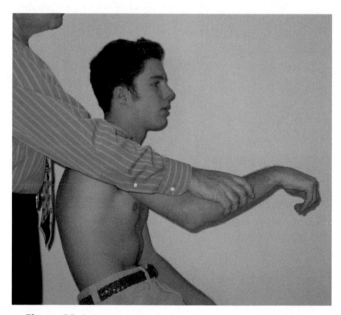

• **Figure 38-1** Hawkins test for shoulder impingement syndrome.

39 The Gerber Subcoracoid Impingement Test

The Gerber subcoracoid impingement test is useful in identifying shoulder impingement caused by impingement between the rotator cuff and the coracoid process (Fig. 39-1). To perform the Gerber subcoracoid impingement test, the patient is placed in the sitting position and the affected upper extremity is flexed forward 90 degrees and then adducted 15 to 20 degrees across the body to bring the lesser tuberosity of the humerus into contact with the coracoid process (Fig. 39-2). Pain during the maneuver is highly suggestive of an impingement syndrome, and imaging of the shoulder is indicated to further delineate the diagnosis.

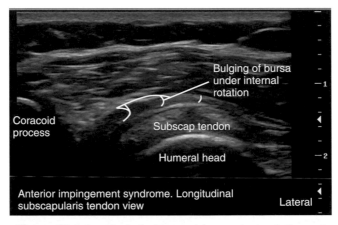

Bulging of bursa under internal rotation

Coracoid process

Subscap tendon

Humeral head

Anterior impingement syndrome. Longitudinal subscapularis tendon view

Lateral

• **Figure 39-1** Longitudinal ultrasound image demonstrating subcoracoid impingement. Note the bulging of the bursa.

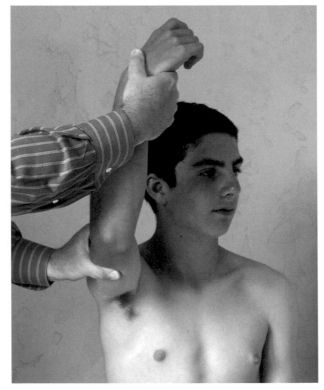

• **Figure 39-2** The Gerber subcoracoid impingement test.

40 The Zaslav Rotation Resistance Test for Shoulder Impingement

The Zaslav rotation resistance test is a useful confirmatory test in patients who exhibit a positive Neer or Hawkins impingement test and may aid the examiner in determining whether the shoulder impingement is occurring at the sub-acromial outlet or is internal, that is, has an intraarticular source. To perform the Zaslav rotation resistance test for shoulder impingement, the patient is placed in the sitting position with the examiner standing behind the patient. The patient's affected upper extremity is then moved to the 90-degree abducted position, and the patient is asked to externally rotate the extremity while the examiner evaluates the patient's muscle strength to approximately 80 degrees (Fig. 40-1). The examiner then repeats the test by asking the patient to internally rotate the affected extremity while the examiner evaluates the patient's muscle strength with internal rotation (Fig. 40-2). If the examiner notes that the patient's external rotation strength is normal and the patient's internal rotation strength is weak, the test suggests internal impingement. If the examiner notes that the patient's internal rotation strength is normal and the patient's external rotation strength is weak, the test suggests a more classic outlet impingement (Fig. 40-3).

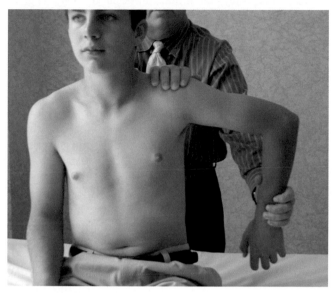

• **Figure 40-2** Step two of the Zaslav rotation resistance test is to assess the patient's muscle strength when internally rotating his or her shoulder.

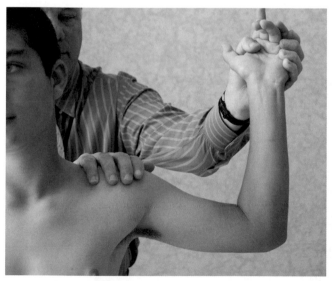

• **Figure 40-1** Step one of the Zaslav rotation resistance test is to assess the patient's muscle strength when externally rotating his or her shoulder.

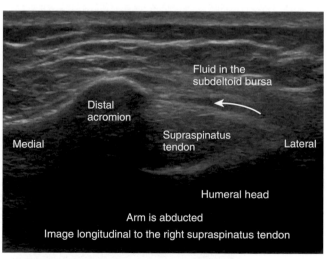

Fluid in the subdeltoid bursa

Distal acromion

Medial

Supraspinatus tendon

Lateral

Humeral head

Arm is abducted
Image longitudinal to the right supraspinatus tendon

• **Figure 40-3** Longitudinal ultrasound image demonstrating subacromial or outlet impingement with the patient's right upper extremity abducted.

Bicipital tendinitis is a common cause of anterior shoulder pain. Although more commonly seen in the fifth and sixth decades, this painful condition can occur at an early age as a result of overuse. Activities that are frequently implicated as inciting factors of bicipital tendinitis include throwing activities, swimming, and golf. Mothers may present with bicipital tendinitis as a result of carrying their infants for long periods of time.

In the absence of acute overuse of the shoulder, bicipital tendinitis rarely exists as an isolated pathologic condition but most often coexists with shoulder instability and shoulder impingement syndromes. This fact is not surprising, given that the long tendon of the biceps works with the rotator cuff to help stabilize the shoulder during movement. This role as shoulder stabilizer is increased in the presence of rotator cuff tendinopathies or complete rotator cuff tears and puts significant additional strain on the biceps tendon.

Bicipital tendinitis may also occur as the result of narrowing or osteophyte formation along the course of the bicipital groove (Fig. 41-1). These changes lead to chronic tendon inflammation and damage and, if untreated, can result in acute tendon rupture, especially during an episode of heavy lifting (Fig. 41-2). Less commonly, rupture of the transverse humeral ligament, which serves as a fulcrum and tether for the biceps tendon, may rupture, allowing the biceps tendon to sublux with resultant greatly magnified forces when the tendon flexes the elbow, leading to damage to the tendon over time.

The patient with bicipital tendinitis most often presents with anterior shoulder pain that is made worse with overhead activities and improved with rest. The patient frequently gives a history of shoulder overuse, although in the cases of narrowing of the bicipital groove or in the setting of chronic shoulder instability, the onset may be more insidious. On physical examination, the patient is exquisitely tender to palpation of the tendon as it passes over the bicipital groove (Fig. 41-3). Shoulder extension and elbow flexion also exacerbate the pain. The Speed and Yergason provocation tests for bicipital tendinitis are specific for this disorder and aid the clinician in diagnosis and treatment (see Figs. 42-1 and 43-1).

As mentioned previously, because bicipital tendinitis frequently coexists with shoulder instability or impingement syndromes, specific physical examination tests including the anterior and posterior drawer signs, the apprehension test, the relocation test, and the jerk test as well as the Neer and Hawkins tests should be performed to identify potential sources of underlying pathology responsible for the evolution of bicipital tendonitis.

Plain radiographs of the shoulder, including special views of the bicipital groove, as well as computed tomographic

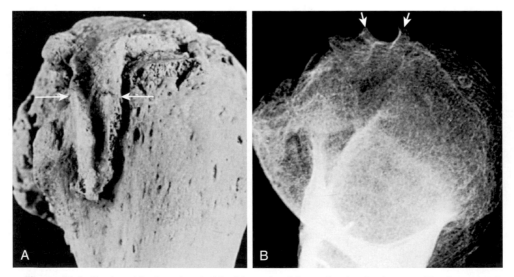

• **Figure 41-1** Tendon of the long head of the biceps brachii muscle, showing bone proliferation around the bicipital groove. Photograph **(A)** and radiograph **(B)** show marked osseous proliferation along the course of the bicipital groove *(arrows)*. (From Cone RO, Danzig G, Resnick D, et al: The bicipital groove: radiographic, anatomic, and pathologic study, *AJR* 141:781, 1983. Copyright 1983 by American Roentgen Ray Society.)

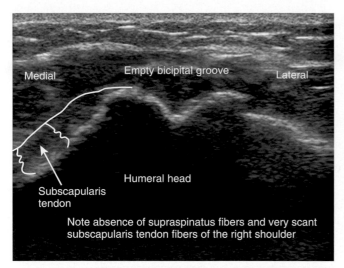

• **Figure 41-2** Ultrasound image demonstrating complete rupture of the biceps tendon as evidenced by the empty bicipital groove. Note abnormalities of the musculotendinous units of the supraspinatus and subscapularis components of the rotator cuff.

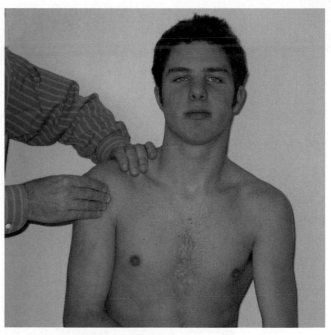

• **Figure 41-3** Palpation of the bicipital tendon.

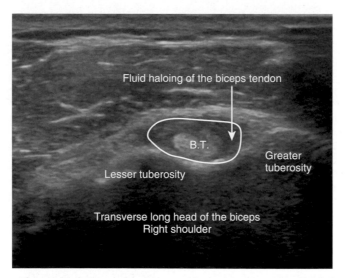

• **Figure 41-4** Transverse ultrasound image demonstrating bicipital tendinitis. Note the haloing of fluid around the inflamed tendon.

images of the humeral head with 3-dimensional reconstruction of the bicipital groove will help to identify narrowing or osteophyte formation that might be irritating and damaging the biceps tendon. Magnetic resonance imaging (MRI) and ultrasound imaging of the shoulder should aid the clinician in identifying abnormalities of the bicipital tendon as well as rotator cuff tendinopathy or complete rotator cuff tears that might be responsible for the patient's bicipital tendinitis (Figs. 41-4 and 41-5). Specialized MRI views of the transverse humeral ligament may identify rupture of the ligament and resultant subluxation of the biceps tendon.

Treatment of bicipital tendinitis should be aimed at treating the underlying pathology whenever it can be

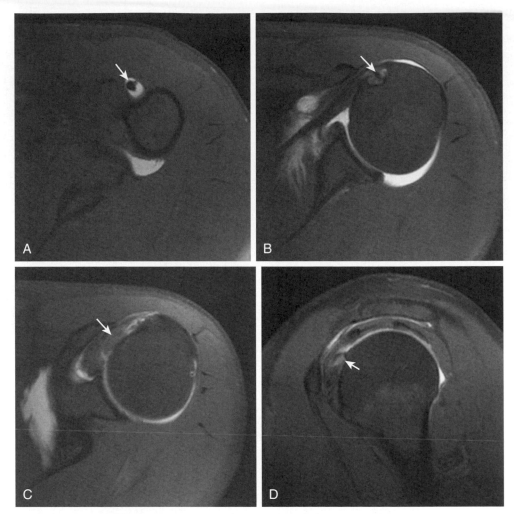

• **Figure 41-5** Axial (**A** to **C**) and sagittal oblique (**D**) T1W with fat suppression (FST1W) magnetic resonance arthogram images of the long head of biceps (LHB) tendon *(white arrows)* in a patient with pain over the biceps. **A,** The LHB tendon in the distal tendon sheath is normal. **B,** More proximally, the tendon is attenuated and is surrounded by intermediate–signal intensity (SI) soft tissue thickening, with osteophytes arising from the lesser tuberosity in the medial aspect of the bicipital groove. **C** and **D,** In the rotator interval, the tendon is thickened and demonstrates areas of increased SI due to tendinopathy. (From Waldman SD, Campbell, RSD: *Imaging of pain,* Philadelphia, 2010, Saunders/Elsevier, fig 96-1.)

identified. Avoidance of activities that provoke or exacerbate the patient's symptoms as well as a short course of antiinflammatory agents will provide symptomatic relief for most patients. Careful injection of corticosteriods around the inflamed tendon may also be of value, although inadvertent injection into the already compromised biceps tendon can lead to acute rupture. To provide long-lasting relief, surgical treatment may ultimately be required in cases of narrowing of the bicipital groove or rupture of the transverse humeral ligament.

To perform the Speed test for bicipital tendinitis, the patient should assume the standing position with his or her elbow fully extended and the arm supinated. The examiner then exerts firm downward force at the level of the antecubital fossa and asks the patient to flex the affected shoulder against resistance (Fig. 42-1). The test is considered positive if the patient complains of pain when flexing the shoulder against resistance (Video 42-1).

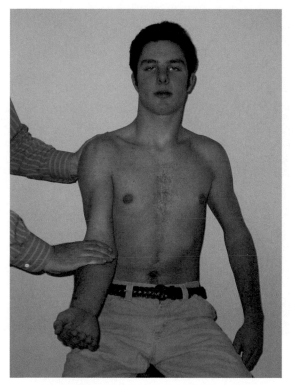

• **Figure 42-1** Speed test for bicipital tendinitis.

To perform the Yergason test for bicipital tendinitis, have the patient assume the standing position with his or her elbow flexed to 90 degrees. The examiner then grasps the wrist of the affected arm and asks the patient to supinate that arm against resistance (Fig. 43-1). The test is considered positive if the patient complains of pain when supinating the arm against resistance (Video 43-1).

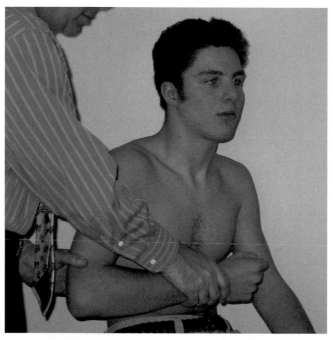

• **Figure 43-1** Yergason test for bicipital tendinitis.

As mentioned in previous chapters, the knowledge gained from advances in magnetic resonance imaging (MRI) and dynamic ultrasound imaging and arthroscopy of the shoulder has led to a greater understanding of the important role that the biceps tendon plays in the maintenance of shoulder stability. When there is irritation or mild displacement of the biceps tendon, the patient frequently first presents with bicipital tendinitis. If the pathologic condition remains untreated, cumulative trauma to the biceps tendon and surrounding structures can lead to scarring with chronic medial displacement of the tendon or, in extreme cases, complete tendon rupture. Such medial displacement puts additional abnormal stress on the coracohumeral ligament and the subscapularis muscle. Over time, both of these structures may tear, allowing further subluxation of the biceps tendon and exacerbation of the patient's shoulder dysfunction (Fig. 44-1). The clinical scenario is known as the subluxing biceps tendon syndrome.

The subluxing biceps tendon syndrome is most often seen in individuals who perform strenuous overhead work, such as drywall hangers, javelin throwers, quarterbacks, and competitive swimmers. The patient with subluxing biceps tendon syndrome most often complains of the combination of pain and a popping or clicking sensation in the shoulder as the biceps tendon moves into and out of the bicipital groove during shoulder abduction, external rotation, and elevation (Fig. 44-2).

These clinical symptoms are by no means pathognomonic for this syndrome, and the clinician will need several sources of information to determine the underlying pathology that is responsible for the subluxation (Fig. 44-3). These sources include specialized physical examination tests, such as the snap test for biceps tendon subluxation and the Gerber lift-off test (see Chapter 45) for subscapularis muscle rupture. Further information can be obtained from targeted MRI of the biceps tendon and bicipital groove, looking at

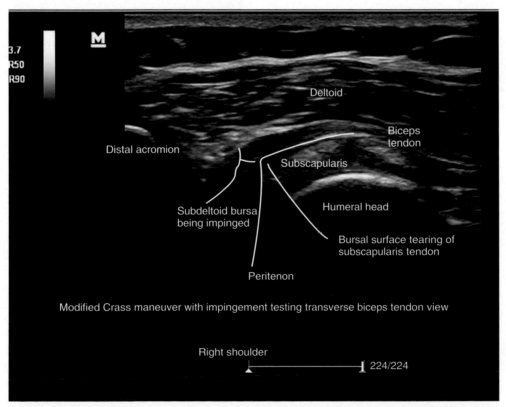

• **Figure 44-1** Ultrasound imaging of the subscapularis muscle and biceps tendon demonstrating the interrelationship between the subscapularis musculotendinous unit and the proximal biceps tendon.

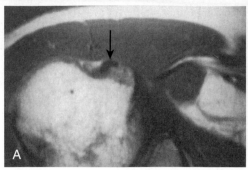
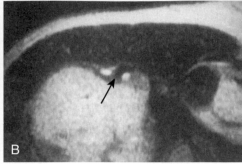

• **Figure 44-2** Biceps tendon subluxation. **A,** This axial (2000/20) image shows the biceps tendon subluxing onto the lesser tuberosity *(arrow)*. **B,** The T2-weighted (2000/80) image shows similar findings *(arrow)*. High-signal fluid is seen adjacent to the tendon at the point of subluxation. Fluid is not seen in the glenohumeral joint or in other portions of the tendon sheath. (From Crues JV, Stoller DW, Ryu RKN: Shoulder. In Stark DD, Bradley WG, editors: *Magnetic resonance imaging*, ed 3, St. Louis, 1999, Mosby, p 714.)

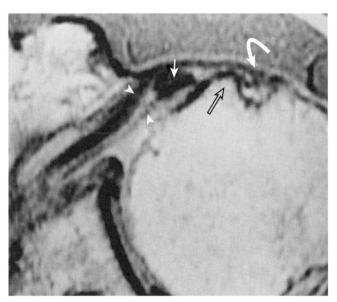

• **Figure 44-3** Tendon of the long head of the biceps brachii muscle: medial dislocation (magnetic resonance [MR] imaging). A 54-year-old man fell on his shoulder while skiing and subsequently was unable to abduct his arm. A transaxial proton density-weighted (TR/TE, 2000/30) spin echo MR image shows that the biceps tendon *(solid straight arrow)* has slipped medially over the lesser tuberosity *(open arrow)* and appears to be lying between the partially displaced fibers *(arrow-heads)* of the subscapularis tendon. The transverse humeral ligament *(curved arrow)* appears intact. (From Resnick D, Kang HS: *Internal derangements of joints: emphasis on MR imaging*, Philadelphia, 1997, Saunders, p 305.)

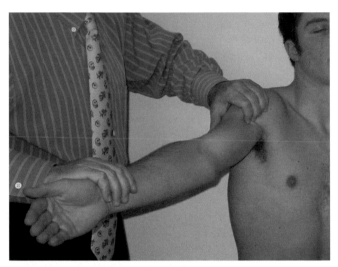

• **Figure 44-4** Snap test for subluxing biceps tendon syndrome.

the special relationships of the two structures as the shoulder is imaged in various degrees of abduction, external rotation, and elevation. This information also gives the orthopedic surgeon a road map for how to surgically repair the underlying pathology that is responsible for the tendon subluxation.

The snap test for subluxing tendon biceps aids the clinician in separating this pathologic condition of the shoulder from other pathologic conditions of the shoulder that

present with the primary symptoms of pain and a clicking or popping sensation with shoulder movement. The snap test is performed with the patient in the standing position. The patient is asked to fully abduct, externally rotate, and elevate the affected shoulder. The examiner then palpates the shoulder as the patient slowly lowers his or her arm. An audible or palpable snap is appreciated as the biceps tendon subluxes back into the bicipital groove (Fig. 44-4).

Unfortunately, a positive snap test for subluxing biceps tendon syndrome does not point the examiner to the specific pathology that is responsible for tendon subluxation, such as a ruptured coracohumeral ligament or a ruptured subscapularis muscle; it indicates only that biceps tendon subluxation is likely. To narrow the potential causes, the examiner should then perform the Gerber lift-off test to identify rupture of the subscapularis muscle. Confirmatory targeted magnetic resonance scanning with the affected shoulder in various stages of abduction, external rotation, and elevation is also indicated.

45 The Gerber Lift-Off Test for Rupture of the Subscapularis Muscle

The Gerber lift-off test will aid the clinician in determining whether the patient's subluxing biceps tendon is due to rupture of the subscapularis muscle. To perform the test, the patient is asked to stand and place his or her fully pronated hand behind his or her back at the level of the belt line (Fig. 45-1). The examiner then puts firm pressure against the patient's hand and asks the patient to push the examiner's hand away (Fig. 45-2). Patients with significant trauma to the subscapularis muscle and its tendinous insertions will be unable to push the examiner's hand away. Confirmatory targeted magnetic resonance imaging and dynamic ultrasound images with the affected shoulder in various stages of abduction, external rotation, and elevation as well as specific images of the musculotendinous units of the rotator cuff, in particular the subscapularis, is also indicated to confirm the diagnosis and guide treatment options (Fig. 45-3 and Video 45-1).

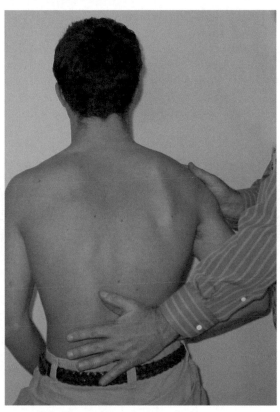

• **Figure 45-2** Gerber lift-off test for rupture of the subscapularis muscle: note placement of examiner's hands.

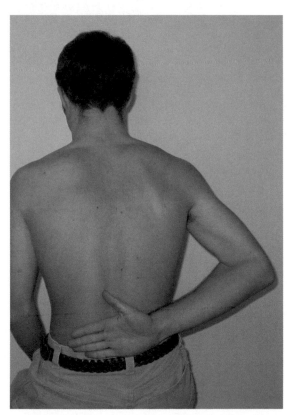

• **Figure 45-1** Gerber lift-off test for rupture of the subscapularis muscle: patient positioning.

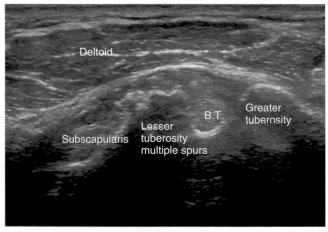

• **Figure 45-3** Transverse ultrasound image demonstrating intersubstance tears of the subscapularis musculotendinous unit. Note osteophytes of the lesser tuberosity of the humerus. *B.T.,* Biceps tendon.

46 The Gerber Belly Press Test for Subscapularis Weakness

Weakness of internal rotation of the shoulder is highly suggestive of weakness of the subscapularis muscle. The Gerber belly press test is an easy way to confirm such weakness. To perform the Gerber belly press test, the patient is placed in the sitting position and instructed to firmly press the palm of the hand of the affected upper extremity against his or her belly while keeping the arm in maximum internal rotation. If internal rotational strength is normal, the patient will be able to keep his or her elbow in front of the trunk (Fig. 46-1). If the strength of internal rotation of the affected upper extremity is diminished, the patient will tend to maintain pressure on the abdomen by externally rotating the shoulder and flexing the wrist, the ipsilateral elbow dropping behind the trunk (Fig. 46-2 and Video 46-1).

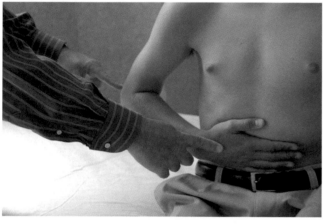

• **Figure 46-1** The Gerber belly press test for subscapularis weakness: if internal rotational strength is normal, the patient will be able to keep his or her elbow in front of the trunk.

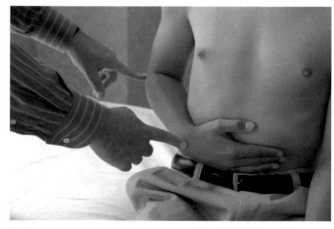

• **Figure 46-2** The Gerber belly press test for subscapularis weakness: if the strength of internal rotation of the affected upper extremity is diminished, the patient will tend to maintain pressure on the abdomen by externally rotating the shoulder and flexing the wrist, the ipsilateral elbow dropping behind the trunk.

47 The Internal Rotation Lag Sign for Rupture of the Subscapularis Tendon

To perform the internal rotation lag sign test for rupture of the subscapularis tendon, the examiner stands behind the patient and the patient's affected upper extremity is held by the examiner in almost maximal internal rotation behind the patient's back. The elbow is then flexed to 90 degrees, and the shoulder is held at 20 degrees of elevation and 20 degrees of extension. The examiner then gently lifts the affected upper extremity away from the patient's lumbar region until maximal internal rotation is reached. The patient is then asked to actively maintain that position with the examiner supporting the patient's elbow but releasing the wrist (Fig. 47-1). The test is considered positive if any significant lag is observed when the examiner releases the patient's wrist (Video 47-1). Such a lag is highly suggestive of rupture of the subscapularis tendon. Rupture of the tendon can be confirmed with ultrasound and/or magnetic resonance imaging (Fig. 47-2).

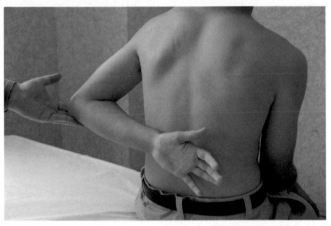

• **Figure 47-1** The internal rotation lag sign test for rupture of the subscapularis tendon. The test is considered positive if any significant lag is observed when the examiner releases the patient's wrist. Such a lag is highly suggestive of rupture of the subscapularis tendon.

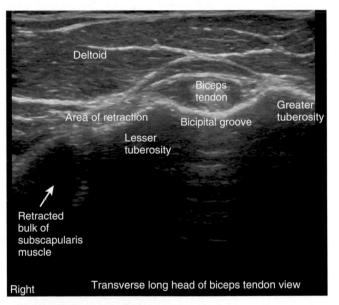

• **Figure 47-2** Transverse ultrasound image demonstrating complete tear and retraction of the subscapularis musculotendinous unit.

Snapping scapula syndrome is an abnormal condition of the shoulder characterized by an audible or tactile snapping or popping associated with movement of the scapula across its thoracic articulation (Fig. 48-1). Snapping scapula syndrome may be associated with pain or may be painless. There are many causes of the snapping scapula syndrome, but all causes find their basis in one of three general pathologic categories: (1) changes in congruence of the anterior scapula where it interfaces with the posterior chest wall, (2) changes in the soft tissues that lie between the anterior scapula and posterior chest wall, and (3) abnormalities of the posterior chest wall.

Changes in the congruence of the anterior scapula can occur as a result of either a physical alteration of the scapula or pathologic processes that alter the way the scapula slides across the posterior chest wall. Examples of physical alterations of the scapula that have been implicated in the evolution of snapping scapula syndrome include scapular fracture, bone tumor (most notably osteochondroma), and the development of bony enthesophytes as a result of chronic shoulder dysfunction (Fig. 48-2). Examples of

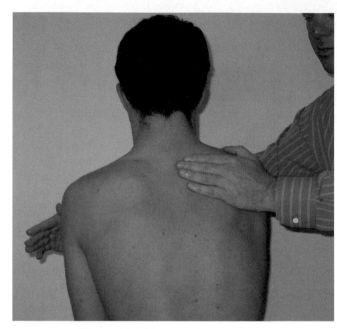

• **Figure 48-1** The snapping scapula test.

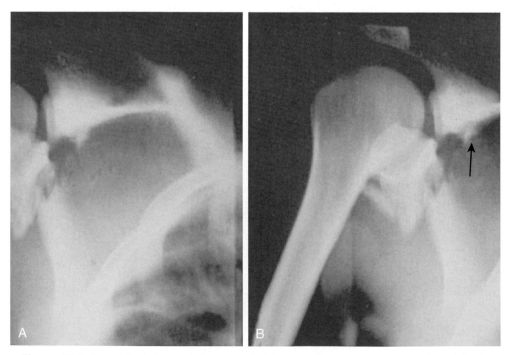

• **Figure 48-2** **A** and **B,** Anteroposterior computed tomography scans show extension of fracture through the scapular spine (*arrow* in **B**) isolating the upper glenoid fragment and coracoid. (From Browner BE, Jupiter JB, Levine AM, et al: *Skeletal trauma,* ed 2, Philadelphia, 1998, Saunders, p 1659.)

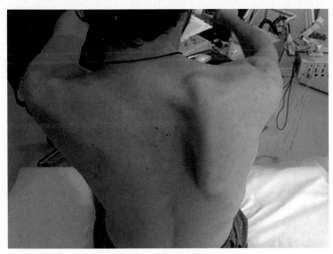

• **Figure 48-3** Winged scapula, typical symptomatology for brachial neuritis or Parsonage-Turner syndrome. (From Deroux A, Brion JP, Hyerle L, et al: Association between hepatitis E and neurological disorders: two case studies and literature review, *J Clin Virol* 60(1):60–62, 2014, fig 1.)

pathologic processes that alter the way the scapula slides against the posterior chest wall that have been implicated in the evolution of snapping scapula syndrome include neurologic compromise of scapular function by cerebrovascular accident, brachial plexopathy, trauma to the long thoracic nerve of Bell, and entrapment of the suprascapular nerve (Fig. 48-3).

Changes in the soft tissues between the scapula and posterior chest wall that have been implicated in the evolution of snapping scapula syndrome include bursitis, muscle hypertrophy, muscle atrophy, and muscle inflammation from polymyositis.

Changes in the posterior chest wall that have been implicated in the evolution of snapping scapula syndrome include chest wall tumor and poorly healed fractured ribs. It should be noted that any one of these three primary pathologic processes can cause a secondary pathologic process to occur, further exacerbating the patient's symptoms, such as secondary bursitis as a result of chronic irritation by a bony enthesophyte.

Because tumors of the thorax and scapula are frequently the cause of snapping scapula syndrome, all patients suffering from this shoulder disorder should undergo careful radiographic evaluation of the scapula and posterior chest wall as well as computed tomography (CT) of the scapula with 3-dimensional reconstruction and CT of the posterior chest wall. Magnetic resonance imaging (MRI) of the affected area with and without contrast should also be performed to help identify potential soft tissue abnormalities that might be serving as the primary or secondary pathologic processes responsible for the development of snapping scapula syndrome. MRI of the brain with and without contrast should be performed on all patients who are thought to have a neurologic process as the source of their scapular dysfunction. The information gleaned from the MRI should then be combined with information obtained from electromyography and nerve conduction velocities of the cervical nerve roots, brachial plexus, suprascapular nerve, and long thoracic nerve of Bell to further characterize the neurologic pathologic process.

Rupture of the long head of the biceps tendon occurs suddenly and often without warning. The pathology responsible for biceps tendon rupture is in most cases a long time in happening, however. Repetitive stress placed on the biceps tendon because of dysfunction of the shoulder joint, in particular shoulder impingement syndromes, rotator cuff tear, and anterior shoulder instability, will initially result in bicipital tendinitis. Left untreated, over time, bicipital tendinitis will cause fibrosis, calcification, and weakening of the biceps tendon (Fig. 49-1). The tendon most commonly ruptures at its weakest point, which is where the long head of the tendon exits the joint capsule. Rarely the long head of the biceps tendon will rupture more distally when subjected to extreme abnormal force. Even more rare is rupture of the short head of the biceps. Rupture of the short head occurs with extremely rapid and forceful adduction and flexion of the elbow.

In most patients over 40 years of age, the long head of the biceps tendon will rupture without obvious provocation. Occasionally, the long head of the biceps tendon will rupture in younger patients during a period of extreme stress on the tendon, such as during power weight lifting.

Clinically, when the long head of the biceps tendon ruptures, the patient will experience a sudden sharp pain in the anterior shoulder accompanied by an audible popping as the tendon ruptures and retracts. The patient with rupture of the long head of the biceps tendon will present with a characteristic soft tissue abnormality known as the "Popeye" sign, as the biceps muscle bunches up as it retracts distally,

giving the arm a "Popeye the Sailor Man" appearance (Fig. 49-2). Ecchymosis running distally into the antecubital fossa is common as blood flows down the empty tendon sheath. Tenderness over the bicipital groove is common, and a defect along the course of the biceps muscle is easily palpable (Fig. 49-3).

The diagnosis of rupture of the biceps tendon can be confirmed by performing the Ludington test for rupture of the long head of the biceps. Any doubt about the diagnosis can be removed by obtaining magnetic resonance imaging (MRI) or ultrasound imaging along the entire course of the biceps tendon (Figs. 49-4 and 49-5).

The Ludington test for ruptured long tendon of the biceps is useful in helping the clinician to confirm the clinical suspicion of biceps tendon rupture. The test is performed by placing the patient in the sitting position and having the patient place the hand of the affected extremity

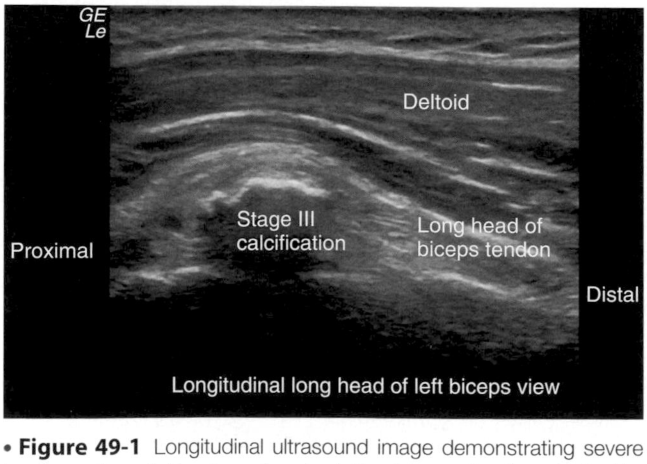

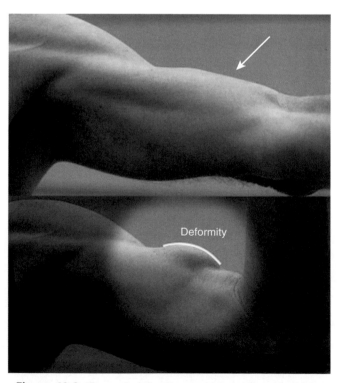

• **Figure 49-1** Longitudinal ultrasound image demonstrating severe tendinopathy of the long head of the biceps tendon. Note the calcification.

• **Figure 49-2** "Popeye" deformity associated with ruptured long tendon of the biceps. (From Shawn Chillag, Kim Chillag: Popeye deformity—an augenblick diagnosis, *Am J Med* 127(5):385, 2014, fig 1.)

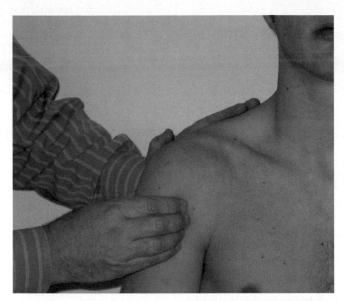

• **Figure 49-3** Palpation of the long tendon of the biceps.

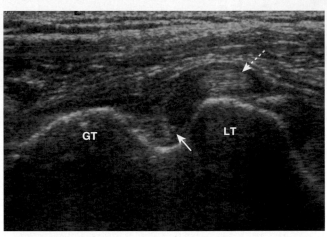

• **Figure 49-5** Transverse ultrasound image of the proximal humerus demonstrating an empty bicipital groove *(white arrow)*. However, the long head of the biceps tendon is subluxated medially and is clearly visible lying on the lesser tuberosity *(broken white arrow)*. When the tendon is dislocated more medially, it can be difficult to identify and can be mistaken for a tendon rupture. *GT,* Greater tuberosity; *LT,* lesser tuberosity.

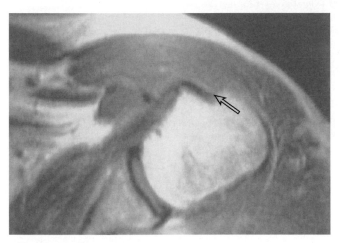

• **Figure 49-4** Long head of the biceps tendon tear. Axial image reveals absence of the biceps tendon in the intertuberous groove *(arrow)*. This patient also has a large rotator cuff tear. (From Stark DD, Bradley WG: *Magnetic resonance imaging,* ed 3, St. Louis, 1999, Mosby, p 712.)

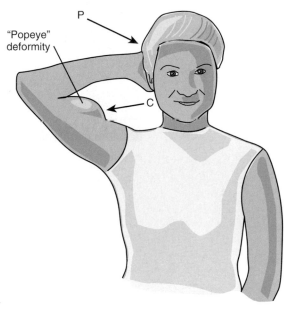

• **Figure 49-6** The Ludington test for ruptured long tendon of the biceps. *C,* Contraction of biceps; *P,* pressure applied.

behind his or her head. The patient is then asked to push against the back of the head and simultaneously contract the affected biceps muscle (Fig. 49-6). If the long tendon of the biceps is ruptured, this maneuver will accentuate the pathognomonic "Popeye" deformity associated with tendon rupture. If the Ludington test is positive, MRI of the affected shoulder and upper extremity along the entire course of the biceps is indicated to delineate the point of rupture and the relative position of the distal end of the biceps tendon.

50 The Squeeze Test for Distal Rupture of the Biceps Tendon

To perform the squeeze test for distal rupture of the biceps tendon, the patient is placed in the seated position with the elbow of the affected extremity flexed approximately 75 degrees to reduce the tension on the brachialis muscle to allow the examiner to focus on the biceps muscle. The forearm is then slightly pronated to increase tension on the biceps brachii tendon. The examiner then places one hand on the distal myotendinous junction and the other hand around the belly of the biceps muscle (Fig. 50-1). The examiner then squeezes both hands simultaneously, which causes the belly of the biceps muscle to retract anteriorly. If the myotendinous unit is intact, the forearm will supinate. If there is rupture of either the tendon or the muscle itself, the forearm will not supinate and the test is considered positive.

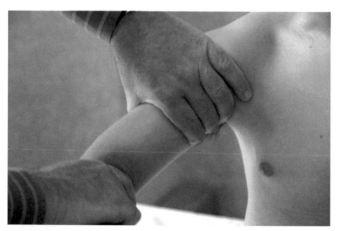

• **Figure 50-1** If the myotendinous unit is intact, the forearm will supinate. If there is rupture of either the tendon or the muscle itself, the forearm will not supinate and the test is considered positive.

51 Clinical Correlates: Diseases of the Rotator Cuff

Ask any physician which muscles make up the rotator cuff, and you will probably get a correct answer. Analogous to cranial nerves "On Old Olympus" and so on, the use of the acronym *SITS* seems to fix the supraspinatus, infraspinatus, teres minor, and subscapularis muscles indelibly in every doctor's mind. Yet ask the same doctor what the rotator cuff does, and beyond vague comments about lifting the shoulder, things quickly become quite muddled. The purpose of this chapter is to clearly define what the rotator cuff is, what it does, and which diseases affect it.

WHAT THE ROTATOR CUFF IS AND WHAT IT DOES

When asked what the rotator cuff is, most physicians would answer that it is a structure of the shoulder made up of the supraspinatus, infraspinatus, teres minor, and subscapularis muscles. This is partially correct, but the answer is in fact significantly more complicated than that. To fully understand the role of the rotator cuff in health and disease, the clinician must first appreciate that the rotator cuff must be thought of as a functional musculotendinous unit rather than four discrete muscles. Although it is true that each of these four muscles contributes to the rotator cuff, it is not only the muscles but also their fasciae and, most important, their tendons that make up the functional unit that we call the rotator cuff (Fig. 51-1).

Arising from the superior aspect of the scapula, the supraspinatus muscle and its covering fascia wrap themselves around the superior humeral head and terminate as a strong tendon that inserts into the uppermost facet of the greater tuberosity of the humerus. The infraspinatus muscle arises from the inferior aspect of the scapula, and its muscle fibers and fascia transform and merge into a dense tendon that passes behind the capsule of the glenohumeral joint to insert into the middle facet of the greater tuberosity of the humerus. The teres minor muscle arises from the mediolateral portion of the scapula and the fascia of the infraspinatus muscle, and its muscle fibers and fascia transform into a tendon that passes behind and below the glenohumeral capsule to insert into the inferior facet of the greater tuberosity of the humerus. The subscapularis muscle arises from the medial portion of the anterior surface of the scapula, and as its muscle fibers transform into a tendon, they extend laterally to attach to the lesser tubercle of the humerus.

One of the primary functions of the musculotendinous units that make up the rotator cuff is to provide stabilization of the glenohumeral joint during shoulder motion as well as to strengthen the relatively weak glenohumeral joint capsule (see Chapter 17). The supraspinatus and infraspinatus musculotendinous unit help to reinforce the superior aspect of the glenohumeral joint capsule; the teres minor musculotendinous unit helps to reinforce the posterior aspect of the joint capsule; and the subscapularis musculotendinous unit helps to reinforce the anterior portion of the joint capsule. The rotator cuff also serves as an important initiator of abduction of the upper extremity. In addition to these functions, the rotator cuff helps to stabilize the shoulder by counterbalancing the inherent upward force of the deltoid muscle during shoulder motion.

In thinking about the role of the rotator cuff in shoulder motion, it is useful to think of all of the muscles and their associated fasciae and tendons actively working as a single unit. They work in concert to maintain the stability of the shoulder joint throughout a wide and varied range of motion. The rotator cuff accomplishes this amazing task by allowing each component muscle to smoothly and subtly vary the strength and velocity of contraction and relaxation as the shoulder moves through its range of motion. It is also important to recognize that the rotator cuff does not function as an isolated structure but works with the other

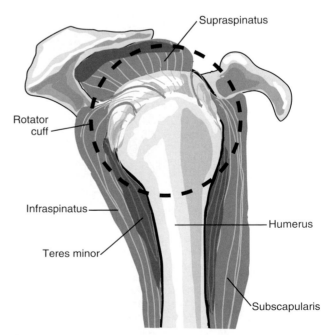

• **Figure 51-1** The rotator cuff is a functional musculotendinous unit composed of four muscles, their fasciae, and tendons.

muscles and structures of the shoulder, including the deltoid muscle, the long tendon of the biceps muscle, and the coracohumeral and glenohumeral ligaments, to allow a complex and unique range of motion of the shoulder relative to the other joints of the body.

Given the complex interaction of these musculotendinous units with each other as well as with their surrounding structures, it should not be surprising that disease of one structure can severely affect the function of the other interdependent structures. Because of the tenuous nature of the blood supply to the tendons of the rotator cuff, these structures are particularly vulnerable to damage. Weakening of the tendons as a result of ischemic changes and chronic inflammation can first lead to rotator cuff tendinopathy and, if left untreated, ultimately to rotator cuff tear.

THE PATHOGENESIS OF ROTATOR CUFF DISEASE

As was mentioned earlier, the poor blood supply to the musculotendinous units that make up the rotator cuff make these structures especially vulnerable to damage. This

hypovascularity is most pronounced in the distal portion of the supraspinatus tendon, which, not surprisingly, is one of the most common locations of complete rotator cuff tear. Although the clinical presentation of acute complete rotator cuff tear is dramatic, the clinician should recognize that there is a continuum of rotator cuff tendinopathy that is responsible for a significant amount of shoulder pain and dysfunction encountered in clinical practice.

At one end of the continuum is mild tendinitis, which is often accompanied by bursitis (Figs. 51-2 and 51-3). Clinically, this can present as diffuse shoulder pain that is made worse with range of motion, nocturnal pain with difficulty sleeping on the affected shoulder, and a catching or grating sensation with shoulder abduction. These symptoms usually respond to conservative therapy consisting of nonsteroidal antiinflammatory agents, local application of heat and ice, physical therapy, and local injection of corticosteroid.

If untreated, this mild tendinitis can worsen, with further degeneration of the tendons leading to calcific tendinitis and ultimately a frozen shoulder (Figs. 51-4 and 51-5). Clinically, the patient will experience extreme pain on range of motion with a limited ability to reach above the head.

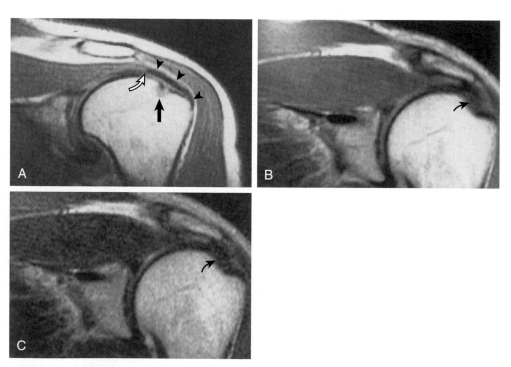

• **Figure 51-2** Early rotator cuff degeneration. **A,** Oblique coronal short-TE image shows normal supraspinatus muscle and tendon, with myotendinous junction near the 12 o'clock position of the humeral head *(curved arrow)*. The tendon is black along its entire course from the myotendinous junction to its attachment on the greater tuberosity *(arrowheads)*. The tendon is uniform in thickness and sharply marginated. The subdeltoid and subacromial fat planes are intact. Despite the normal supraspinatus muscle and tendon, a small erosion is seen at the insertion of the infraspinatus tendon *(straight arrow)*. **B,** Short-TE images show early degenerative changes in the rotator cuff with high signal intensity within the cuff *(arrow)*. **C,** Long-TE images reveal low signal intensity within the cuff *(arrow)*. (From Crues JV, Stoller DW, Ruy RKN: Shoulder. In Stark DD, Bradley WG, editors: *Magnetic resonance imaging*, ed 3, St. Louis, 1999, Mosby, p 708.)

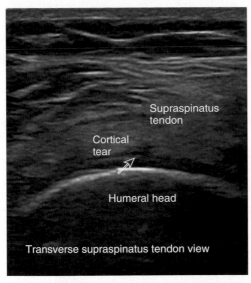

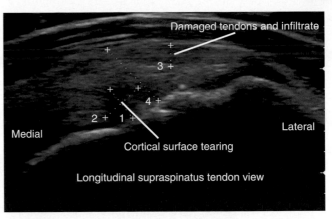

• **Figure 51-5** Severe tendinopathy of the supraspinatus tendon is demonstrated on this longitudinal ultrasound image of a patient with chronic shoulder pain. Note the loss of the normal sonographic tendon architecture as well as significant cortical tearing.

• **Figure 51-3** Longitudinal ultrasound image demonstrating mild tendinopathy of the supraspinatus tendon. Note the small cortical tear.

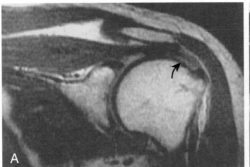

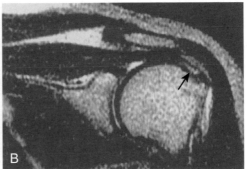

• **Figure 51-4** Severe degenerative changes within the rotator cuff. Increased signal intensity within the rotator cuff on short-TE images (*arrow* in **A**) is as bright as or brighter than fat on long-TE images (*arrow* in **B**). This finding is compatible with severe degenerative changes and poor mechanical properties of the cuff. (From Crues JV, Stoller DW, Ruy RKN: Shoulder. In Stark DD, Bradley WG, editors: *Magnetic resonance imaging*, ed 3, St. Louis, 1999, Mosby, p 709.)

Careful examination of the posterior shoulder might also reveal atrophy of the supraspinatus and infraspinatus muscles from disuse. At this point, treatment not only must be aimed at treating the inflammatory aspect of the disease and trying to restore function but also must include a careful evaluation for other inciting causes of rotator cuff dysfunction, including impingement syndromes, shoulder instability, and diseases of the surrounding structures. Extreme care must be taken in injecting corticosteroids around the rotator cuff at this stage of the disease, as the already damaged and weakened tendons are extremely susceptible to rupture.

Untreated, chronic rotator cuff tendinopathy will progress to partial thickness or complete rotator cuff tears (Figs. 51-6 and 51-7). These tears can occur acutely as a result of a specific traumatic event (Figs. 51-8 and 51-9) or spontaneously without an obvious inciting event as the weakened tendon suddenly fails (Figs. 51-10 and 51-11). Such spontaneous ruptures usually occur in the over-51 age group, and the sudden and dramatic nature of the event can be quite upsetting to the patient.

On clinical examination, the patient with a complete rotator cuff tear will be able only to shrug or hike the affected shoulder. The patient will exhibit a positive drop arm sign, which is highly suggestive of complete rotator cuff tear (see Fig. 50-1). Magnetic resonance imaging (MRI), ultrasound imaging, or arthrography of the shoulder will confirm the diagnosis of complete rotator cuff tear and distinguish this diagnosis from other internal derangements of the shoulder. Complete rotator cuff tears require surgery,

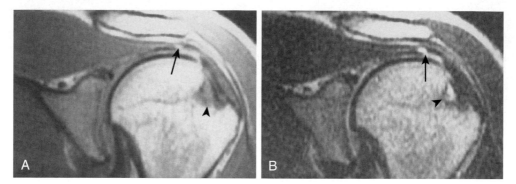

• **Figure 51-6** Partial rotator cuff tear. Small and partial rotator cuff tears present with increased signal within the cuff on short-TE (*arrow* in **A**) and long-TE (*arrow* in **B**) images. The erosion at the insertion of the infraspinatus and supraspinatus tendons results from chronic trauma during the deceleration phase of throwing *(arrowheads)*. (From Crues JV, Stoller DW, Ruy RKN: Shoulder. In Stark DD, Bradley WG, editors: *Magnetic resonance imaging*, ed 3, St. Louis, 1999, Mosby, p 710.)

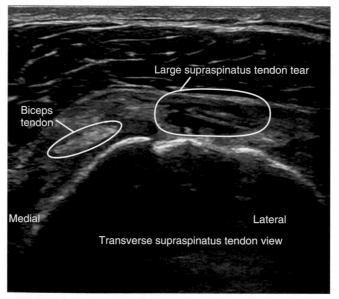

• **Figure 51-7** Transverse ultrasound image demonstrating a large tear of the supraspinatus tendon in a patient with acute shoulder trauma.

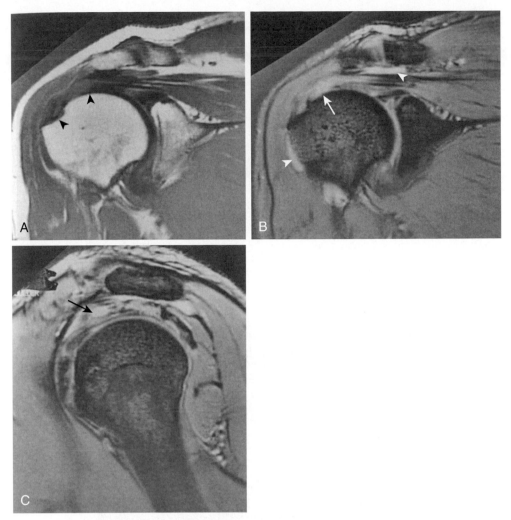

• **Figure 51-8** Complete supraspinatus tear. **A,** T1 coronal oblique image, shoulder. The distal 2 cm of the supraspinatus tendon (between *arrowheads*) is intermediate, rather than the normal low signal intensity, and thickened. **B,** T2* coronal oblique image, shoulder. High-signal fluid *(arrow)* fills the defect in the supraspinatus tendon. Fluid is present in the subacromial/subdeltoid bursa *(arrowheads)*. There is no retraction of the musculotendinous junction. **C,** T2* sagittal oblique image, shoulder. There is focal high signal *(arrow)* in the defect of the torn supraspinatus tendon, where normally a low-signal oval tendon should be evident. (From Kaplan PA, Helms CA, Dussault R, et al: *Musculoskeletal MRI*, Philadelphia, 2001, Saunders, p 187.)

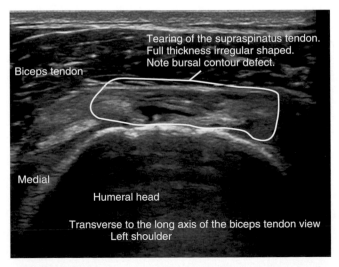

• **Figure 51-9** Transverse ultrasound image demonstrating a complex full thickness tear of the supraspinatus tendon without significant retraction.

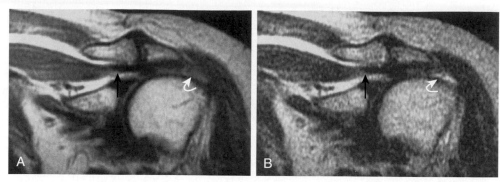

• **Figure 51-10** Proximal retraction of the myotendinous junction of the supraspinatus muscle. **A,** Short-TE image. **B,** Long-TE image. A characteristic finding in large rotator cuff tears is retraction of the myotendinous junction from unopposed traction of the muscle *(arrow)*. The extent of retraction is helpful in estimating the size of the tear. At surgery, the tear in this cuff measured approximately 2.5 cm. The extent of high signal intensity in the region of the distal cuff is also compatible with a 2.5-cm tear *(curved arrow)*. (From Crues JV, Stoller DW, Ruy RKN: Shoulder. In Stark DD, Bradley WG, editors: *Magnetic resonance imaging*, ed 3. St. Louis, 1999, Mosby, p 711.)

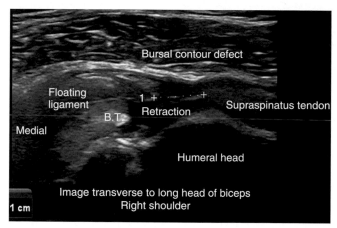

• **Figure 51-11** Transverse ultrasound image demonstrating a complete rupture of the supraspinatus tendon with retraction.

which can usually be performed arthroscopically if done within a short time after the tear. If surgical treatment is delayed, an open procedure might be required to retrieve the retracted ends of the torn tendon.

The clinician should be aware of two caveats when diagnosing and treating diseases of the rotator cuff: (1) rotator cuff disease rarely exists as an isolated pathologic process and is usually associated with other shoulder pathology, such as bursitis, impingement syndromes, and shoulder instability, and (2) shoulder pain and dysfunction that mimics rotator cuff disease may arise from diseases occurring outside the shoulder, such as brachial plexopathies and tumors and Pancoast tumor; failure to assiduously search for such problems can yield disastrous results.

52 The Drop Arm Test for Complete Rotator Cuff Tear

The drop arm test is useful in helping the clinician to identify those patients with complete rotator cuff tear. As mentioned in Chapter 51, complete rotator cuff tear can occur spontaneously and without an obvious inciting event. The sudden and dramatic presentation of this problem can be quite upsetting and perplexing to the patient. In the drop arm test for complete rotator cuff tear, the patient is asked to assume the standing position and relax the affected shoulder with the arm resting comfortably at the patient's side. The clinician then gently abducts the affected extremity to 90 degrees and holds the arm in this position (Fig. 52-1). The clinician then informs the patient that the clinician is going to release the arm and the patient must try to hold the arm at 90 degrees abduction. If the patient has a complete rotator cuff tear, he or she will be unable to hold the arm in the abducted position, and the arm will fall to the patient's side. The patient will often shrug or hitch the shoulder forward to use the intact muscles of the rotator cuff and the deltoid to keep the arm in the abducted position (Fig. 52-2). If the drop arm test is positive, the clinician should obtain a magnetic resonance image, ultrasound imaging, or arthrogram of the affected shoulder to confirm the diagnosis of complete rotator cuff tear (Video 52-1).

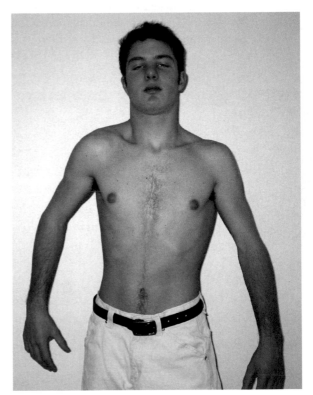

• **Figure 52-2** A patient with a complete rotator cuff tear will be unable to hold the arm in the abducted position, and it will fall to the patient's side. The patient will often shrug or hitch the shoulder forward to use the intact muscles of the rotator cuff and the deltoid to keep the arm in the abducted position.

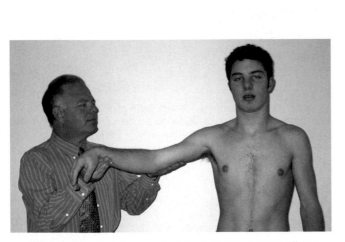

• **Figure 52-1** The drop arm test for complete rotator cuff tear.

53 The External Rotation Lag Sign for Rupture of the Supraspinatus or Infraspinatus Tendon

The external rotation lag sign test is useful in identifying rupture of the supraspinatus or infraspinatus tendon. To perform the external rotation lag sign test, the patient is placed in the sitting position and the examiner passively flexes the elbow of the patient's affected extremity to 90 degrees and elevates the patient's shoulder approximately 20 degrees. The patient's affected shoulder is then rotated externally to within 5 degrees of maximal external rotation. The examiner supports the patient's wrist and elbow and then asks the patient to maintain the position of the affected extremity (Fig. 53-1). The examiner continues to support the elbow and releases the wrist (Fig. 53-2). If there is a rupture of the supraspinatus or infraspinatus tendon or both, the examiner will observe a lag or drop (Video 53-1).

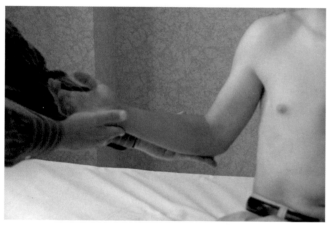

• **Figure 53-1** The external rotation lag sign test for rupture of the supraspinatus or infraspinatus tendon: the examiner supports the patient's wrist and elbow and then asks the patient to maintain the position of the affected extremity.

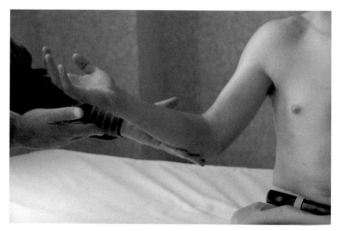

• **Figure 53-2** The external rotation lag sign test for rupture of the supraspinatus or infraspinatus tendons: the examiner continues to support the elbow and releases the wrist. If there is a rupture of the supraspinatus or infraspinatus tendon or both, the examiner will observe a lag or drop.

The musculotendinous unit of the shoulder joint is susceptible to the development of tendinitis for several reasons. First, the joint is subjected to a wide range of motions that are often repetitive in nature. Second, the space in which the musculotendinous unit functions is restricted by the coracoacromial arch, making impingement a likely possibility with extreme movements of the joint. Third, the blood supply to the musculotendinous unit is poor, making healing of microtrauma more difficult. All of these factors can contribute to tendinitis of one or more of the tendons of the shoulder joint, and the supraspinatus tendon is no exception.

Supraspinatus tendinitis can present as either an acute or chronic painful condition of the shoulder. Acute supraspinatus tendinitis will usually occur in a younger group of patients following overuse or misuse of the shoulder joint. Inciting factors may include carrying heavy loads in front and away from the body, throwing injuries, or the vigorous use of exercise equipment. Chronic supraspinatus tendinitis tends to occur in an older group of patients and to present in a more gradual or insidious manner without a single specific event of antecedent trauma. The pain of supraspinatus tendinitis will be constant and severe, with sleep disturbance often reported. The pain of supraspinatus tendinitis is felt primarily in the deltoid region. It is moderate to severe in intensity and may be associated with a gradual loss of range of motion of the affected shoulder. The patient will often awaken at night when he or she rolls over onto the affected shoulder.

The patient suffering from supraspinatus tendinitis may attempt to splint the inflamed tendon by elevating the scapula to remove tension from the ligament, giving the patient a "shrugging" appearance. There is usually point tenderness over the greater tuberosity. The patient will exhibit a painful arc of abduction and will complain of a catch or sudden onset of pain in the midrange of the arc due to subacromial impingement and/or impingement of the humeral head onto the supraspinatus tendon (Figs. 54-1 to 54-4). Patients with supraspinatus tendinitis will exhibit a positive Dawbarn sign.

The Dawbarn sign test for supraspinatus tendonitis is performed by having the patient assume the standing position. The clinician then palpates the superior aspect of the greater tuberosity of the humerus. In patients who suffer from supraspinatus tendonitis, this maneuver will reproduce the pain that the patient experiences with range of motion of the shoulder. The affected arm is then gradually abducted to its fullest extent. As the arm approaches the top of the painful arc, the pain will disappear, suggesting a supraspinatus tendonitis (Fig. 54-5). The clinician should be aware that the Dawbarn sign may also be positive in patients who suffer from subacromial bursitis. Magnetic resonance imaging (MRI) and/or ultrasound testing of the affected shoulder should be performed in patients who are

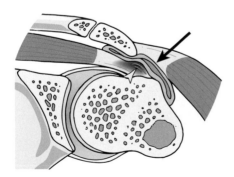

• **Figure 54-1** Drawing (coronal plane, cut section) of left shoulder during active elevation of arm halfway between flexion and abduction with hand in pronation explicitly depicts pooling of fluid in lateral aspect of subacromial-subdeltoid bursa *(arrow)* and alteration of normally convex surface of supraspinatus tendon *(arrowhead)* as arm is elevated. Supraspinatus tendon is not always involved in grade 2 subacromial impingement. There is also evidence of supraspinatus tendinosis and inflammatory changes in bursa. (From El-Liethy N, Kamal H, Abdelwahab N, et al: Value of dynamic sonography in the management of shoulder pain in patients with rheumatoid arthritis, *Egyptian J Radiol Nuclear Med* 45(4):1171–1182, fig 5.)

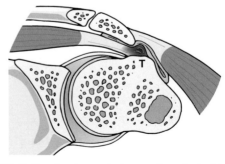

• **Figure 54-2** Drawing (coronal plane, cut section) of left shoulder during active elevation of arm halfway between flexion and abduction with hand in pronation shows upward migration of humeral head in relation to glenoid cavity, which prevents passage of greater tuberosity *(T)* and soft-tissue structures of supraspinatus outlet beneath acromion. (From El-Liethy N, Kamal H, Abdelwahab N, et al: Value of dynamic sonography in the management of shoulder pain in patients with rheumatoid arthritis, *Egyptian J Radiol Nuclear Med* 45(4):1171–1182, fig 6.)

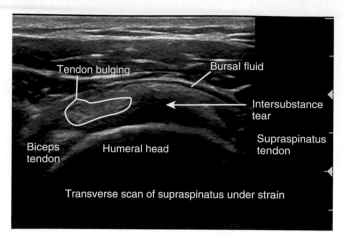

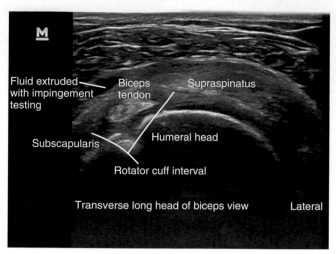

• **Figure 54-3** Transverse ultrasound image obtained during dynamic ultrasound imaging demonstrating impingement of the supraspinatus musculotendinous unit in a patient with a positive Dawbarn sign. Note the bunching up of the tendon and extruded bursal fluid as well as significant tendinopathy.

• **Figure 54-4** Transverse ultrasound image obtained during dynamic ultrasound imaging demonstrating impingement of the supraspinatus musculotendinous unit in a patient with a positive Dawbarn sign. Note the pooling of fluid with abduction.

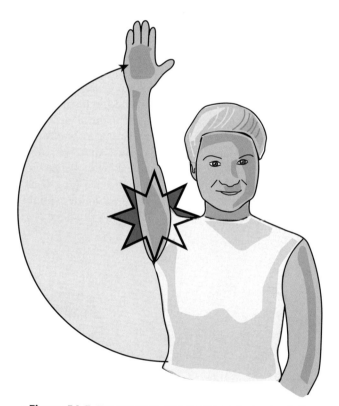

• **Figure 54-5** The Dawbarn sign for supraspinatus tendinitis.

thought to be suffering from supraspinatus tendonitis, to help differentiate these clinically distinct entities as well as to rule out rotator cuff tear.

Early in the course of the disease, passive range of motion is full and without pain. As the disease progresses, patients who suffer from supraspinatus tendinitis will often experience a gradual decrease in functional ability with decreasing shoulder range of motion, making simple everyday tasks, such as hair combing, fastening a brassiere, or reaching overhead, quite difficult. With continued disuse, muscle wasting may occur, and a frozen shoulder might develop.

55 The Empty Can Test for Supraspinatus Tendinitis

The musculotendinous unit of the shoulder joint is susceptible to the development of tendinitis for several reasons. First, the joint is subjected to a wide range of motions that are often repetitive in nature. Second, the space in which the musculotendinous unit functions is restricted by the coracoacromial arch, making impingement a likely possibility with extreme movements of the joint (Fig. 55-1). Third, the blood supply to the musculotendinous unit is poor, making healing of microtrauma more difficult. All of these factors can contribute to tendinitis of one or more of the tendons of the shoulder joint, and the supraspinatus tendon is no exception.

Supraspinatus tendinitis can present as either an acute or chronic painful condition of the shoulder. Acute supraspinatus tendinitis will usually occur in a younger group of patients following overuse or misuse of the shoulder joint. Inciting factors may include carrying heavy loads in front and away from the body, throwing injuries, or the vigorous use of exercise equipment. Chronic supraspinatus tendinitis tends to occur in an older group of patients and to present in a more gradual or insidious manner without a single specific event of antecedent trauma. The pain of supraspinatus tendinitis will be constant and severe, with sleep disturbance often reported. The pain of supraspinatus tendinitis is felt primarily in the deltoid region. It is moderate to severe in intensity and may be associated with a gradual loss of range of motion of the affected shoulder. The patient will often awaken at night when he or she rolls over onto the affected shoulder.

The patient suffering from supraspinatus tendinitis may attempt to splint the inflamed tendon by elevating the scapula to remove tension from the ligament, giving the patient a "shrugging" appearance. There is usually point tenderness over the greater tuberosity. The patient will exhibit a painful arc of abduction and will complain of a catch or sudden onset of pain in the midrange of the arc due to subacromial impingement and/or impingement of the humeral head onto the supraspinatus tendon (Figs. 55-2 and 55-3). Patients with supraspinatus tendinitis will exhibit a positive empty can test.

The empty can test for supraspinatus tendonitis is performed by having the patient assume the standing position.

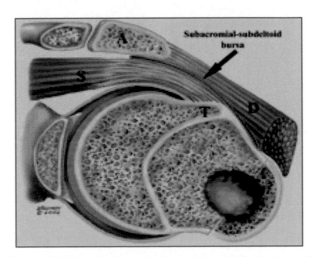

• **Figure 55-1** Drawing (coronal plane, cut section) of subacromial space of the left shoulder during active elevation of arm halfway between flexion and abduction with hand in pronation shows normal relationships between acromion (A), greater tuberosity (T) of humeral head, and intervening soft tissues—namely, supraspinatus tendon (S) and subacromial-subdeltoid bursa (arrow). D, Deltoid muscle. (From El-Liethy N, Kamal H, Abdelwahab N, et al: Value of dynamic sonography in the management of shoulder pain in patients with rheumatoid arthritis, *Egyptian J Radiol Nuclear Med* 45(4):1171–1182, 2014.)

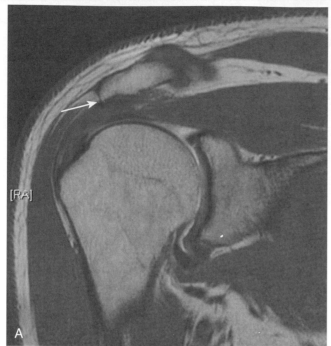

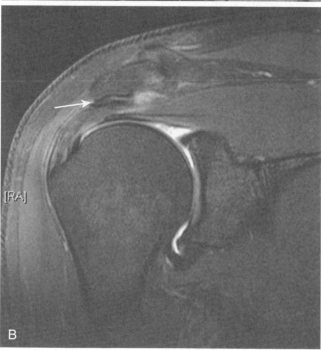

• **Figure 55-2** Coronal T1-weighted (T1W) **(A)** and T2W with fat suppression (FST2W) **(B)** magnetic resonance arthrogram images demonstrating enthesopathy of the acromion *(white arrows)* with impingement of the supraspinatus tendon, which is thickened and tendinopathic. There is early subacromial bursitis. (From Waldman SD, Campbell, RSD: *Imaging of pain,* Philadelphia, 2010, Saunders/Elsevier, p 250, fig 98-2.)

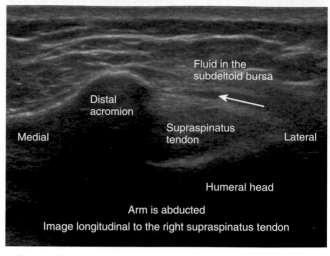

• **Figure 55-3** Ultrasound image longitudinal to the supraspinatus tendon obtained during dynamic ultrasound imaging in a patient with a positive empty can test demonstrating subacromial impingement of the supraspinatous musculotendinous unit. Note fluid in the subdeltoid bursa.

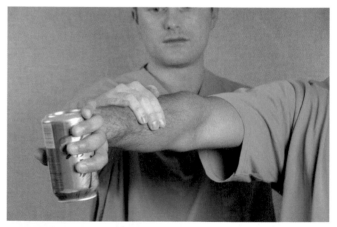

• **Figure 55-4** The empty can test for supraspinatus tendonitis is performed by having the patient assume the standing position. The affected arm is then gradually elevated to 90 degrees in the scapular plan with the elbow fully extended, the arm in full internal rotation, and the forearm pronated, as if the patient is trying to shake the last few drops out of an empty can. The examiner then exerts downward pressure to the affected arm. The test is considered positive if the patient experiences a significant increase in pain or demonstrates weakness.

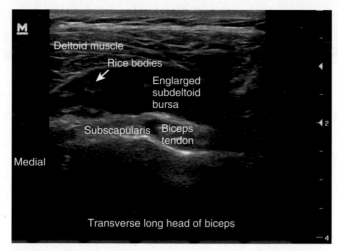

• Figure 55-5 Transverse ultrasound image demonstrating subdeltoid bursitis.

The affected arm is then gradually elevated to 90 degrees in the scapular plan with the elbow fully extended, the arm in full internal rotation, and the forearm pronated, as if the patient is trying to shake the last few drops out of an empty can (Fig. 55-4). The examiner then exerts downward pressure to the affected arm. The test is considered positive if the patient experiences a significant increase in pain or demonstrates weakness.

The clinician should be aware that the empty can test may also be positive in patients who suffer from subacromial bursitis (Fig. 55-5). Magnetic resonance imaging and/or ultrasound testing of the affected shoulder should be performed in patients who are thought to be suffering from supraspinatus tendonitis, to help differentiate these clinically distinct entities as well as to rule out rotator cuff tear.

56 The Jobe Supraspinatus Test

To perform the Jobe supraspinatus test, the patient is placed in the seated position and is asked to abduct both shoulders to 90 degrees. The patient then is asked to rotate both arms internally so the thumbs point downward and to forward flex his or her shoulders 30 degrees. The patient is then asked to maintain this position while the examiner exerts firm downward pressure to assess and compare the strength of the supraspinatus muscle on both sides (Fig. 56-1). The test is positive if the examiner identifies weakness or insufficiency on either side (Video 56-1).

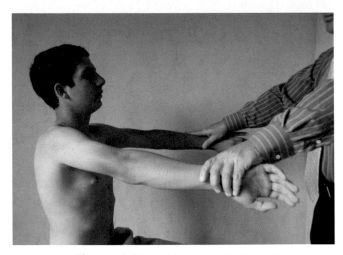

• **Figure 56-1** The Jobe supraspinatus test.

57 The Midarc Abduction Test for Infraspinatus Tendinitis

The musculotendinous unit of the shoulder joint is susceptible to the development of tendinitis for several reasons. First, the joint is subjected to a wide range of motions, which are often repetitive in nature. Second, the space in which the musculotendinous unit functions is restricted by the coracoacromial arch, making impingement a likely possibility with extreme movements of the joint. Third, the blood supply to the musculotendinous unit is poor, making healing of microtrauma more difficult. All of these factors can contribute to tendinitis of one or more of the tendons of the shoulder joint, and the infraspinatus tendon is no exception (Fig. 57-1).

Infraspinatus tendinitis can present as either an acute or chronic painful condition of the shoulder. Acute infraspinatus tendinitis will usually occur in a younger group of patients following overuse or misuse of the shoulder joint. Inciting factors may include activities that require repeated abduction and lateral rotation of the humerus, such as installing brake pads during assembly line work. The vigorous use of exercise equipment has also been implicated.

The pain of infraspinatus tendinitis is constant and severe and is localized in the deltoid area. Significant sleep disturbance is often reported. Patients with infraspinatus tendinitis will exhibit pain with lateral rotation of the humerus and on active abduction and will exhibit a painful midarc abduction test. Chronic infraspinatus tendinitis tends to occur in an older group of patients and to present in a more gradual or insidious manner without a single specific event of antecedent trauma. The pain of infraspinatus tendinitis

may be associated with a gradual loss of range of motion of the affected shoulder. The patient will often awaken at night when he or she rolls over onto the affected shoulder.

The patient might attempt to splint the inflamed infraspinatus tendon by rotating the scapula posteriorly to remove tension from the tendon (Fig. 57-2). There is usually point tenderness over the greater tuberosity. The patient will exhibit a painful arc of abduction and will complain of a catch or sudden onset of pain in the midrange of the arc with the pain improving as the patient reaches the top of the arc of abduction (Fig. 57-3). Early in the course of the disease, passive range of motion is full and without pain. As the disease progresses, patients who suffer from infraspinatus tendinitis will often experience a gradual decrease in functional ability, with decreasing shoulder range of motion making simple everyday tasks, such as hair combing, fastening a brassiere, or reaching overhead, quite difficult. With continued disuse, muscle wasting may occur, and a frozen shoulder might develop.

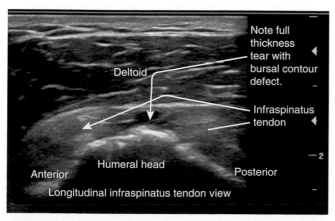

• **Figure 57-1** Longitudinal ultrasound image demonstrating a full thickness tear of the infraspinatus tendon in a patient with an acute shoulder injury.

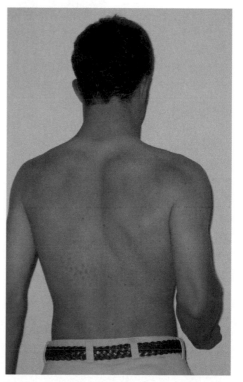

• **Figure 57-2** Patients might attempt to rotate the scapula posteriorly to relieve tension from the inflamed infraspinatus tendon.

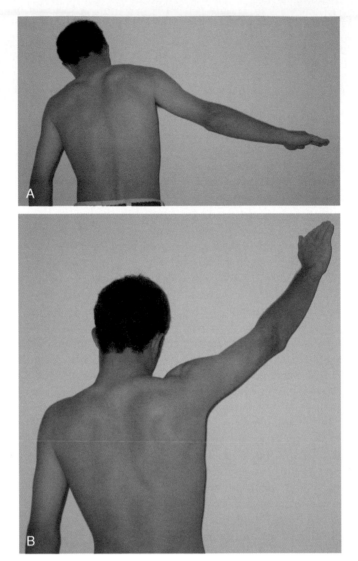

• **Figure 57-3 A** and **B,** Midarc abduction test for infraspinatus tendinitis.

58 The External Rotation Stress Test for Impairment of the Infraspinatus and Teres Minor Muscles

The external rotation stress test is useful in helping the examiner identify impairment of the infraspinatus and teres minor muscles, which serve as the primary external rotators of the shoulder. To perform the external rotation test, the patient is placed in the sitting position with his or her shoulders in neutral position and externally rotated 50 to 60 degrees. The examiner then applies internal rotational force against the dorsum of the patient's hands with the patient resisting the examiner's efforts to rotate the shoulders internally to neutral (Fig. 58-1). The test is considered positive if pain or weakness is identified (Video 58-1).

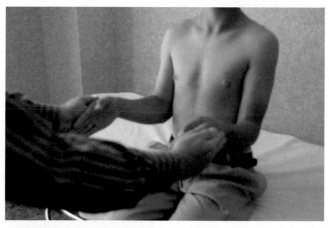

• **Figure 58-1** The external rotation stress test for impairment of the infraspinatus and teres minor muscles.

In the drop arm test for subdeltoid bursitis, the patient is placed in the standing position with the affected arm resting at the patient's side. The examiner then slowly abducts the affected arm, watching for signs of pain. When the arm is abducted as far as the patient will tolerate, it is supported there for a few seconds and then suddenly released (Figs. 59-1 and 59-2). If the patient has a complete rotator cuff tear, he or she will be unable to support the affected extremity, and it will fall to the patient's side (see Chapter 52). If the patient has subdeltoid bursitis, the patient will wince and cry out in pain when the arm is released. It should be remembered that partial rotator cuff tear and subdeltoid bursitis can coexist; for this reason, magnetic resonance imaging and/or ultrasound imaging of the shoulder should be performed on all patients with a positive drop arm test for subdeltoid bursitis to avoid missing this potentially problematic coexistent pathology (Fig. 59-3).

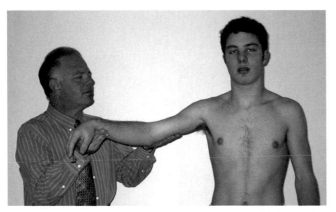

• **Figure 59-1** The drop arm test for subdeltoid bursitis: the examiner supports the abducted arm.

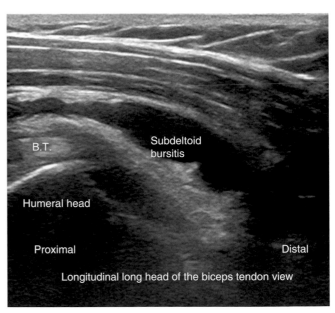

• **Figure 59-3** Longitudinal ultrasound image demonstrating subdeltoid bursitis and tears and tendinosis of the supraspinatus musculotendinous unit. *B.T.,* Biceps tendon.

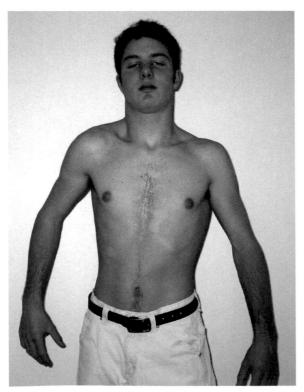

• **Figure 59-2** The drop arm test for subdeltoid bursitis: the abducted arm is released.

60 The Adduction Release Test for Subcoracoid Bursitis

The subcoracoid bursa is vulnerable to injury from both acute trauma and repeated microtrauma. Acute injuries frequently take the form of direct trauma to the shoulder when a person plays sports or falls on the shoulder. The repeated strain associated with repetitive motion can result in inflammation of the subcoracoid bursa. If the inflammation of the subcoracoid bursa becomes chronic, calcification of the bursa can occur.

The subcoracoid bursa lies between the joint capsule and the coracoid process. It is susceptible to irritation by pressure from the coracoid process against the head of the humerus during extreme arm movement or when previous damage to the musculotendinous unit of the shoulder allows abnormal movement of the head of the humerus in the glenoid fossa.

The patient who suffers from subcoracoid bursitis frequently complains of pain with forward movement with adduction of the shoulder. The pain is localized to the area over the coracoid process, with referred pain noted at the medial shoulder. Often the patient is unable to sleep on the affected shoulder and may complain of a sharp, "catching" sensation when abducting the shoulder, especially on first awakening. Physical examination might reveal point tenderness over the coracoid process. Subcoracoid bursitis can be distinguished from subdeltoid bursitis in that the pain of subcoracoid bursitis is reproduced with palpation directly over the coracoid process, whereas the pain of subdeltoid bursitis is reproduced with palpation of a point more inferior to the coracoid on the deltoid muscle (Fig. 60-1). Patients who suffer from subcoracoid bursitis will also exhibit a positive adduction release test.

The adduction release test for subcoracoid bursitis is performed by having the patient assume the standing position with the affected arm at his or her side. The patient is then asked to internally rotate the affected arm until the pain the patient has been experiencing is reproduced (Fig. 60-2). The examiner then supports the affected arm and asks the patient to begin adducting the arm against the examiner's resistance (Fig. 60-3). The examiner suddenly releases the resistance to adduction (Fig. 60-4). If the patient is suffering from subcoracoid bursitis, the patient will experience a marked increase in pain (Video 60-1). The clinical impression of subcoracoid bursitis can then be confirmed by magnetic resonance and/or ultrasound imaging (Fig. 60-5).

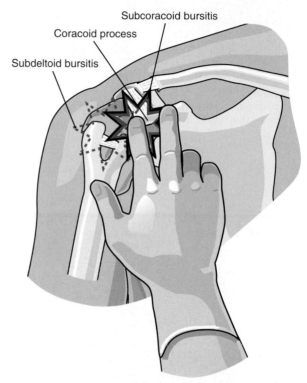

Subcoracoid bursitis
Coracoid process
Subdeltoid bursitis

• **Figure 60-1** Subcoracoid bursitis can be reproduced with palpation directly over the coracoid process.

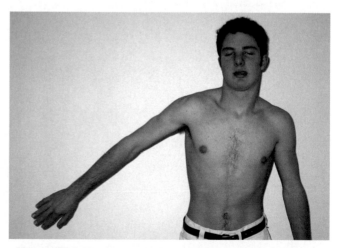

• **Figure 60-2** The adduction release test for subcoracoid bursitis: the patient is asked to internally rotate the affected arm until the pain is reproduced.

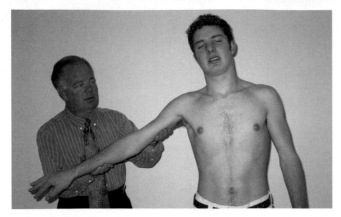

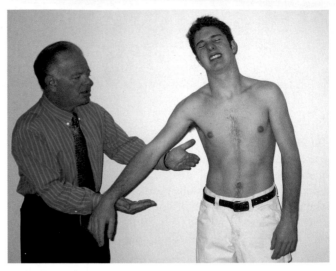

• **Figure 60-3** The adduction release test for subcoracoid bursitis: the examiner supports the affected arm and asks the patient to begin adducting the arm against the examiner's resistance.

• **Figure 60-4** The adduction release test for subcoracoid bursitis: if the patient is suffering from subcoracoid bursitis, he or she will experience a marked increase in pain following a sudden release of the resistance to adduction.

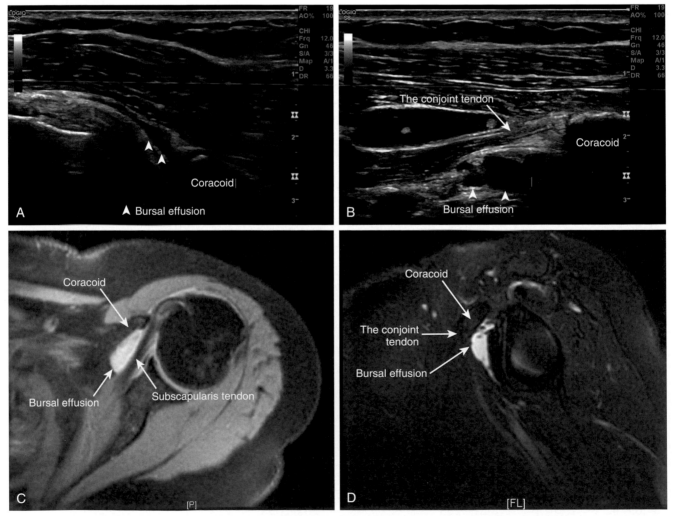

• **Figure 60-5** Transverse ultrasound view **(A)** of subcoracoid bursitis with effusion between the coracoid process and subscapularis tendon. Longitudinal view **(B)** of conjoined tendon attached to the coracoid process demonstrates the subcoracoid bursal effusion under the coracoid process and surrounding conjoined tendon. Fat-suppressed axial **(C)** and sagittal **(D)** magnetic resonance images demonstrate distension of subcoracoid bursa with effusion. (From Drakes S, Thomas S, Kim S, et al: Ultrasonography of subcoracoid bursal impingement syndrome, *PM R* 7(3):329–333, 2015, fig 3.)

61 The Adduction Stress Test for Acromioclavicular Joint Dysfunction

The acromioclavicular joint is vulnerable to injury from both acute trauma and repeated microtrauma. Acute injuries frequently take the form of falls directly onto the shoulder in playing sports or falling from bicycles. Repeated strain from throwing injuries or working with the arm raised across the body can also result in trauma to the joint. Following trauma, the joint may become acutely inflamed, and if the condition becomes chronic, arthritis of the acromioclavicular joint might develop. Injuries to the acromioclavicular joint can range from sprains and strains of the acromioclavicular joint with all ligaments remaining intact (Fig. 61-1, *A*) to situations in which only the acromioclavicular ligament is disrupted (Fig. 61-1, *B*) to complete disruption of the ligaments of the acromioclavicular joint with dislocation of the joint (Fig. 61-1, *C*).

The patient who suffers from acromioclavicular joint dysfunction will frequently complain of pain when reaching across the chest (Fig. 61-2). Often the patient will be unable to sleep on the affected shoulder and might complain of a grinding sensation in the joint, especially on first awakening. Physical examination may reveal enlargement or swelling of the joint with tenderness to palpation. Patients with acromioclavicular joint dysfunction will often exhibit a positive adduction stress test and a positive chin adduction test (see Chapter 62). If there is significant disruption of the ligaments of the acromioclavicular joint, these maneuvers might reveal joint instability, and obvious deformity of the affected shoulder will be evident. With disruption of the ligaments, elevation of the clavicle with widening of the distance between the clavicle and acromion as well as a positive step-off sign will be noted on plain radiography, magnetic resonance, and ultrasound imaging (Figs. 61-3 and 61-4).

To perform the adduction stress test for acromioclavicular joint dysfunction, the patient is asked to remove his or her shirt. The patient is asked to assume the standing position, and the examiner stands behind the patient examining the shoulders for any asymmetry that might be suggestive of disruption of the acromioclavicular ligaments. The examiner then has the patient maximally extend the affected shoulder and arm behind him or her while the examiner exerts forward pressure on the scapula (Fig. 61-5). The affected arm is then slowly adducted behind the back. Patients with acromioclavicular joint dysfunction will experience a marked increase in pain with this passive adduction, and the examiner might notice an increase in shoulder deformity as stress is placed on the joint (Fig. 61-6). The examiner should avoid sudden or forceful movements when adducting the affected arm to avoid further damage to the ligaments.

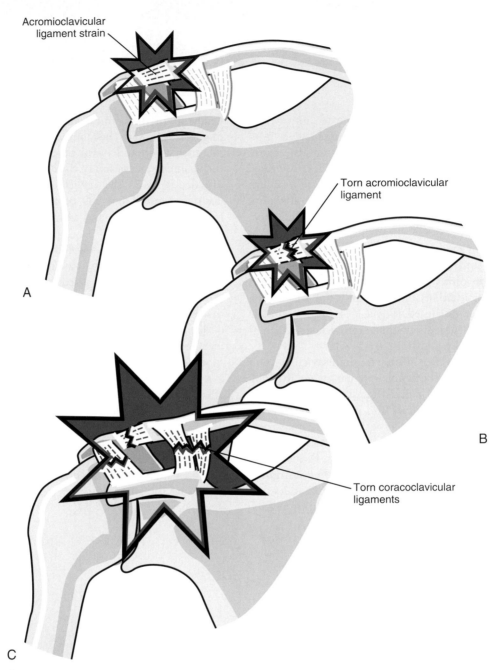

Acromioclavicular ligament strain

Torn acromioclavicular ligament

Torn coracoclavicular ligaments

A

B

C

• **Figure 61-1** Acromioclavicular joint injuries range from sprains and strains with all ligaments remaining intact **(A)** to situations in which only the acromioclavicular ligament is disrupted **(B)** to complete disruption of the ligaments of the acromioclavicular joint with dislocation of the joint **(C)**.

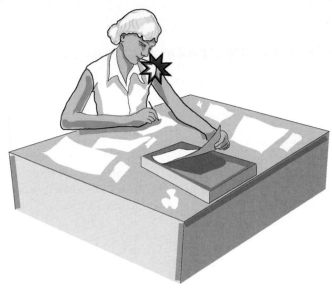

• **Figure 61-2** The patient suffering from acromioclavicular joint dysfunction will frequently complain of pain when reaching across the chest.

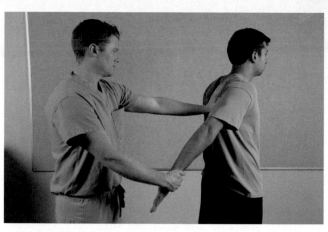

• **Figure 61-5** To perform the adduction stress test for acromioclavicular joint dysfunction, the examiner has the patient maximally extend the affected shoulder and arm behind him or her while the examiner exerts forward pressure on the scapula.

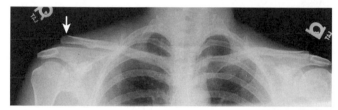

• **Figure 61-3** Widening of the acromioclavicular joint after disruption of the acromioclavicular ligament: type 3 injury—stress radiography. Compare the radiographic findings on the normal left side and the abnormal right side. The involved clavicle *(arrow)* is elevated, with an increased distance between the coracoid process and the inferior surface of the clavicle. (From Resnick D, Kang HS: *Internal derangements of joints: emphasis on MR imaging*, Philadelphia, 1997, Saunders, p 286.)

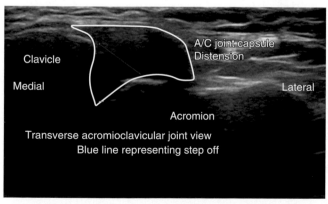

• **Figure 61-4** Transverse ultrasound image demonstrating complete acromioclavicular separation. Note the positive step-off sign.

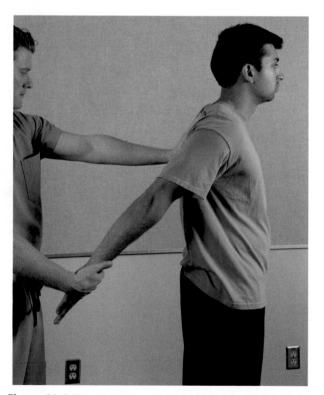

• **Figure 61-6** The affected arm is then slowly adducted behind the back.

62 The Chin Adduction Test for Acromioclavicular Joint Dysfunction

The chin adduction test for acromioclavicular joint dysfunction is performed by having the patient assume the standing position with his or her shirt off. The examiner stands in front of the patient and examines the acromioclavicular joints for any evidence of asymmetry with the patient's arms in neutral position. The examiner then has the patient abduct the affected arm to 90 degrees. The patient is then instructed to adduct the affected arm and shoulder directly under the chin and grasp the contralateral shoulder (Fig. 62-1). Patients who suffer from acromioclavicular joint dysfunction will experience a marked increase in pain with adduction (Video 62-1).

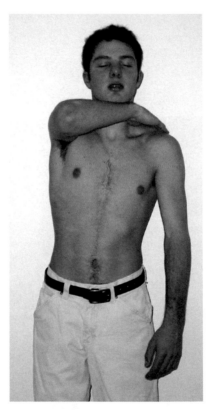

• **Figure 62-1** The chin adduction test for acromioclavicular joint dysfunction.

To perform the Paxino test for acromioclavicular joint dysfunction, the patient is asked to remove his or her shirt. The patient is asked to assume the standing position, and the examiner stands behind the patient examining the shoulders for any asymmetry that might be suggestive of disruption of the acromioclavicular ligaments. The examiner then places his or her thumb under the posteriolateral aspect of the acromion and the index finger of the same hand is placed superior to the mid clavicle (Fig. 63-1). The examiner then squeezes the palpating fingers together. The test is considered positive if pain is elicited or increased at the acromioclavicular joint.

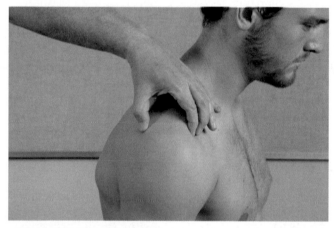

• **Figure 63-1** To perform the Paxino test for acromioclavicular joint dysfunction, the examiner places his or her thumb under the posteriolateral aspect of the acromion and the index finger of the same hand is placed superior to the mid clavicle. The examiner then squeezes the palpating fingers together. The test is considered positive if pain is elicited or increased at the acromioclavicular joint.

The axillary nerve is susceptible to injury from fracture of the proximal humerus, shoulder dislocation, or inflammatory conditions involving the brachial plexus. The axillary nerve arises from the posterior cord of the brachial plexus and provides motor innervation to the teres minor and deltoid muscles. Compromise of the motor division of the axillary nerve will result in weakness of shoulder abduction between 15 and 90 degrees. If the lesion persists, clinically apparent wasting of the deltoid muscle will result. The axillary nerve also provides cutaneous innervation to an ovoid area of the skin overlying the approximate area of where a sergeant's chevron would be placed, thus giving the basis for the name of the sergeant's chevron test (Fig. 64-1).

To perform the sergeant's chevron test, the clinician identifies the imaginary area that would underlie a sergeant's chevron and then, working from the center of the area outward, checks for diminished cutaneous sensation with a sterile needle (Fig. 64-2). The patient's crying out in pain as the needle moves from the area of diminished sensation in the distribution of the axillary nerve into the intact area supplied by the posterior, lateral, or medial cutaneous branches of the radial nerves constitutes a positive sergeant's chevron test. A positive test should direct the clinician to obtain careful electromyographic testing to determine the exact anatomic site of the lesion that is responsible for the axillary nerve deficit, with careful attention being paid to the brachial plexus. If brachial plexus lesions are identified, chest radiographs with apical lordotic views to rule out superior sulcus (Pancoast) tumor and magnetic resonance and ultrasound imaging of the shoulder should be carried out.

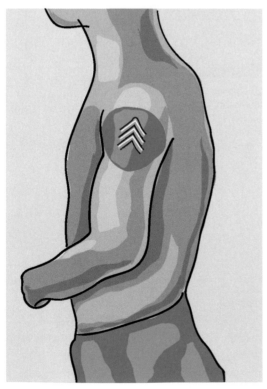

• **Figure 64-1** Cutaneous distribution of the axillary nerve.

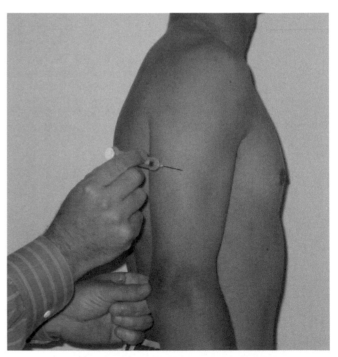

• **Figure 64-2** The sergeant's chevron test.

65 The Adson Maneuver for Thoracic Outlet Syndrome

Like the Homan sign, the Adson maneuver is one of the most maligned tests in clinical medicine because of its high incidence of false positive results in otherwise normal individuals. In spite of this fact, the Adson maneuver provides useful additional clinical information when combined with the subjective information that is gleaned from a careful history and physical examination as well as objective information obtained from electromyography and imaging modalities. It is thought that the Adson maneuver identifies compression of the subclavian artery and vein and the lower cord of the brachial plexus by the anterior scalene muscles and the other structures that might be causing compromise of the scalene triangle and is useful in the diagnosis of thoracic outlet syndrome.

Thoracic outlet syndrome is the name that is given to a number of sometimes overlapping clinical entities that have in common the ability to produce a constellation of symptoms, including numbness and paresthesia radiating into the affected upper extremity (most commonly in the distribution of the ulnar nerve) combined with a deep aching pain in the neck, shoulder, and arm that is made worse with prolonged abduction of the shoulder. Sometimes clumsiness and weakness of the affected extremity are also present, especially if the arm is abducted for long periods of time, such as when painting a ceiling. What all of these clinical entities have in common is compression of the nerves or arteries and veins as they pass through the closed space known as the thoracic outlet (Fig. 65-1).

The thoracic outlet can be thought of as a series of narrow rapids or cataracts through which the subclavian artery and vein and the lower trunk of the brachial plexus must pass on their way to the arm. The first narrowing and point of possible entrapment is where these structures pass between the anterior scalene and medial scalene muscles at their point of attachment on the first rib. A rudimentary cervical rib may be present in some patients and may further complicate the anatomic entrapment at this level (Fig. 65-2). The second potential site of entrapment is where these structures pass between the clavicle anteriorly, the first rib posteromedially, and the superior edge of the scapula posterolaterally. The final point of possible neural compromise is where the subclavian artery and vein and fibers from the lower trunk of the brachial plexus pass under the coracoid process and beneath the tendinous insertion of the pectoralis minor muscle. These neurovascular elements may be compromised at any and all points along their path, and the compromise may on rare occasions be limited to just one of these structures, leaving the others apparently unharmed.

Thoracic outlet syndrome has historically been both misdiagnosed and overdiagnosed owing to the myriad pathologic conditions that can cause the constellation of symptoms

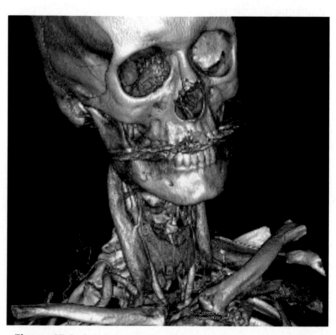

• **Figure 65-2** Computed tomographic reconstruction of a right cervical rib, which is a common cause of thoracic outlet syndrome. Note how the cervical rib articulates with the first rib. (From Pindrik J, Allan J: Belzberg, Peripheral nerve surgery: primer for the imagers, *Neuroimaging Clin N Am* 24(1):193–210, 2014, fig 1.)

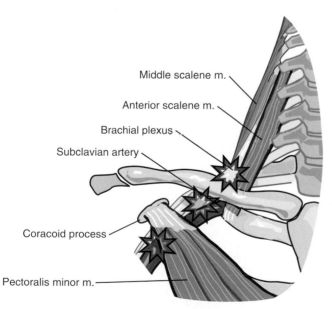

Middle scalene m.
Anterior scalene m.
Brachial plexus
Subclavian artery
Coracoid process
Pectoralis minor m.

• **Figure 65-1** Possible sites of nerve and artery compression in thoracic outlet syndrome.

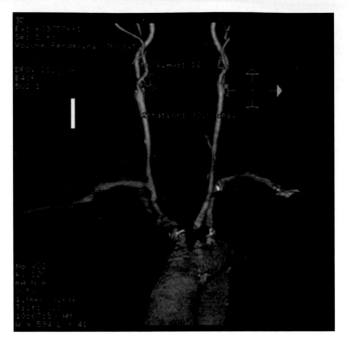

• **Figure 65-3** Computed tomography of an 18-year-old basketball player with arterial thoracic outlet syndrome identified bilateral subclavian artery aneurysms. (From de Mooij T, Duncan AA, Kakar S: Vascular injuries in the upper extremity in athletes, *Hand Clinics* 31(1):39–52, 2015, fig 4.)

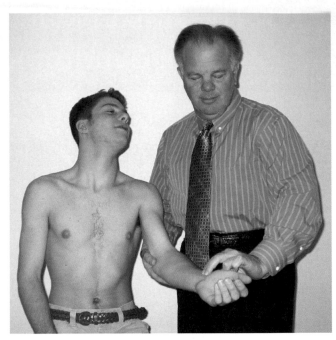

• **Figure 65-4** The Adson maneuver for thoracic outlet syndrome.

thought of as thoracic outlet syndrome, such as cervical radiculopathy, brachial plexopathies, aneurysms, and vasculitides (Fig. 65-3). This was especially true in the days before electromyography, computed tomography ultrasound, and magnetic resonance imaging. For this reason, thoracic outlet syndrome as a discrete clinical diagnosis should be thought of as a diagnosis of exclusion.

To perform the Adson maneuver, the patient is placed in the sitting position and asked to turn his or her head toward the side being examined. The examiner then palpates the patient's radial pulse at the wrist to obtain a baseline reading. The patient is then asked to extend his or her head fully and inhale as deeply as possible while the examiner monitors the radial pulse for any diminution of the pulse pressure (Fig. 65-4 and Video 65-1).

The Adson maneuver should be considered positive only if *two* criteria are met: (1) there is a diminution of the patient's radial pulse at the wrist when the maneuver is performed, and (2) the maneuver recreates the patient's symptoms. If only one of these positive findings is present, the clinician should look for causes other than thoracic outlet syndrome as an explanation of the patient's symptoms.

66 The Costoclavicular Test for Thoracic Outlet Syndrome

The costoclavicular test for thoracic outlet syndrome provides the clinician with useful additional clinical information when combined with the subjective information that is gleaned from a careful history and physical examination as well as objective information obtained from electromyography and imaging modalities (see Chapter 65). It is thought that the costoclavicular test identifies compression of the subclavian artery and vein and the lower cord of the brachial plexus by the clavicle and first rib, which will present clinically as thoracic outlet syndrome (see Fig. 65-1).

In the costoclavicular test, the patient is placed in the sitting position and asked to assume a position of extreme military attention. The examiner then palpates the patient's radial pulse at the wrists to obtain a baseline reading. The patient is then asked to thrust his or her shoulders fully backward and downward while the examiner monitors the radial pulse for any diminution of the pulse pressure (Fig. 66-1).

The costoclavicular test should be considered positive only if *two* criteria are met: (1) there is a diminution of the patient's radial pulse at the wrist when the maneuver is performed, and (2) the maneuver recreates the patient's symptoms. If only one of these positive findings is present, the clinician should look for causes other than thoracic outlet syndrome as an explanation of the patient's symptoms.

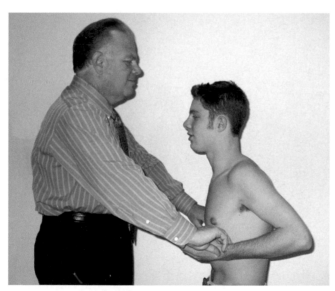

• **Figure 66-1** The costoclavicular test.

The hyperabduction test for thoracic outlet syndrome provides the clinician with useful additional clinical information when combined with the subjective information that is gleaned from a careful history and physical examination as well as objective information obtained from electromyography and imaging modalities (see Chapters 65 and 66). It is believed that this test will help identify compression of the subclavian artery and vein and lower cord of the brachial plexus by the pectoralis minor muscle and the coracoid process, which will present clinically as thoracic outlet syndrome (see Fig. 65-1).

In the hyperabduction test, the patient is placed in the sitting position. The examiner then palpates the patient's radial pulse at the wrists to obtain a baseline reading. The patient is then asked to raise both arms above the head with the elbows flexed approximately 10 degrees and the arms slightly extended out from the body while the examiner monitors the radial pulse for any diminution of the pulse pressure (Fig. 67-1 and Video 67-1).

The hyperabduction test should be considered positive only if *two* criteria are met: (1) there is a diminution of the patient's radial pulse at the wrist when the maneuver is performed, and (2) the maneuver recreates the patient's symptoms. If only one of these positive findings is present, the clinician should look for causes other than thoracic outlet syndrome as an explanation of the patient's symptoms.

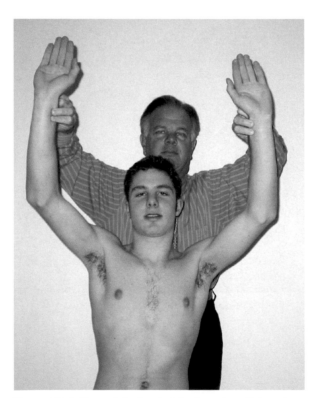

• **Figure 67-1** Hyperabduction test for thoracic outlet syndrome.

SECTION 3

The Elbow

The proper functioning of the elbow is essential for successfully carrying out the activities of daily living. One only has to ask anyone who has suffered from a seemingly minor elbow malady such as tennis elbow to confirm this fact. With elbow dysfunction, bathing, getting dressed, and even using the toilet become problematic. For this reason, the clinician needs a clear understanding of the functional anatomy of this complex joint, as clinical diagnosis of elbow problems (e.g., lateral epicondylitis, pronator syndrome) is based in the anatomic structure that is dysfunctional.

Although conventionally thought of as a hinge joint analogous to the knee, the elbow in fact has a unique compound range of motion that is due to the interplay between the hinge-type function and the rotational pronation and supination that allows precise positioning of the hand with its highly mobile fingers and opposing thumb. Each of the three bones that make up the joint—the humerus, the ulna, and the radius—has specialized ends to facilitate the elbow function and strength (Fig. 68-1).

From a functional anatomy viewpoint, the elbow has three areas that are involved in the majority of elbow disorders: (1) the humeral-ulnar interface, (2) the humeral-radial interface, and (3) the radial-ulnar interface. The humeral-ulnar interface comprises the area surrounding and including the trochlea of the humerus and the trochlear notch, coronoid process, and olecranon of the ulna (Fig. 68-2). The humeral-radial interface comprises the area surrounding and including the capitulum of the humerus and the radial head (Fig. 68-3). The radial-ulnar interface comprises the area surrounding and including the head of the radius and the radial notch of the ulna (Fig. 68-4).

The humeral-radial interface and the humeral-ulnar interface allow for the elbow's hinge-type movement. These articular interfaces and the joint surrounding ligaments contribute to the stability of the elbow in flexion and, to a lesser extent, extension. In health, this hinge portion of the elbow can traverse approximately 150 degrees. Because of the shape of the humeral trochlea and the ulnar trochlear notch, the arm moves into a valgus position of the forearm in extension. This valgus position is called the carrying angle and is 10 to 15 degrees in men and up to 18 degrees in women. When the arm flexes, it moves into a more varus

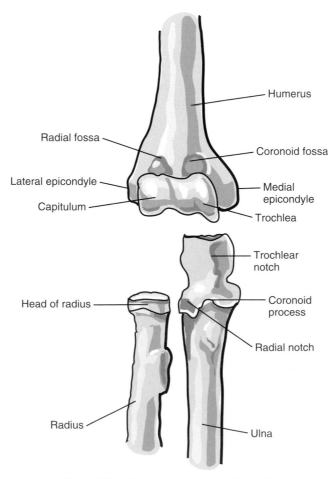

• **Figure 68-1** Bony anatomy of the elbow joint.

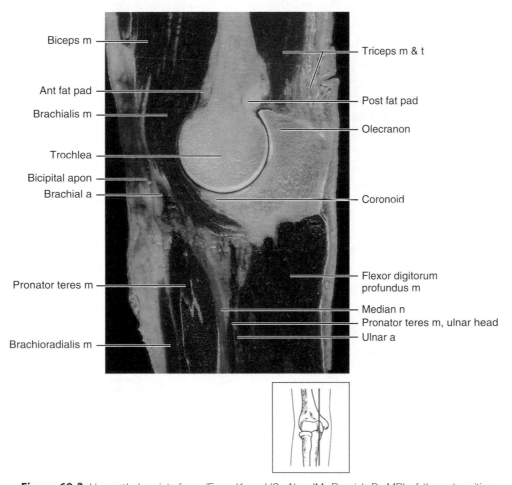

• **Figure 68-2** Humeral-ulnar interface. (From Kang HS, Ahn JM, Resnick D: *MRI of the extremities*, ed 2, Philadelphia, 2002, Saunders, p 113.)

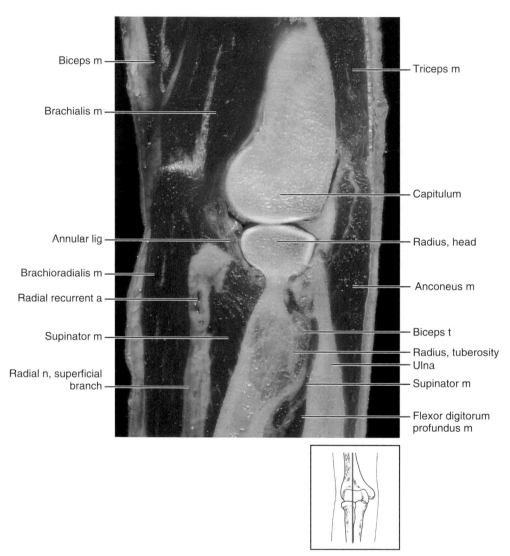

• **Figure 68-3** Humeral-radial interface. (From Kang HS, Ahn JM, Resnick D: *MRI of the extremities*, ed 2, Philadelphia, 2002, Saunders, p 123.)

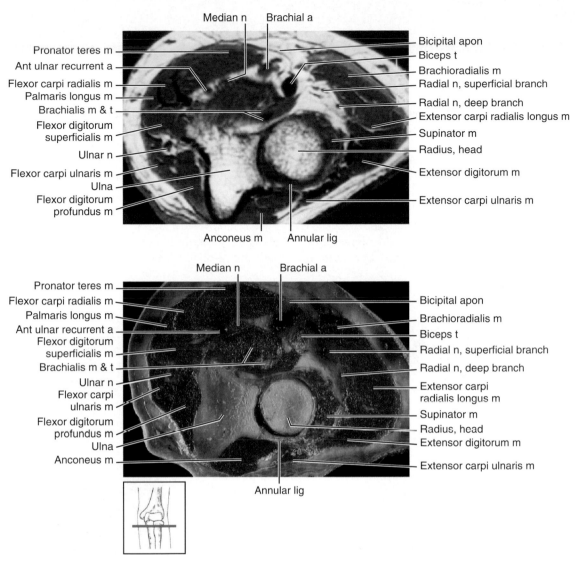

Median n   Brachial a

Pronator teres m
Ant ulnar recurrent a
Flexor carpi radialis m
Palmaris longus m
Brachialis m & t
Flexor digitorum superficialis m
Ulnar n
Flexor carpi ulnaris m
Ulna
Flexor digitorum profundus m

Bicipital apon
Biceps t
Brachioradialis m
Radial n, superficial branch
Radial n, deep branch
Extensor carpi radialis longus m
Supinator m
Radius, head
Extensor digitorum m
Extensor carpi ulnaris m

Anconeus m   Annular lig

Median n   Brachial a

Pronator teres m
Flexor carpi radialis m
Palmaris longus m
Ant ulnar recurrent a
Flexor digitorum superficialis m
Brachialis m & t
Ulnar n
Flexor carpi ulnaris m
Flexor digitorum profundus m
Ulna
Anconeus m

Bicipital apon
Brachioradialis m
Biceps t
Radial n, superficial branch
Radial n, deep branch
Extensor carpi radialis longus m
Supinator m
Radius, head
Extensor digitorum m
Extensor carpi ulnaris m

Annular lig

• **Figure 68-4** Radial-ulnar interface. (From Kang HS, Ahn JM, Resnick D: *MRI of the extremities*, ed 2, Philadelphia, 2002, Saunders, p 104.)

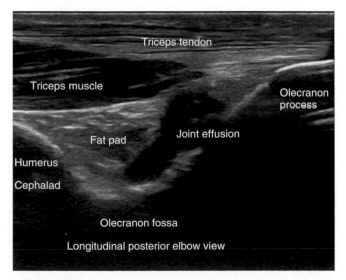

Triceps tendon
Triceps muscle
Olecranon process
Fat pad
Joint effusion
Humerus
Cephalad
Olecranon fossa
Longitudinal posterior elbow view

• **Figure 68-5** Longitudinal ultrasound image demonstrating the insertion of the triceps musculotendinous unit into the olecranon process. Note the mild tendinosis and posterior joint effusion.

position, which functionally puts the hand in closer proximity to the mouth to aid in feeding. Flexion of the arm at the elbow is carried out primarily by the biceps and brachialis muscles, with extension carried out primarily by the opposing triceps muscle. The insertion points of the musculotendinous units are common sites of elbow pain and dysfunction (Fig. 68-5).

In addition to the bony architecture and surrounding ligaments, the elbow is richly endowed with bursae to facilitate the joint's varied movements. These bursae are extremely susceptible to overuse, inflammation, and even infection and are also common sites of elbow pain and dysfunction. Most notably, the olecranon and cubital bursae are commonly affected (Fig. 68-5). When these bursae become inflamed, they can impinge on and irritate their associated tendons and tendinous insertions, with resultant tendinitis and occasionally nerve entrapment.

Because of the lack of soft tissue overlying the elbow joint, many of the structures that are susceptible to disease are easily visualized on inspection. The anterior and posterior elbow should be inspected in the neutral, flexed, and extended positions. The examiner should note the carrying angle; the normal valgus position is 10 to 15 degrees in men and up to 18 degrees in women (Figs. 69-1 and 69-2). An increased carrying angle is seen following ligamentous injury or fracture and with congenital disorders such as Turner syndrome. The examiner should also look for diffuse swelling of the joint that might be suggestive of arthritis or rubor that might be suggestive of a crystal arthropathy, an inflammatory process, or infection (Fig. 69-3). Areas of special interest should include the antecubital fossa, where careful inspection for needle marks that might be suggestive of intravenous drug abuse or localized swelling that might be suggestive of cubital bursitis should be carried out. The area surrounding the olecranon process should be observed for edema or localized swelling that might be suggestive of an olecranon bursitis (Fig. 69-4). Subcutaneous nodules along the posterior ulna are highly suggestive of rheumatoid arthritis (see Fig. 69-4).

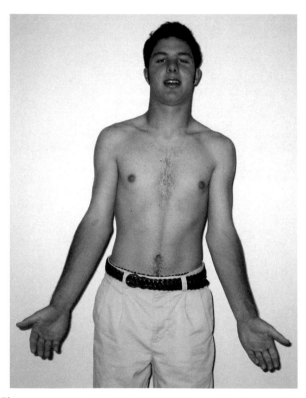

• **Figure 69-1** The carrying angle of the normal valgus position in males should be 10 to 15 degrees.

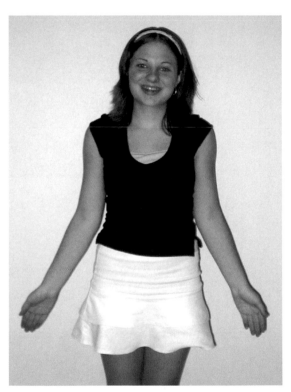

• **Figure 69-2** The carrying angle of the normal valgus position in females should not exceed 18 degrees.

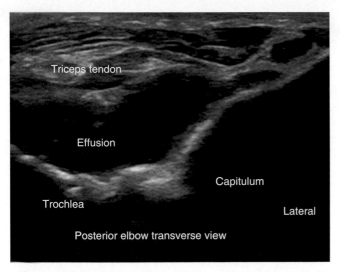

• **Figure 69-3** Transverse ultrasound image demonstrating a significant effusion of the elbow joint.

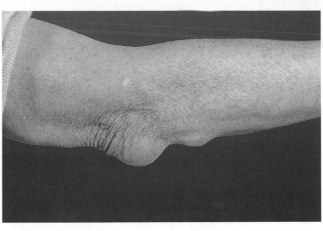

• **Figure 69-4** Olecranon bursitis in a patient with rheumatoid arthritis. A rheumatoid nodule is also shown. (From Careet S, Canoso J: The spine. In Klippel JH, Dieppe PA editors: *Rheumatology*, ed 2, London, 1998, Mosby, p 84.)

Because of the subcutaneous nature of many of the structures within the elbow joint that are prone to disease, careful palpation of the joint and surrounding tissues is extremely important in the diagnosis of elbow pain and dysfunction. The antecubital fossa should be palpated to identify any swelling or soft tissue mass. Bursitis or lipoma should be readily identifiable, as should phlebitic veins or arterial aneurysm from previous arterial puncture. The lateral epicondyle should be palpated to identify tennis elbow (Figs. 70-1 and 70-2). The area just distal and lateral to the lateral epicondyle is then palpated to identify radial tunnel syndrome, which is caused by entrapment of the posterior interosseous branch of the radial nerve (Fig. 70-3). The medial epicondyle should then be palpated to identify golfer's elbow (Figs. 70-4 and 70-5). The examiner should then turn his or her attention to the posterior elbow, and the area surrounding the olecranon should be carefully palpated to identify gouty tophi, loose bodies from previous fracture, and boggy edema and soft tissue mass that might suggest olecranon bursitis.

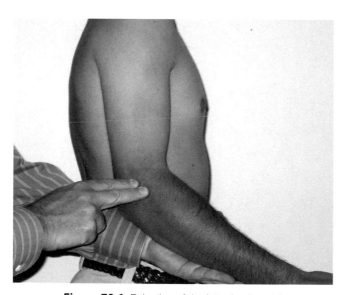

• **Figure 70-1** Palpation of the lateral epicondyle.

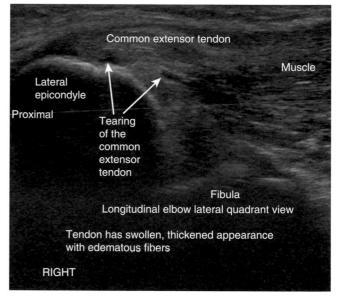

• **Figure 70-2** Longitudinal ultrasound image demonstrating lateral epicondylitis (tennis elbow). Note the tearing of the common extensor tendon and the loss of the normal sonographic fibular tendon architecture.

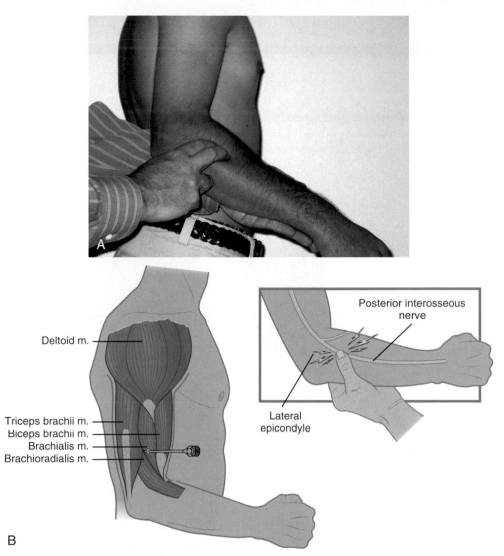

A

B

Deltoid m.

Triceps brachii m.
Biceps brachii m.
Brachialis m.
Brachioradialis m.

Posterior interosseous nerve

Lateral epicondyle

• **Figure 70-3 A** and **B,** Palpation of the area distally and laterally from the lateral epicondyle. (**B** from Waldman SW: *Atlas of pain management techniques,* Philadelphia, 2000, Saunders, p 85.)

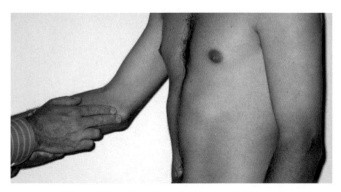

• **Figure 70-4** Palpation of the medial epicondyle.

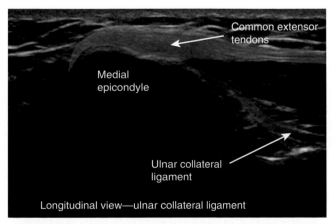

Common extensor tendons

Medial epicondyle

Ulnar collateral ligament

Longitudinal view—ulnar collateral ligament

• **Figure 70-5** Longitudinal ultrasound image demonstrating mild tendinosis of the common flexor tendon in a patient suffering from golfer's elbow.

The range of motion of the elbow should be assessed in flexion, extension, and forearm pronation and supination. Although young children can extend their elbows 10 to 15 degrees, most adults have little if any elbow extension (Fig. 71-1, *A*). Normal elbow flexion in adults is approximately 135 to 140 degrees, although most of the activities of daily living require less than complete elbow flexion (Fig. 71-1, *B*).

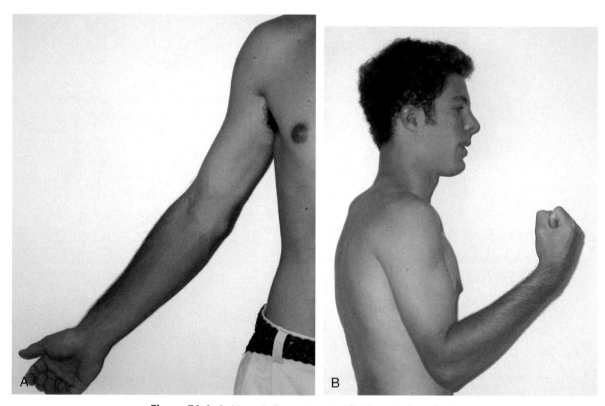

• **Figure 71-1 A,** Normal elbow extension. **B,** Normal elbow flexion.

Supination and pronation of the elbow are essential for humans to carry out their essential activities of daily living, including feeding. The complex movement of forearm rotation requires movement both at the radiohumeral joint and at the proximal and distal radioulnar joints. Fortunately, because of the wide range of motion of the shoulder, compromise of rotation of the forearm can be partially compensated for, albeit in a functionally inefficient way, by increased reliance on shoulder movement.

To assess the range of motion of the elbow in supination, the patient is asked to assume the standing position with the arms against the chest wall and the elbows flexed to 90 degrees. The patient is then asked to place his or her thumbs in alignment with the humerus (Fig. 72-1, *A*). The patient is then asked to turn his or her palms upward (Fig. 72-1, *B*). Normal elbow supination is 75 to 80 degrees.

To assess the range of motion of the elbow in pronation, the patient is asked to assume the standing position with the arms against the chest wall and the elbows flexed to 90 degrees. The patient is then asked to place his or her thumbs in alignment with the humerus (Fig. 72-2, *A*). The patient is then asked to turn his or her palms downward (Fig. 72-2, *B*). Normal elbow pronation is 75 to 80 degrees.

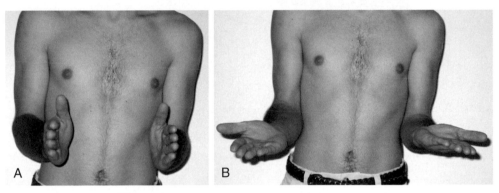

• **Figure 72-1** **A** and **B,** Assessment of elbow supination.

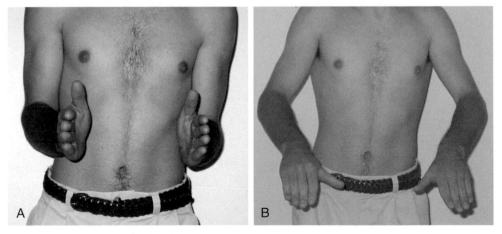

• **Figure 72-2** **A** and **B,** Assessment of elbow pronation.

73 The Valgus Stress Flexion Test for Medial Ligamentous Incompetence

The valgus stress flexion test is useful in the identification of medial ligamentous incompetence of the elbow. To perform the valgus stress flexion test, the patient is asked to assume the standing position and to abduct the shoulder to approximately 75 to 80 degrees. The patient is then asked to flex his or her elbow to approximately 30 degrees. The examiner then exerts valgus stress on the elbow (Fig. 73-1). The test is considered positive if medial laxity is identified.

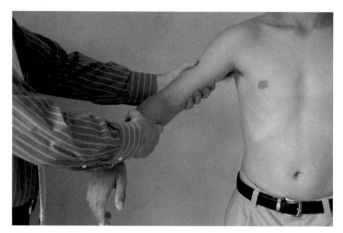

• **Figure 73-1** The valgus stress flexion test for medial ligamentous incompetence.

74 The Varus Stress Flexion Test for Lateral Ligamentous Incompetence

The varus stress flexion test is useful in the identification of lateral ligamentous incompetence of the elbow. To perform the varus stress flexion test, the patient is asked to assume the standing position and to abduct the shoulder to approximately 75 to 80 degrees. The patient is then asked to flex his or her elbow to approximately 30 degrees. The examiner then exerts varus stress on the elbow (Fig. 74-1). The test is considered positive if lateral laxity is identified.

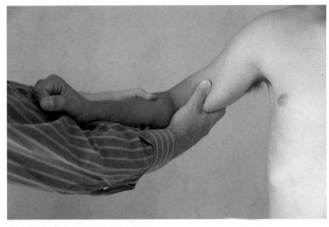

• **Figure 74-1** The varus stress flexion test for lateral ligamentous incompetence.

The lateral pivot-shift test helps the examiner to identify laxity of the ulnar part of the lateral collateral ligament. When there is laxity of the ulnar part of the lateral collateral ligament, the resulting instability allows the humeroulnar joint to sublux, with secondary dislocation of the humeroradial joint. To perform the lateral pivot-shift test for posterolateral insufficiency, the patient is placed in the supine position. The affected extremity is then extended back over the patient's head, and the shoulder is rotated externally (Fig. 75-1). While standing at the head of the table, the examiner then supinates the patient's forearm and simultaneously applies valgus stress and axial compression and flexion of the elbow (Fig. 75-2). Apprehension in the awake patient indicates a positive test and is highly suggestive of insufficiency of the ulnar part of the lateral collateral ligament of the elbow.

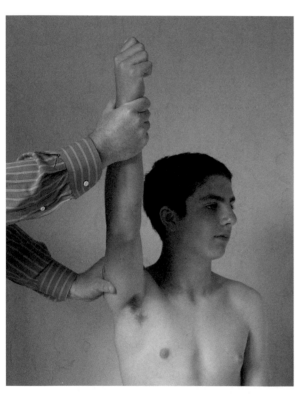

• **Figure 75-1** The lateral pivot-shift test for posterolateral insufficiency: the examiner extends the affected extremity up over the patient's head and externally rotates the shoulder.

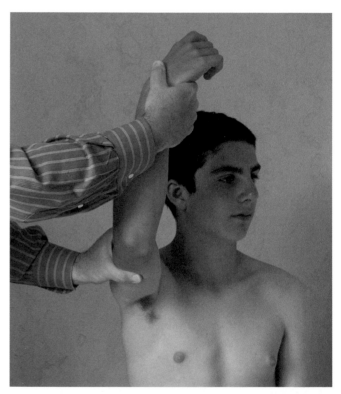

• **Figure 75-2** The lateral pivot-shift test for posterolateral insufficiency: the examiner supinates the patient's forearm and applies valgus stress and axial compression and flexion of the elbow.

Ulnar nerve entrapment at the elbow is the second most common upper extremity nerve entrapment syndrome, after carpal tunnel syndrome. The patient presenting with ulnar nerve entrapment at the elbow will frequently complain of difficulty turning a key, using a hammer, or holding a fishing rod. These disabilities are due to a combination of factors, including: (1) loss of pinch strength between the thumb and adjacent fingers, (2) loss of synchronization of finger flexion while trying to grasp, and (3) loss of coordination between the thumb and digits while trying to grasp.

Unfortunately, the nomenclature of ulnar nerve entrapment at the elbow is sometimes confusing because of a lack of consistency in associating the underlying pathologic process with the naming of the clinical syndrome. For the purposes of the clinician trying to utilize physical examination to identify the source of upper extremity neurologic dysfunction or pain, the following clinical syndromes will present in an essentially identical manner:

- Cubital tunnel syndrome
- Tardy ulnar palsy
- Ulnar palsy

Once the clinician has identified compromise of ulnar nerve function and suspects one of these clinical syndromes, electromyography and magnetic resonance imaging (MRI) and/or ultrasound imaging will be required to pinpoint the anatomic site and cause of ulnar nerve entrapment at the elbow.

The Froment paper sign for ulnar nerve entrapment at the elbow is an elegant test that reveals a classic deformity of the thumb while trying to pinch caused by weakness of the adductor pollicis brevis and the flexor pollicis brevis, which stabilize the metacarpophalangeal joint of the thumb. This loss of stabilization of the metacarpophalangeal joint causes a hyperextension of this joint with compensatory flexion of the interphalangeal joint of the thumb. As the patient tries to increase pinch strength to overcome the weakness of the adductor pollicis brevis and the flexor pollicis brevis, this loss of the compensatory flexion deformity increases, producing a positive Froment paper sign.

To perform this test, the patient is asked to lightly grasp a piece of paper between the thumb and index finger of each hand. If ulnar entrapment is present, the examiner will notice that the interphalangeal joint of the thumb of the affected extremity will flex in an effort to grasp the paper (Fig. 76-1). The examiner then asks the patient to more tightly grasp the paper. If ulnar nerve entrapment is present, the flexion deformity should increase in comparison to the thumb of the unaffected extremity (Fig. 76-2). This increased flexion is considered a positive Froment paper sign and is highly suggestive of ulnar nerve entrapment at the elbow. In a small subset of patients, lesions of the brachial plexus or entrapment of the ulnar nerve above the elbow or in the forearm or wrist can also produce a positive Froment paper sign. For this reason, careful electromyography, MRI, and ultrasound imaging at the level of suspected ulnar nerve entrapment should be carried out.

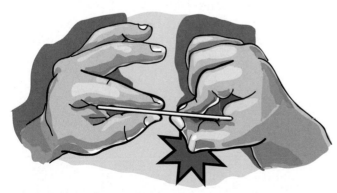

• **Figure 76-1** The Froment paper test is performed by asking the patient to lightly grasp a piece of paper between the thumb and index finger of each hand and monitoring the flexion of the thumb interphalangeal joint on the affected side. Increased pinch strength is required to compensate for weakness, causing an increased flexion deformity.

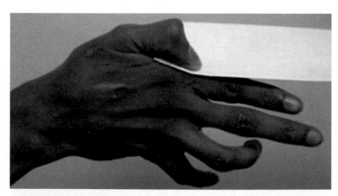

• **Figure 76-2** Positive Forment paper sign as indicated by the flexion deformity.

Ulnar nerve entrapment at the elbow is the second most common upper extremity nerve entrapment syndrome, after carpal tunnel syndrome. The patient presenting with ulnar nerve entrapment at the elbow will frequently complain of difficulty turning a key, using a hammer, or holding a fishing rod. These disabilities are due to a combination of factors, including: (1) loss of pinch strength between the thumb and adjacent fingers, (2) loss of synchronization of finger flexion while trying to grasp, and (3) loss of coordination between the thumb and digits while trying to grasp.

Unfortunately, the nomenclature of ulnar nerve entrapment at the elbow is sometimes confusing because of a lack of consistency in associating the underlying pathologic process with the naming of the clinical syndrome. For the purposes of the clinician trying to utilize physical examination to identify the source of upper extremity neurologic dysfunction or pain, the following clinical syndromes will present in an essentially identical manner:

- Cubital tunnel syndrome
- Tardy ulnar palsy
- Ulnar palsy

Once the clinician has identified compromise of ulnar nerve function and suspects one of these clinical syndromes, electromyography and magnetic resonance imaging (MRI)

and/or ultrasound imaging will be required to pinpoint the anatomic site and cause of ulnar nerve entrapment at the elbow.

The Jeanne sign for ulnar nerve entrapment at the elbow is similar to the Froment paper sign. In addition to the compensatory flexion of the interphalangeal joint seen in Froment paper sign, with Jeanne sign, there is hyperextension of the metacarpophalangeal joint of the thumb due to denervation-induced weakness of the flexor pollicis brevis muscle. The positive test for Jeanne sign is often seen in conjunction with a positive test for Froment paper sign.

To perform the test for Jeanne sign, the patient is asked to lightly grasp a key between the thumb and radial aspect of the index finger of the affected hand (Fig. 77-1). The patient is then asked to grasp the key more tightly. If ulnar entrapment is present, the examiner will note that the metacarpophalangeal joint of the thumb hyperextends to help stabilize the weakened joint to increase the grasp pressure (Fig. 77-2). In a small subset of patients, lesions of the brachial plexus or entrapment of the ulnar nerve above the elbow or in the forearm or wrist can also produce a positive Jeanne and/or Froment paper sign. For this reason, careful electromyography, MRI, and ultrasound imaging at the level of suspected ulnar nerve entrapment should be carried out.

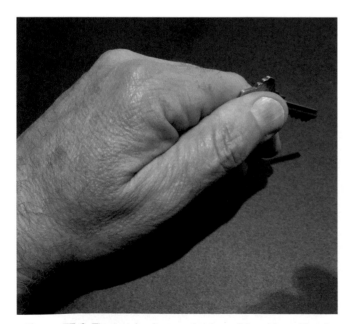

• **Figure 77-1** The test for Jeanne sign is performed by asking the patient to lightly grasp a key between the thumb and radial aspect of the index finger of each hand and monitoring the flexion of the thumb interphalangeal joint on the affected side.

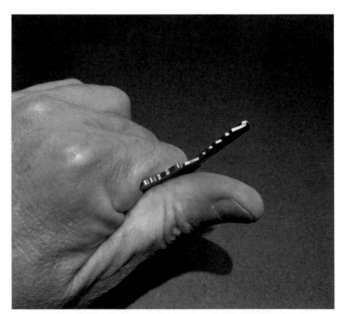

• **Figure 77-2** The patient is then asked to grasp the key more tightly. The test for Jeanne sign is positive if the metacarpophalangeal joint of the affected thumb hyperextends in order to stabilize the joint to increase grasp pressure.

The Wartenberg Sign for Ulnar Nerve Entrapment at the Elbow

Patients suffering from ulnar nerve entrapment at the elbow often complain of an inability to reach into their pockets because the little finger catches on the opening of the pockets. This disability, while seemingly mild, causes a significant amount of distress and is caused by the weakness of the adductors of the little finger.

The Wartenberg sign for ulnar nerve entrapment at the elbow is a simple way to identify the inability to adduct the little finger. Such weakness primarily results from the compromise of the third palmar interosseous muscle combined with the other functional disabilities associated with ulnar nerve entrapment discussed in Chapter 76. Clinically, this weakness presents as a chronically abducted posture of the little finger when the forearm is pronated and the fingers are fully extended, which is also known as a positive Wartenberg sign (Fig. 78-1).

To perform the test for Wartenberg sign for ulnar nerve entrapment at the elbow, the patient is asked to place an object such as a ring of keys into the pants pocket on the affected side (Video 78-1). The patient is then asked to reach into the pocket and retrieve the object. If there is weakness of the adductors of the affected little finger, the finger will catch on the opening of the pocket, and the patient will not be able to get his or her hand fully into the pocket to retrieve the object (Fig. 78-2). Such weakness can be confirmed by performing a little finger adduction test (see Chapter 79). A positive test for Wartenberg sign and a positive little finger adduction test are highly suggestive of ulnar nerve entrapment at the elbow.

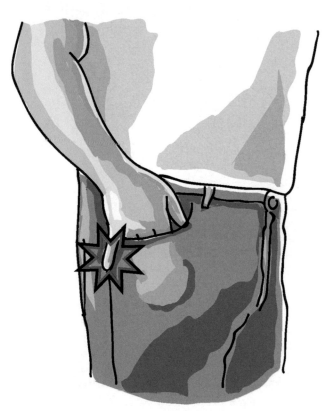

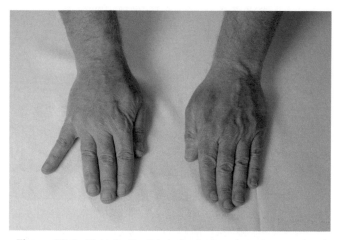

• **Figure 78-1** Clinically, the Wartenberg sign presents as a chronically abducted posture of the little finger when the forearm is pronated and the fingers are fully extended.

• **Figure 78-2** The test for Wartenberg sign for ulnar nerve entrapment at the elbow.

The little finger adduction test for ulnar nerve entrapment at the elbow is a simple way to identify an inability to adduct the little finger. Such weakness primarily results from the compromise of the interosseous muscles combined with the other functional disabilities associated with ulnar nerve entrapment discussed in Chapters 76, 77, and 78.

To perform the little finger adduction test for ulnar nerve entrapment at the elbow, the patient is asked to touch his or her little finger to the index finger (Fig. 79-1 and Video 79-1). This maneuver requires that the strength of the interosseous muscles be relatively intact, and an inability to perform such a task constitutes a positive little finger adduction test.

A positive little finger adduction test as well as a positive Froment paper sign (see Chapter 76) or a positive Wartenberg sign (see Chapter 78) are highly suggestive of ulnar nerve entrapment at the elbow. As discussed previously, in some patients, lesions of the brachial plexus or entrapment of the ulnar nerve above the elbow or in the forearm or wrist may produce similar physical findings. Careful electromyography and magnetic resonance and ultrasound imaging at the level of suspected ulnar nerve entrapment should be carried out (Fig. 79-2).

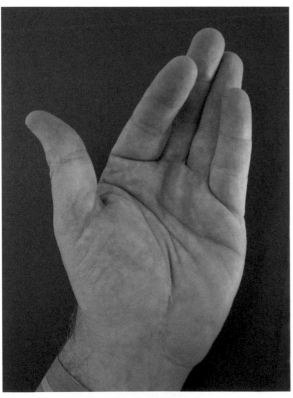

• **Figure 79-1** Little finger adduction test.

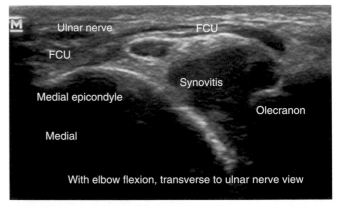

• **Figure 79-2** Transverse ultrasound image demonstrating compression of the ulnar nerve at the elbow by exuberant synovitis in a patient suffering from rheumatoid arthritis. *FCU,* Flexor carpi ulnaris.

80 The Valgus Extension Overload Test for Olecranon Impingement

The valgus extension overload test aids the examiner in identifying the presence of a posteromedial olecranon osteophyte or olecranon fossa overgrowth or compression by calcification due to inflammatory processes (Fig. 80-1). To perform the valgus extension overload test, the examiner stabilizes the humerus with one hand and, with the opposite hand, pronates the forearm while simultaneously applying a firm valgus force and quickly maximally extending the elbow (Fig. 80-2). The test is considered positive if the rapid extension of the elbow causes posteromedial pain, presumably due to the tip of the olecranon osteophyte or calcification being forced into engagement into the olecranon fossa.

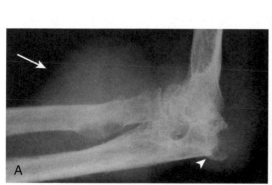
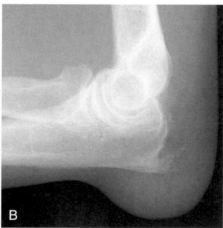

• **Figure 80-1** Elbow abnormalities in gout. **(A)** Olecranon changes consisting of soft tissue swelling and subajacent osseous erosion *(arrowhead)* are seen. Additional soft tissue swelling is also evident *(arrow)*. **(B)** Similar changes in another patient with a tophus containing calcification. (From Resnick D, Kransdorf MJ, editors: *Bone and joint imaging,* ed 3, Philadelphia, 2005, Saunders, p 451.)

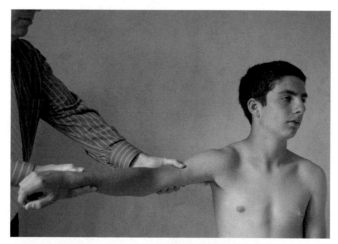

• **Figure 80-2** The valgus extension overload test. The examiner stabilizes the humerus with one hand, and with the opposite hand, pronates the forearm while simultaneously applying a firm valgus force and quickly maximally extending the elbow.

81 The Compression Test for Lateral Antebrachial Cutaneous Nerve Entrapment Syndrome

Lateral antebrachial cutaneous nerve entrapment syndrome is caused by entrapment of the lateral antebrachial cutaneous nerve by the biceps tendon or the brachialis muscle. Clinically, the patient who suffers from lateral antebrachial cutaneous nerve entrapment syndrome complains of pain and paresthesias radiating from the elbow to the base of the thumb. Dull aching of the radial aspect of the forearm, which often worsens if the arm is left in a partially flexed position, is also a common complaint. The lateral antebrachial cutaneous nerve is a continuation of the musculocutaneous nerve. The musculocutaneous nerve passes through the fascia lateral to the biceps tendon before it continues into the forearm as the lateral antebrachial cutaneous nerve (Fig. 81-1). The nerve is susceptible to entrapment at this point. The lateral antebrachial cutaneous nerve passes behind the cephalic vein, where it divides into a volar branch that continues along the radial border of the forearm, providing sensory innervation to the skin over the lateral half of the volar surface of the forearm. It passes anterior to the radial artery at the wrist to provide sensation to the base of the thumb. The dorsal branch provides sensation to the dorsal lateral surface of the forearm.

The pain of lateral antebrachial cutaneous nerve entrapment syndrome may develop after an acute twisting injury to the elbow or direct trauma to the soft tissues overlying the lateral antebrachial cutaneous nerve, or the onset of pain may be more insidious, without an obvious inciting factor. The carrying of heavy purses or grocery bags in the crook of the elbow has also been implicated in compression of the nerve. The pain is constant and is made worse with use of the elbow. Patients with lateral antebrachial cutaneous nerve entrapment syndrome often note increasing pain while keyboarding or playing the piano. Sleep disturbance is common. On physical examination, there is tenderness to palpation of the lateral antebrachial cutaneous nerve at the elbow at a point just lateral to the biceps tendon. Elbow range of

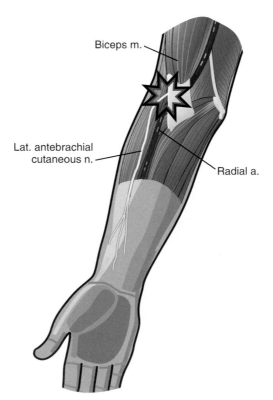

Biceps m.

Lat. antebrachial cutaneous n.

Radial a.

• **Figure 81-1** Lateral antebrachial cutaneous nerve entrapment: relevant soft tissue anatomy.

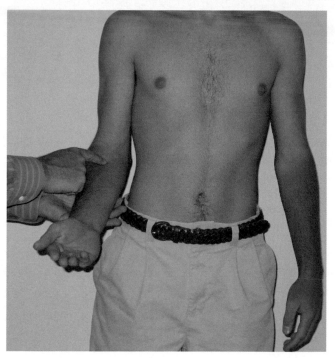

• **Figure 81-2** Compression test for lateral antebrachial cutaneous nerve entrapment.

motion is normal. Patients with lateral antebrachial cutaneous nerve entrapment syndrome exhibit pain on active resisted flexion or rotation of the forearm. Patients with antebrachial cutaneous nerve entrapment syndrome will usually exhibit a positive compression test.

The compression test for antebrachial cutaneous nerve entrapment syndrome is performed by having the patient assume the seated position with the affected arm partially flexed (Fig. 81-2). The examiner compresses the area lateral to the biceps tendon at the elbow tightly for 30 seconds. Patients suffering from antebrachial cutaneous nerve entrapment syndrome will note an increase in pain and paresthesias in the distribution of the antebrachial cutaneous nerve (Video 81-1).

Because cervical radiculopathy and tennis elbow can sometimes mimic lateral antebrachial cutaneous nerve entrapment syndrome, careful electromyography should be performed to distinguish C6 radiculopathy from entrapment of the antebrachial cutaneous nerve and to rule out a double crush syndrome. Magnetic resonance imaging and/or ultrasound imaging of the elbow is indicated if joint instability or mass is suspected. Injection of the lateral antebrachial cutaneous nerve with local anesthetic can serve as both a diagnostic and a therapeutic maneuver.

82 The Snap Sign for Snapping Triceps Syndrome

The causes of ulnar nerve entrapment of the elbow are many and include thickening of the retinaculum of the roof of the cubital tunnel (the Osborne lesion), thickening of the floor of the cubital tunnel, osteophyte development of the bones surrounding the ulnar nerve, compression of the ulnar nerve by soft tissue mass or tumor, and abnormal subluxation of the ulnar nerve out of the cubital tunnel (Fig. 82-1). This abnormal movement may be caused by a hypoplastic retinaculum or with subluxation of the medial head of the triceps muscle during flexion of the elbow. When subluxation of the triceps muscle occurs, a palpable and at times audible snapping of the elbow can be identified. These findings form the basis for the snap sign for snapping triceps syndrome.

To elicit the snap sign for snapping triceps syndrome, the patient is placed in a seated position and is asked to repeatedly flex the affected arm rapidly while the examiner cups the elbow in his or her hand (Fig. 82-2). An audible or palpable snap constitutes a positive snap sign, and magnetic resonance imaging of the elbow in both the flexed and extended positions should be obtained to ascertain the anatomic abnormality responsible for the snapping triceps syndrome (Video 82-1). Electromyography and cross-elbow nerve conduction studies can help to identify the anatomic site of ulnar nerve entrapment and to rule out radiculopathy and plexopathy that may be confusing the clinical picture.

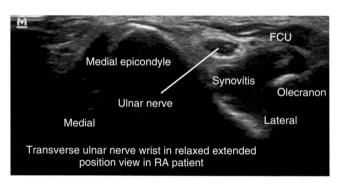

• **Figure 82-1** Transverse ultrasound image demonstrating compromise of the ulnar nerve by synovitis formation in a patient with rheumatoid arthritis. *FCU,* Flexor carpi ulnaris; *RA,* rheumatoid arthritis.

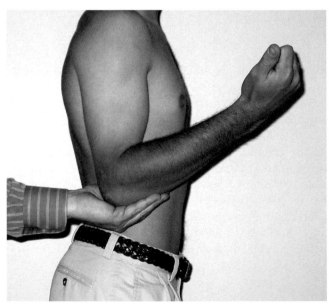

• **Figure 82-2** Eliciting the snap sign for snapping triceps syndrome.

83 The Creaking Tendon Sign for Triceps Tendinitis

Olecranon bursitis is by far the most common cause of posterior elbow pain. Less common, although as painful, is triceps tendinitis. Triceps tendinitis can occur from a repetitive stress injury such as repeated resisted extension when using exercise equipment, direct trauma to the posterior elbow with the elbow in extension (e.g., a quarterback sack while passing a football), or a sudden decelerating counterforce during active extension of the arm (e.g., warding off a blow during kickboxing). Triceps tendinitis presents with pain on extension of the elbow. In contradistinction to olecranon bursitis, there is minimal joint effusion or swelling, and the main physical finding is a tender, hot distal triceps tendon that may creak during extension of the affected extremity. The creaking forms the basis for the creaking tendon sign.

To identify the creaking tendon sign for triceps tendinitis, the patient is placed in the sitting position and asked to perform active resisted extension of the arm while the examiner places his or her index finger over the distal triceps tendon (Fig. 83-1). If triceps tendinitis is present, pressure exerted by the examiner on the distal tendon may increase the patient's pain, and the examiner may appreciate a creaking of the tendon as the arm extends. These findings constitute a positive creaking tendon test for triceps tendinitis and should lead the examiner to obtain magnetic resonance imaging of the elbow to identify any bony or soft tissue abnormality that is responsible for the tendinopathy and to rule out partial tears of the triceps tendon.

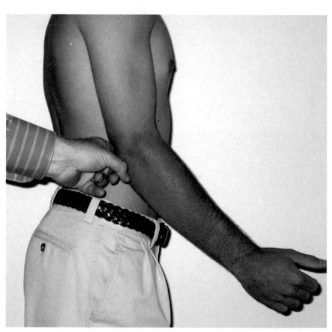

• **Figure 83-1** Creaking tendon sign for triceps tendinitis.

84 The Ballottement Test for Olecranon Bursitis

The olecranon bursa is vulnerable to injury from both acute trauma and repeated microtrauma. Acute injuries frequently take the form of direct trauma to the elbow when playing sports such as hockey or falling directly onto the olecranon process. Repeated pressure from leaning on the elbow to rise or from working long hours at a drafting table can result in inflammation and swelling of the olecranon bursa (Fig. 84-1). Gout or bacterial infection rarely may precipitate acute olecranon bursitis. If the inflammation of the olecranon bursa becomes chronic, calcification of the bursa may occur, with residual nodules called gravel.

The patient who suffers from olecranon bursitis will frequently complain of pain and swelling with any movement of the elbow but especially with extension. The pain is localized to the olecranon area, with referred pain often noted above the elbow joint. Often, the patient is more concerned about the swelling around the bursa than about the pain because the swelling is dramatic and its onset is abrupt. Physical examination reveals point tenderness over the olecranon and swelling of the bursa, which at times can be quite extensive. Passive extension and resisted shoulder flexion reproduce the pain, as does any pressure over the bursa.

Patients suffering from olecranon bursitis will also exhibit a positive ballottement test.

To perform the ballottement test for olecranon bursitis, the patient is asked to assume the sitting position, and the affected extremity is allowed to rest lightly in the examiner's arm. The examiner then gently ballottes the swollen area over the olecranon. The ballottement should reveal a soft, nonfluctuant fluid-filled swelling that ballots easily. Lack of ballottement suggests abscess or another pathologic process. Magnetic resonance and/or ultrasound imaging can help clarify the cause of the posterior elbow swelling if the diagnosis is in doubt (Figs. 84-2 and 84-3).

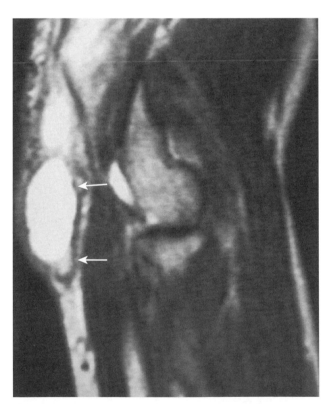

• **Figure 84-2** Olecranon bursitis. Sagittal T2-weighted magnetic resonance image shows a focal fluid collection posteriorly (arrows) in a patient with triceps tendon tear (not shown in this image). (From Kaplan PA, Helms CA, Dussault R, et al: *Musculoskeletal MRI*, Philadelphia, 2001, Saunders, p 235.)

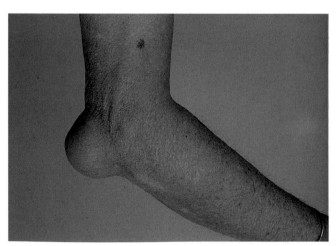

• **Figure 84-1** Olecranon bursitis in early rheumatoid arthritis. (From Groff GD: Axial and peripheral joints: olecranon bursitis. In Klippel JH, Dieppe PA, editors: *Rheumatology*, ed 2, London, 1998, Mosby, p 143.)

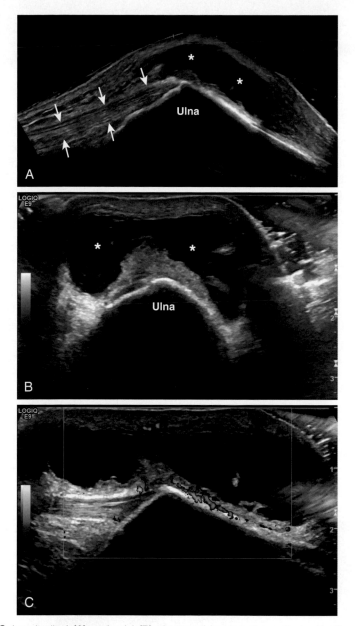

• **Figure 84-3** Longitudinal **(A)** and axial **(B)** ultrasound images of a patient with olecranon bursitis. There is a low-echo, fluid-filled bursa *(asterisks)* superficial to the proximal ulna, and the distal triceps tendon is visualized on the longitudinal image *(white arrows)*. **(C)** The Doppler ultrasound image demonstrates increased vascularity in the periphery of the bursa consistent with mild inflammatory synovitis. (From Waldman SD, Campbell, RSD: *Imaging of pain,* Philadelphia, 2010, Saunders/Elsevier, p 275, fig 108-1.)

Tennis elbow (also known as lateral epicondylitis) is caused by repetitive microtrauma to the extensor tendons of the forearm. The pathophysiology of tennis elbow is initially caused by microtearing at the origin of extensor carpi radialis and extensor carpi ulnaris. Secondary inflammation may occur and can become chronic as the result of continued overuse or misuse of the extensors of the forearm. Coexistent bursitis, arthritis, and gout also may perpetuate the pain and disability of tennis elbow.

Tennis elbow occurs in patients who engage in repetitive activities that include hand grasping, such as politicians shaking hands, or high-torque wrist turning, such as scooping ice cream at an ice cream parlor. Tennis players develop tennis elbow by two separate mechanisms: increased pressure grip strain as a result of playing with too heavy a racquet and making backhand shots with a leading shoulder and elbow rather than keeping the shoulder and elbow parallel to the net (Fig. 85-1). Other racquet sport players also are susceptible to the development of tennis elbow.

The pain of tennis elbow is localized to the region of the lateral epicondyle. It is constant and is made worse with active contraction of the wrist. Patients note the inability to hold a coffee cup or hammer. Sleep disturbance is common.

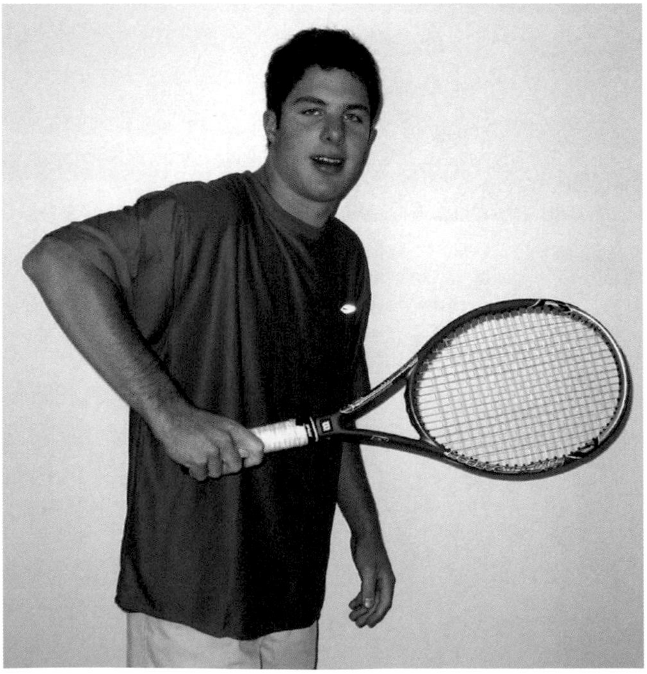

On physical examination, there is tenderness along the extensor tendons at or just below the lateral epicondyle. Many patients with tennis elbow exhibit a bandlike thickening within the affected extensor tendons. Elbow range of motion is normal. Grip strength on the affected side is diminished. Patients with tennis elbow demonstrate a positive tennis elbow test. The test is performed by stabilizing the patient's forearm and then having the patient clench his or her fist and actively extend the wrist (Video 85-1). The examiner then attempts to force the wrist into flexion (Fig. 85-2). Sudden, severe pain is highly suggestive of tennis elbow.

Radial tunnel syndrome and occasionally C6-C7 radiculopathy can mimic tennis elbow. Radial tunnel syndrome is an entrapment neuropathy that results from entrapment of the radial nerve below the elbow (see Chapter 91). Radial tunnel syndrome can be distinguished from tennis elbow in that with radial tunnel syndrome, the maximal tenderness to palpation is distal to the lateral epicondyle over the radial nerve, whereas with tennis elbow, the maximal tenderness to palpation is over the lateral epicondyle (Fig. 85-3). Electromyography helps to distinguish cervical radiculopathy and radial tunnel syndrome from tennis elbow. Plain radiographs are indicated in all patients who present with tennis elbow to rule out joint mice and other occult bony pathology. Magnetic resonance imaging and/or ultrasound imaging of the elbow is indicated to confirm the diagnosis and when joint instability is suspected (Figs. 85-4 and 85-5).

• **Figure 85-1** Mechanism of elbow injury in tennis players.

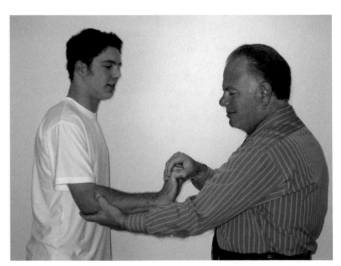

• **Figure 85-2** Test for tennis elbow.

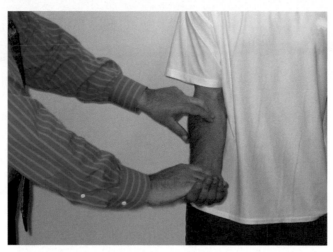

• **Figure 85-3** Patients who suffer from radial tunnel syndrome will experience maximal tenderness over the radial nerve.

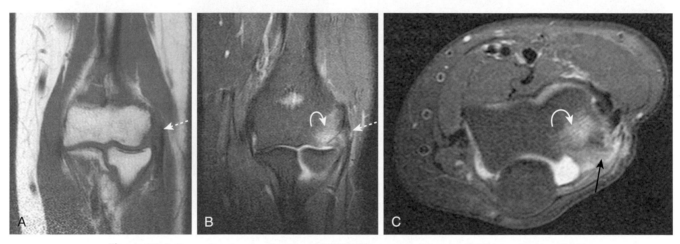

• **Figure 85-4** Coronal proton density **(A)** and FST2W **(B)** magnetic resonance (MR) images of a patient with tennis elbow. There are thickening and increased SI within the common extensor tendon *(broken white arrow)* along with associated underlying bone marrow edema *(curved arrow)*. **C,** The bone marrow is also seen on the axial FST2W MR image *(curved arrow)* and the soft tissue thickening and increased SI posterior to the extensor tendon probably reflect associated soft tissue impingement *(black arrow)*. (From Waldman SD, Campbell, RSD: *Imaging of pain,* Philadelphia, 2010, Saunders/Elsevier, fig 103-2.)

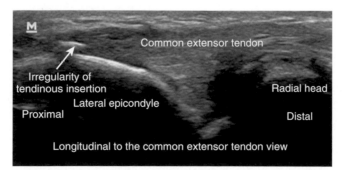

• **Figure 85-5** Longitudinal ultrasound image demonstrating irregularity of the insertion of the common extensor tendon, a classic sonographic finding in patients suffering from tennis elbow.

To perform the Maudsley test for lateral epicondylitis, the patient is placed in the sitting position with the patient's forearm resting comfortably on a table and the hand and wrist hanging off the edge of the table (Fig. 86-1). The examiner then stabilizes the forearm and asks the patient to forcefully extend his or her middle finger against examiner resistance (Fig. 86-2). The test is positive if the patient experiences pain at the lateral epicondyle. The pain elicited by this test is believed to be caused by inflammation of the insertion extensor digitorum communis muscle into the lateral epicondyle.

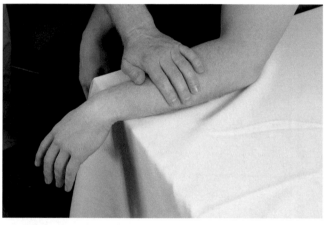

• **Figure 86-1** To perform the Maudsley test for lateral epicondylitis, the patient is placed in the sitting position with the patient's forearm resting comfortably on a table and the hand and wrist hanging off the edge of the table.

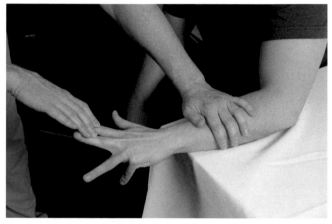

• **Figure 86-2** The examiner then stabilizes the forearm and asks the patient to forcefully extend his or her middle finger against examiner resistance.

To perform the chair lift test for lateral epicondylitis, the patient is asked to stand behind a chair with his or her elbows fully extended and the forearms pronated (Fig. 87-1). The patient is then asked to grasp the back of the chair with a 3-finger pinch using the thumb, index, and long fingers (Fig. 87-2). The patient is then asked to lift the chair (Fig. 87-3). The test is positive if the patient experiences sharp pain at the insertion of the common extensor tendon on the lateral epicondyle when lifting the chair.

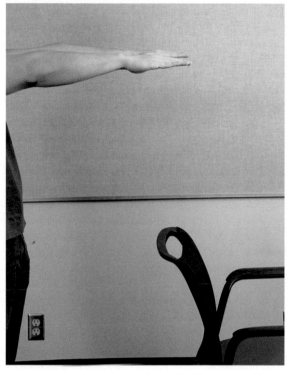

• **Figure 87-1** To perform the chair lift test for lateral epicondylitis, the patient is asked to stand behind a chair with his or her elbows fully extended and the forearms pronated.

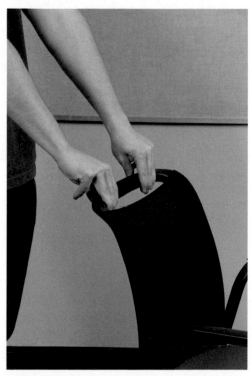

• **Figure 87-2** The patient is then asked to grasp the back of the chair with a 3-finger pinch using the thumb, index, and long fingers.

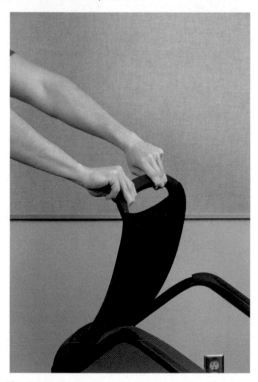

• **Figure 87-3** The patient is then asked to lift the chair.

Golfer's elbow (also known as medial epicondylitis) is caused by repetitive microtrauma to the flexor tendons of the forearm in a manner analogous to tennis elbow. The pathophysiology of golfer's elbow is initially caused by microtearing at the origin of the pronator teres, flexor carpi radialis and flexor carpi ulnaris, and palmaris longus. Secondary inflammation may occur and can become chronic as the result of continued overuse or misuse of the flexors of the forearm. Coexistent bursitis, arthritis, and gout may also perpetuate the pain and disability of golfer's elbow.

Golfer's elbow occurs in patients who engage in repetitive flexion activities, including throwing baseballs, carrying heavy suitcases, and driving golf balls. These activities have in common repetitive flexion of the wrist and strain on the flexor tendons caused by excessive weight or sudden arrested motion. Many of the activities that can cause tennis elbow can also cause golfer's elbow.

The pain of golfer's elbow is localized to the region of the medial epicondyle. It is constant and is made worse with active contraction of the wrist. Patients note the inability to hold a golf club. Sleep disturbance is common. On physical examination, there is tenderness along the flexor tendons at or just below the medial epicondyle. Many patients with golfer's elbow exhibit a bandlike thickening within the affected flexor tendons. Elbow range of motion is normal. Grip strength on the affected side is diminished. Patients with golfer's elbow demonstrate a positive golfer's elbow test. The test is performed by stabilizing the patient's forearm and then having the patient actively flex the wrist. The examiner then attempts to force the wrist into extension (Fig. 88-1). Sudden, severe pain is highly suggestive of golfer's elbow.

Occasionally, C6-C7 radiculopathy can mimic golfer's elbow. The patient suffering from cervical radiculopathy usually has neck pain and proximal upper extremity pain in addition to symptoms below the elbow. Electromyography helps to distinguish radiculopathy from golfer's elbow. Plain radiographs are indicated for all patients who present with golfer's elbow to rule out joint mice and other occult bony pathology. Magnetic resonance imaging and/or ultrasound imaging of the elbow is indicated to confirm the diagnosis and when joint instability is suspected (Fig. 88-2).

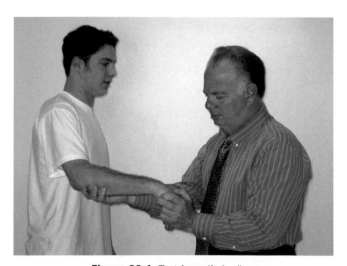

• **Figure 88-1** Test for golfer's elbow.

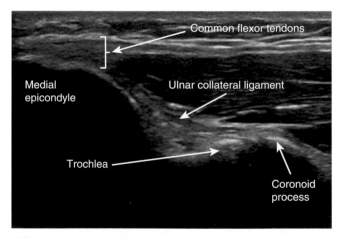

• **Figure 88-2** Longitudinal ultrasound image of the common flexor tendons. Note mild tendinosis.

89 The Polk Test to Differentiate Lateral and Medial Epicondylitis

Some patients find it difficult to localize the specific anatomic location of their elbow pain, especially if the source of pain is from multiple pathologic processes. The Polk test is helpful in accurately differentiating lateral from medial epicondylitis. To perform the test, the patient is asked to assume the seated position and flex the elbows 90 degrees (Fig. 89-1). The patient is then asked to turn his or her palm downward (pronation of the forearm and hand) so that the palm is facing the floor (Fig. 89-2). The patient is then asked to grasp the handles of a reusable shopping bag with contents that weigh at least 6 pounds and then lift the bag (Fig. 89-3). If the lifting of the bag produces sudden pain

over the lateral epicondyle, the diagnosis is most likely tennis elbow. The patient is then asked to turn his or her palm upward (supination of the forearm and hand) so that the palm is facing the ceiling (Fig. 89-4). The patient is then

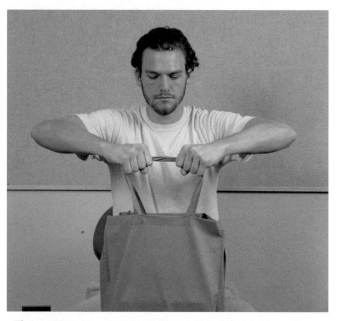

• **Figure 89-3** Step 3 of the Polk test. The patient is then asked to grasp the handles of a reusable shopping bag with contents that weigh at least 6 pounds and then lift the bag.

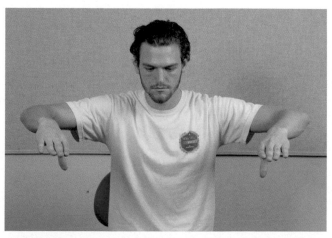

• **Figure 89-1** Step 1 of the Polk test. The patient is asked to assume the seated position and flex the elbows 90 degrees.

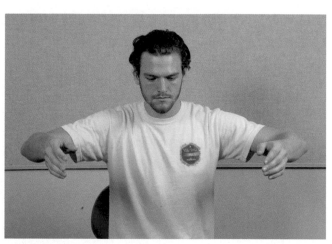

• **Figure 89-2** Step 2 of the Polk test. The patient is then asked to turn his or her palm downward (pronation of the forearm and hand) so that the palm is facing the floor.

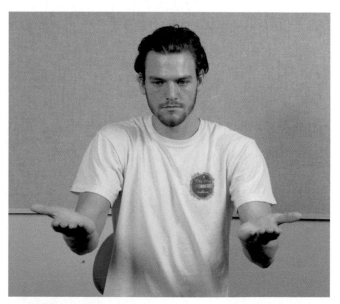

• **Figure 89-4** Step 4 of the Polk test. The patient is then asked to turn his or her palm upward (supination of the forearm and hand) so that the palm is facing the ceiling.

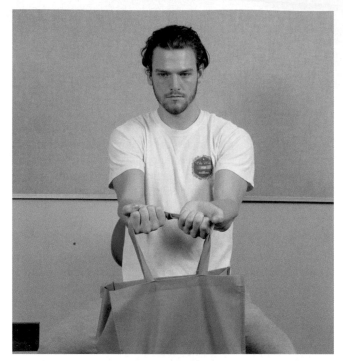

• **Figure 89-5** Step 5 of the Polk test. The patient is then again asked to grasp the handles of a reusable shopping bag with contents that weigh at least 6 pounds and then lift the bag.

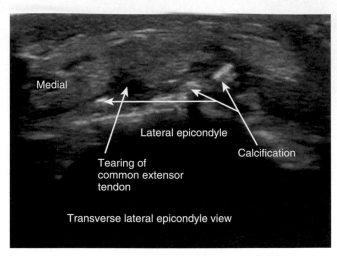

• **Figure 89-6** Transverse ultrasound image demonstrating calcific tendinitis and lateral epicondylitis in a patient with diffuse elbow pain.

again asked to grasp the handles of a reusable shopping bag with contents that weigh at least 6 pounds and then lift the bag (Fig. 89-5). If the lifting of the bag produces sudden pain over the medial epicondyle, the diagnosis is most likely golfer's elbow. It should be remembered that patients who

have difficulty localizing their pain often suffer from more than one pathologic process. In this setting, magnetic resonance imaging and/or ultrasound imaging of the elbow is almost always indicated to confirm the diagnosis and if joint instability is suspected (Fig. 89-6).

90 The Brachialis Jump Test for Climber's Elbow

Because of its more protected nature relative to the distal biceps musculotendinous unit, which is the most commonly injured tendon of the elbow, the distal musculotendinous unit of the brachialis muscle is injured much less commonly. Inciting factors include repetitive stress injuries from pull-ups, sudden extension against a fully contracted brachialis muscle during competitive arm wrestling, and, most commonly, strain during rock climbing (Fig. 90-1).

To perform the brachialis jump test for climber's elbow, the patient is placed in the standing position with the elbow slightly flexed. The patient is then asked to contract the forearm against resistance. The examiner then palpates the distal musculotendinous unit of the muscle in a manner analogous to the palpation of a trigger point (Fig. 90-2). If the distal musculotendinous unit is strained or inflamed, the palpation will elicit a positive jump sign. Magnetic resonance and/or ultrasound imaging will reveal injury or inflammation on fast STIR and T2-weighted images (Fig. 90-3).

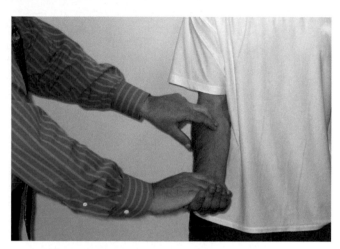

• **Figure 90-2** Brachialis jump test for climber's elbow.

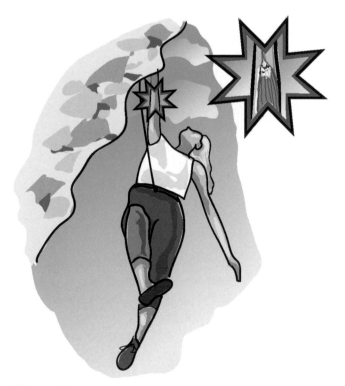

• **Figure 90-1** Strain during rock climbing is a common cause of injury to the distal musculotendinous unit of the brachialis muscle (climber's elbow).

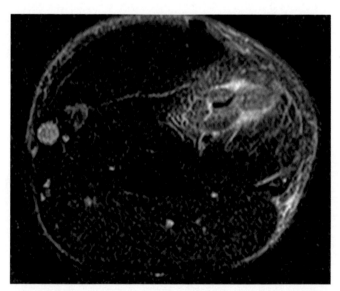

• **Figure 90-3** Climber's elbow. Axial STIR imaging shows abnormal feathery hyperintensity in the brachialis muscle belly in this patient who suffered an injury while doing pull-ups. (From Wenzke DR: MR imaging of the elbow in the injured athlete, *Radiol Clin North Am* 51(2):195–213, 2013.)

SECTION 4

The Forearm

Radial tunnel syndrome is an entrapment neuropathy of the radial nerve that is often clinically misdiagnosed as resistant tennis elbow. In radial tunnel syndrome, the posterior interosseous branch of the radial nerve is entrapped by a variety of mechanisms that have a similar clinical presentation in common. These mechanisms include aberrant fibrous bands in front of the radial head, anomalous blood vessels that compress the nerve, and a sharp tendinous margin of the extensor carpi radialis brevis (Fig. 91-1). These entrapments can exist alone or in combination.

Regardless of the mechanism of entrapment of the radial nerve, the common clinical feature of radial tunnel syndrome is pain just below the lateral epicondyle of the humerus. The pain of radial tunnel syndrome may develop after an acute twisting injury or direct trauma to the soft tissues overlying the posterior interosseous branch of the radial nerve, or the onset may be more insidious, without an obvious inciting factor. The pain is constant and made worse with active supination of the wrist. Patients often note the inability to hold a coffee cup or hammer. Sleep disturbance is common. On physical examination, there is tenderness to palpation of the posterior interosseous branch of the radial nerve just below the lateral epicondyle. Elbow range of motion is normal. Grip strength on the affected side may be diminished. Patients with radial tunnel syndrome exhibit pain on active resisted supination of the forearm.

Cervical radiculopathy and tennis elbow can mimic radial tunnel syndrome. Radial tunnel syndrome can be distinguished from tennis elbow in that with radial tunnel syndrome, the maximal tenderness to palpation is distal to the lateral epicondyle over the posterior interosseous branch of the radial nerve, whereas with tennis elbow, the maximal tenderness to palpation is over the lateral epicondyle (Fig. 91-2). Patients with radial tunnel syndrome will exhibit a positive compression test for radial tunnel syndrome.

To perform the compression test for radial tunnel syndrome, the examiner tightly compresses the area over the radial nerve for 30 seconds (Fig. 91-3). The test is

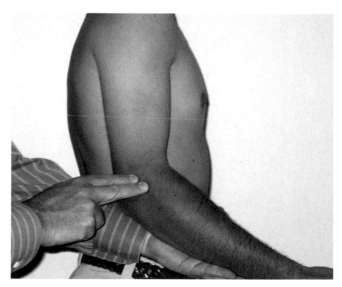

• **Figure 91-2** Palpation of the lateral epicondyle.

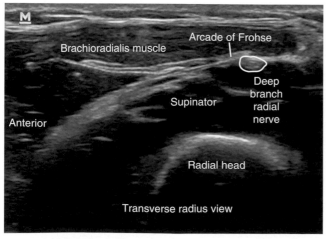

• **Figure 91-1** Transverse ultrasound image demonstrating the relationship of the deep branch of the radial nerve to the arcade of Frohse and the supinator and brachioradialis muscles.

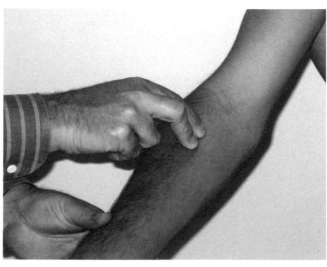

• **Figure 91-3** The compression test for radial tunnel syndrome.

considered positive if the patient complains of pain and paresthesias into the distribution of the radial nerve and increasing weakness of grip strength as the compression of the nerve continues (Video 91-1).

Electromyography helps to distinguish cervical radiculopathy and radial tunnel syndrome from tennis elbow.

Magnetic resonance and/or ultrasound imaging of the elbow and forearm is indicated to confirm the diagnosis and may help elucidate the exact cause of radial nerve compression.

Pronator syndrome is due to median nerve compression by the pronator teres muscle. The onset of symptoms usually occurs after repetitive elbow motions such as chopping wood, sculling, or cleaning fish. It has also been reported in musicians such as harpists and violinists. Clinically, pronator syndrome presents as a chronic aching sensation localized to the forearm with pain occasionally radiating into the elbow. Patients with pronator syndrome may complain about a tired or heavy sensation in the forearm with minimal activity as well as clumsiness of the affected extremity. In contradistinction to carpal tunnel syndrome, nighttime symptoms are uncommon with pronator syndrome.

Physical findings include tenderness over the forearm in the region of the pronator teres muscle. Unilateral hypertrophy of the pronator teres muscle may be identified (Fig. 92-1). A positive Tinel sign over the median nerve as it passes beneath the pronator teres muscle also may be present. Weakness of the intrinsic muscles of the forearm and hand that are innervated by the median nerve may be identified with careful manual muscle testing. A positive pronator syndrome test—pain on forced pronation of the patient's fully supinated arm—is highly suggestive of compression of the median nerve by the pronator teres muscle (Fig. 92-2 and Video 92-1).

Median nerve entrapment by the ligament of Struthers presents clinically as unexplained persistent forearm pain caused by compression of the median nerve by an aberrant ligament that runs from a supracondylar process to the medial epicondyle. Clinically, it is difficult to distinguish from pronator syndrome. The diagnosis is made by electromyography and nerve conduction velocity testing, which demonstrate compression of the median nerve at the elbow, combined with the radiographic and sonographic finding of a supracondylar process.

Both of these entrapment neuropathies can be differentiated from isolated compression of the anterior interosseous nerve, which occurs some 6 to 8 cm below the elbow. These syndromes also should be differentiated from cervical radiculopathy involving the C6 or C7 roots, which may at times mimic median nerve compression. Furthermore, it should be remembered that cervical radiculopathy and median nerve entrapment can coexist as the so-called double crush syndrome. The double crush syndrome is seen most commonly with median nerve entrapment at the wrist or carpal tunnel syndrome.

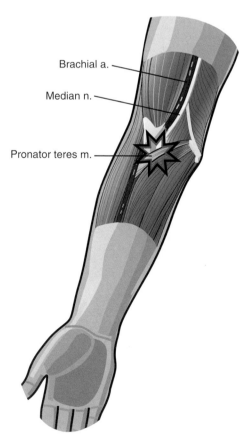

• **Figure 92-1** Pronator syndrome: relevant soft tissue anatomy.

Brachial a.

Median n.

Pronator teres m.

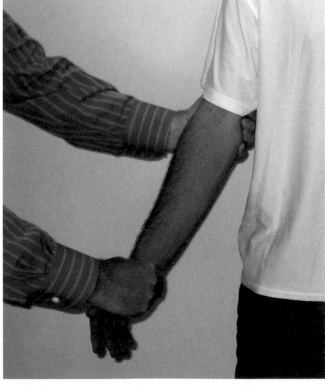

• **Figure 92-2** The forced pronation test for pronator syndrome.

Anterior interosseous syndrome is an uncommon condition that is occasionally encountered by the pain practitioner. Although the condition is uncommon, the characteristic physical findings of anterior interosseous syndrome make it easy to diagnose. The pain and weakness of anterior interosseous syndrome is caused by median nerve compression below the elbow by the tendinous origins of the pronator teres muscle and flexor digitorum superficialis muscle of the long finger or by aberrant blood vessels. The onset of symptoms usually occurs after acute trauma to the forearm or after repetitive forearm and elbow motions such as using an ice pick. An inflammatory cause analogous to Parsonage-Turner syndrome also has been suggested as a cause of anterior interosseous syndrome.

Clinically, anterior interosseous syndrome presents as an acute pain in the proximal forearm. As the syndrome progresses, patients with anterior interosseous syndrome may complain about a tired or heavy sensation in the forearm with minimal activity, as well as the inability to pinch items between the thumb and index fingers because of paralysis of the flexor pollicis longus and the flexor digitorum profundus.

Physical findings include the inability to flex the interphalangeal joint of the thumb and the distal interphalangeal joint of the index finger caused by paralysis of the flexor pollicis longus and the flexor digitorum profundus (Fig. 93-1). Tenderness over the forearm in the region of the pronator teres muscle is seen in some patients who suffer from anterior interosseous syndrome. A positive Tinel sign over the anterior interosseous branch of the median nerve approximately 6 or 8 cm below the elbow also may be present. Patients who suffer from anterior interosseous syndrome will exhibit a positive pinch test. To perform the pinch test for anterior interosseous syndrome, the patient is asked to tightly pinch a key between the thumb and index finger. If compromise of the anterior interosseous nerve is present, the examiner will note flattening of the pinch pattern consistent with weakness of the flexor pollicis longus and flexor digitorum profundus (Fig. 93-2).

The anterior interosseous syndrome also should be differentiated from cervical radiculopathy involving the C6 or C7 roots, which may at times mimic median nerve compression. Furthermore, it should be remembered that cervical radiculopathy and median nerve entrapment can coexist as the so-called double crush syndrome. The double crush syndrome is seen most commonly with median nerve entrapment at the wrist or with carpal tunnel syndrome.

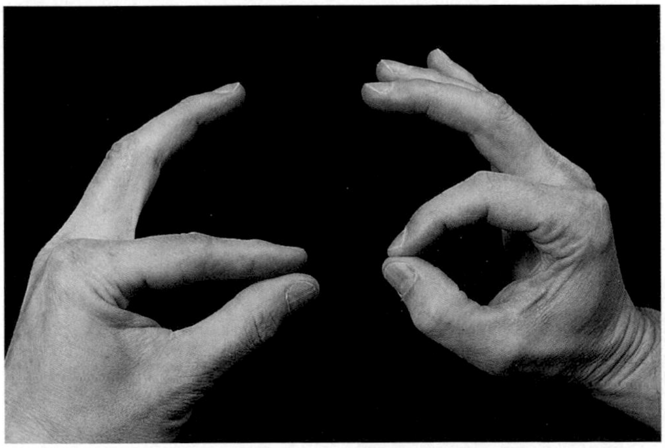

• **Figure 93-1** Anterior interosseous nerve paralysis. The hand on the left demonstrates loss of function of flexor pollicis longus and flexor digitorum profundus muscles, resulting in a characteristic flattened pinch pattern. (From Nashel DJ: Entrapment neuropathies. In Klippel JH, Dieppe PA, editors: *Rheumatology*, ed 2, London, 1998, Mosby, p 164.)

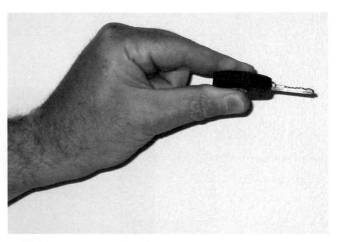

• **Figure 93-2** The pinch test for anterior interosseous syndrome.

Intersection syndrome is an overuse syndrome characterized by pain and swelling at the crossing point of the abductor pollicis longus and extensor pollicis brevis and the extensor carpi radialis longus and extensor carpi radialis brevis (Fig. 94-1). The intersection of these muscle groups is approximately 8 to 10 cm above the radiocarpal joint. The syndrome is commonly precipitated by vigorous use of rowing machines and aggressive weight training. The pain of intersection syndrome can be quite debilitating.

On physical examination, patients suffering from intersection syndrome will have a swollen, diffusely tender area approximately 8 to 10 cm above the radiocarpal joint. These patients will exhibit a positive creaking tendon test caused by tenosynovitis. To perform the creaking tendon test for intersection syndrome, the patient rests his or her arm in the examiner's, and the examiner palpates the point of intersection of the inflamed tendons (Fig. 94-2). The patient is then asked to move his or her thumb and flex and extend the wrist. The test is positive if the examiner appreciates a creaking or crepitant sensation as the inflamed tendons pass over one another.

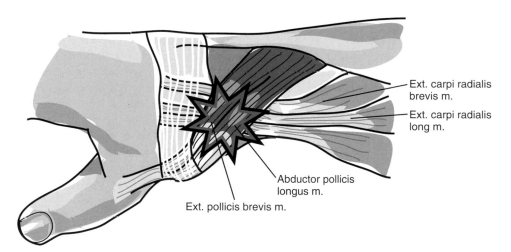

Ext. carpi radialis brevis m.

Ext. carpi radialis long m.

Abductor pollicis longus m.

Ext. pollicis brevis m.

• **Figure 94-1** Intersection syndrome: relevant soft tissue anatomy.

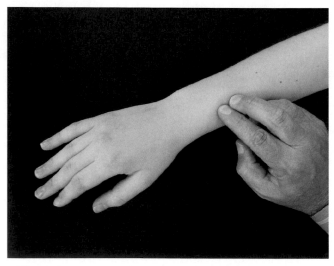

• **Figure 94-2** The creaking tendon test for intersection syndrome.

SECTION 5

The Wrist and Hand

In humans, the wrist functions to transfer the forces and motions of the hand to the forearm and proximal upper extremity. The wrist allows movement in three planes:

- Flexion/extension
- Radial/ulnar deviation
- Pronation/supination

To understand the functional anatomy of the wrist, it is important for the clinician to understand that the wrist is not a single joint, but in fact a complex of five separate joints or compartments that work in concert to allow one to carry out activities of daily living (Fig. 95-1). These five joints are:

- The distal radioulnar joint, which comprises the distal radius and ulna and their interosseous membrane
- The radiocarpal joint, which comprises the distal radius and the proximal surfaces of the scaphoid and lunate bones
- The ulnar carpal joint, which comprises the distal ulna and the triangular fibroelastic cartilage whose function is to connect the distal ulna with the lunate and triquetrum
- The proximal carpal joints, which connect the scaphoid, lunate, and triquetrum via the dorsal, palmar, and interosseous ligaments
- The midcarpal joints, which comprise the capitate, hamate, trapezium, and trapezoid bones

The interaction of the many osseous elements that make up the wrist is made possible by a complex collection of ligamentous structures and a unique structure called the triangular fibroelastic cartilage (TFC). A comprehensive review of the ligaments of the wrist is beyond the scope and purpose of this chapter, but it is helpful for the clinician to understand the basic anatomy. In general, the ligaments can be thought of as being intrinsic to the wrist, that is, having their origin and insertion on the carpal bones, or extrinsic to the wrist, that is, having their origin on the distal radius or ulna and insertion on the carpal bones. All of the ligaments of the wrist have in common a close proximity to the bones of the wrist, which increases their ability to transfer force to the forearm and proximal upper extremity. This lack of interposing muscle or soft tissue also makes the ligamentous structures of the wrist—and the nerves, blood vessels, and bones beneath them—more susceptible to injury.

Located primarily between the distal ulna and the lunate and triquetrum, the TFC is a unique structure that in ways functions in a manner analogous to an intervertebral disc and in ways more like a ligament (Fig. 95-2). The TFC is made up of very strong fibroelastic fibers, and it acts like an intervertebral disc in that it serves as the primary shock absorber of the wrist and acts like a ligament in that it serves as the primary stabilizer for the distal radioulnar joint. The TFC is susceptible to trauma and, because of its poor vascular supply, often heals poorly after injury or surgical interventions, especially on its radial surface.

The musculotendinous units that are responsible for wrist movement find their origins at the elbow and insert on the metacarpals. They can be grouped as flexors, extensors, and deviators. The primary wrist flexors are the flexor

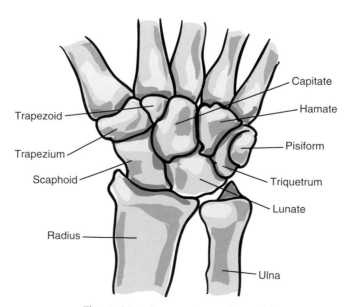

• **Figure 95-1** Bony anatomy of the wrist.

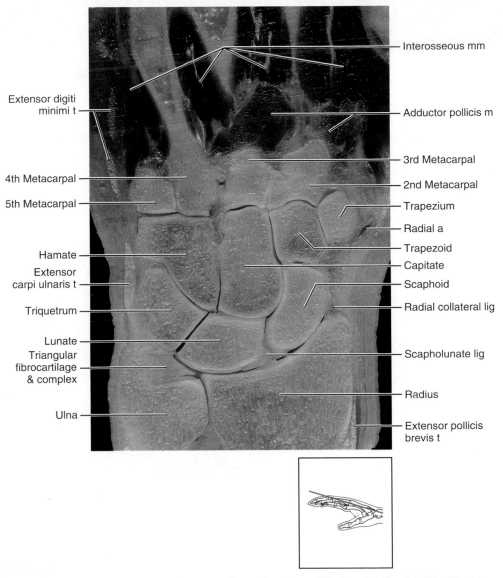

Interosseous mm

Extensor digiti
minimi t

Adductor pollicis m

3rd Metacarpal

4th Metacarpal

2nd Metacarpal

5th Metacarpal

Trapezium

Radial a

Hamate

Trapezoid

Extensor
carpi ulnaris t

Capitate

Scaphoid

Triquetrum

Radial collateral lig

Lunate

Triangular
fibrocartilage
& complex

Scapholunate lig

Radius

Ulna

Extensor pollicis
brevis t

• **Figure 95-2** The triangular fibroelastic cartilage. (From Kang HS, Ahn JM, Resnick D: *MRI of the extremities*, ed 2, Philadelphia, 2002, Saunders, p 163.)

carpi radialis and the flexor carpi ulnaris. The primary wrist extensors are the extensor carpi radialis longus and the extensor carpi radialis brevis. The primary radial deviator is the abductor pollicis longus, and the primary ulnar deviator is the extensor carpi ulnaris. The flexor tendons are held in place by the flexor retinaculum, which extends laterally from the trapezium and scaphoid to the pisiform and hook of the hamate bone. It is estimated that, by preventing bowing of the flexor tendons under load, the flexor retinaculum increases the force of the flexor tendons fivefold.

DORSAL ASPECT

The patient is asked to place the hands with the palms downward, and the examiner inspects the fingers and wrists for any swelling or rubor that might suggest an inflammatory or infectious process (Fig. 96-1). The examiner then looks for ulnar deviation of the fingers and wrists that might suggest rheumatoid arthritis. Degenerative changes, including Heberden and Bouchard nodes of the fingers, are sought out. The presence or absence of any characteristic swelling over the wrists that might suggest ganglion cyst is also noted. Atrophy of the muscles between the metacarpals, which suggests nerve compromise, is also looked for.

PALMAR ASPECT

The patient is then asked to place the palms upward toward the ceiling (Fig. 96-2). The examiner looks for atrophy of the thenar muscles that might be suggestive of a median nerve lesion or atrophy of the hypothenar muscles that might be suggestive of an ulnar lesion. Degenerative changes, especially of the carpometacarpal joint of the thumb, are looked for, as is the classic thickening of the palmar fascia indicative of Dupuytren contracture.

SIDE VIEW

The patient is then asked to position his or her hands with the thumbs pointing toward the ceiling (Fig. 96-3). A careful assessment of the thenar eminence will sometimes lead the examiner to a diagnosis of median nerve entrapment. The position also allows the examiner to assess the carpometacarpal joint of the thumb for degenerative changes.

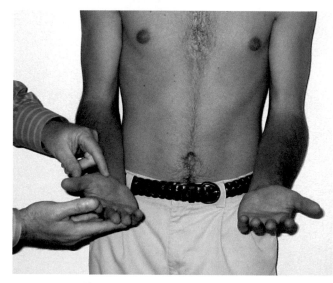

• **Figure 96-2** Palmar view of the hands.

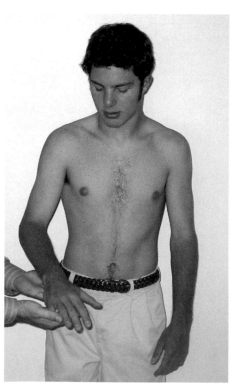

• **Figure 96-1** Dorsal view of the hands.

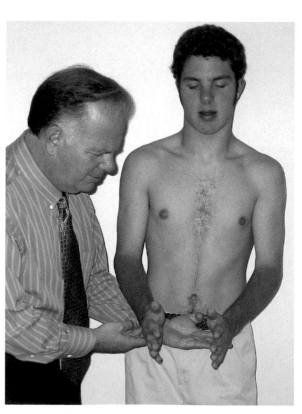

• **Figure 96-3** Side view of the hands.

Palpation of the wrist often leads the examiner to an accurate diagnosis. The patient is asked to relax the wrist and forearm and rest it in the examiner's hands. Because of the dense network of flexor tendons and the flexor retinaculum, subtle pathology of the palmar surface may be missed. Having the patient place the wrist in slight palmar flexion will help. The dorsal surface of the wrist is palpated for synovial thickening, swelling, effusion, and color that might suggest an inflammatory or infectious disease (Fig. 97-1). Crepitus of the wrist may be appreciated when the wrist is passively moved through its range of motion if tenosynovitis is present. Palpation of the dorsal aspect of the wrist for ganglion cyst and the plantar surface of the hand for

Dupuytren contracture is then carried out (Fig. 97-2). Special attention is paid to the carpometacarpal joint of the thumbs, as this is a common site for degenerative arthritis. Attention is then turned to the proximal and distal interphalangeal joints. Each joint is palpated for effusion and synovial swelling and is stressed for instability. Finger tenosynovitis is identified by crepitus, volar swelling, and tendon thickening.

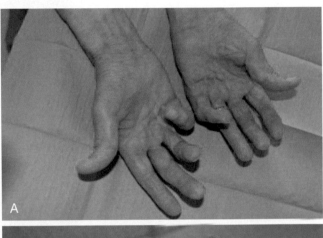

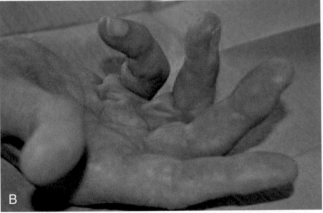

• **Figure 97-2 A** and **B,** Classic findings of Dupuytren contracture. (From Sibaud V, Chevreau C: Abrupt development of Dupuytren's contractures with the BRAF inhibitor vemurafenib, *Joint Bone Spine* 81(4):373–374, 2014.)

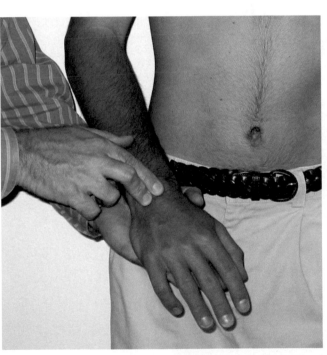

• **Figure 97-1** Palpation of the dorsal surface of the wrist.

To assess wrist extension, the patient is asked to place the arms at the side and flex the elbows to 98 degrees. The patient is then asked to maximally extend or dorsiflex his or her wrists (Fig. 98-1). The normal wrist will extend to approximately 75 degrees. Arthritis, ganglion cysts, or tenosynovitis as well as joint effusions will limit the patient's ability to extend the wrist, as will abnormalities of any of the joints associated with wrist movement (Fig. 98-2) (see Chapter 95).

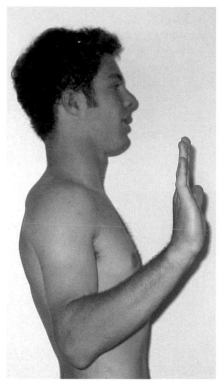

• **Figure 98-1** Lateral view of the extended wrist.

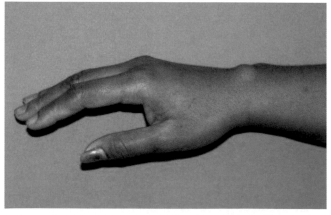

• **Figure 98-2** Dorsal or volar ganglion may limit the ability to extend the wrist. (From Meena S, Gupta A: Dorsal wrist ganglion: current review of literature, *J Clin Orthop Trauma* 5(2):59–64, 2014.)

99 Flexion of the Wrist and Hand

To assess wrist flexion, the patient is asked to place the arms at the side and flex the elbows to 90 degrees. The patient is then asked to maximally flex his or her wrists (Fig. 99-1). The normal wrist will flex to approximately 80 degrees.

Arthritis, ganglion cysts, or tenosynovitis as well as joint effusions will limit the patient's ability to flex the wrist, as will abnormalities of any of the joints associated with wrist movement (Fig. 99-2) (see Chapter 95).

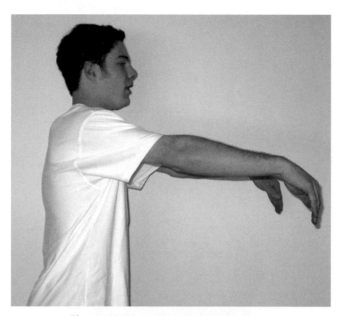

• **Figure 99-1** Lateral view of the flexed wrist.

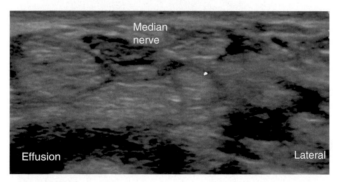

• **Figure 99-2** Transverse ultrasound image demonstrating a significant wrist effusion.

100 Adduction of the Wrist and Hand

When the wrists are fully flexed or extended, little adduction is possible. However, in neutral position, the normal wrist will allow approximately 45 degrees of adduction. To assess wrist adduction, the patient is asked to place his or her arms at the side and flex the elbows to approximately 90 degrees. The patient is then asked to maximally adduct his or her wrists (Fig. 100-1). Arthritis, ganglion cysts, or tenosynovitis as well as joint effusions will limit the patient's ability to adduct the wrist, as will abnormalities of any of the joints associated with wrist movement (see Chapter 95).

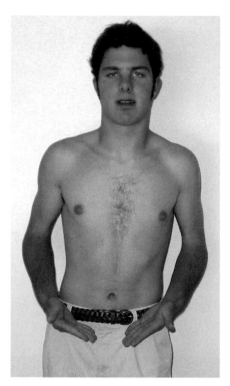

• **Figure 100-1** Lateral view of the adducted wrist.

When the wrists are fully flexed or extended, little abduction is possible. However, in neutral position, the normal wrist will allow approximately 18 degrees of abduction. To assess wrist abduction, the patient is asked to place his or her arms at the sides and flex the elbows to approximately 90 degrees. The patient is then asked to maximally abduct his or her wrists (Fig. 101-1). Arthritis, ganglion cysts, or tenosynovitis as well as joint effusions will limit the patient's ability to abduct the wrist, as will abnormalities of any of the joints associated with wrist movement (Fig. 101-2) (see Chapter 95).

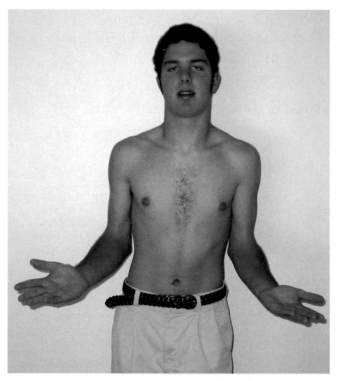

• **Figure 101-1** Lateral view of the abducted wrist.

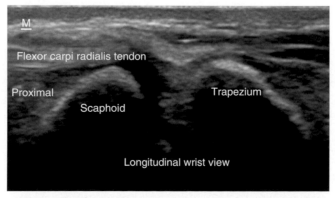

• **Figure 101-2** Longitudinal ultrasound image demonstrating flexor tenosynovitis at the wrist. Note the effusion beneath the tendon.

102 Painful Conditions of the Wrist and Hand

The wrist and hand are susceptible to a variety of painful conditions. More than 90% of them fall into the following categories:
- Carpal tunnel syndrome
- Carpometacarpal arthritis of the thumb
- Ganglion cyst
- Radiocarpal arthritis
- Trigger finger

It is important for the clinician to recognize that pain perceived in the wrist or hand may have its origin in a distant anatomic region or pathologic process, such as Pancoast tumor or pronator syndrome. Pain in the wrist and hand may also be referred, and the clinician should always be aware that angina may present as a dull aching in the wrist and hand. Table 102-1 provides the clinician with an organizational framework on painful conditions of the hand and wrist.

TABLE 102-1 Common Painful Conditions of the Wrist and Hand

Bony Abnormalities	Neurologic Abnormalities
Fracture	Median nerve entrapment
Tumor	Carpal tunnel syndrome
Osteomyelitis	Pronator syndrome
Osteonecrosis	Anterior interosseous nerve syndrome
Kienböck disease and Preiser disease	Ulnar nerve entrapment
Articular Abnormalities	Ulnar tunnel syndrome
Osteoarthritis	Cubital tunnel syndrome
Rheumatoid arthritis	Cheiralgia paresthetica
Collagen Vascular Diseases	Lower brachial plexus lesions
Reiter syndrome	Cervical nerve root lesions
Psoriatic arthritis	Spinal cord lesions
Crystal Deposition Diseases	Syringomyelia
Gout	Spinal cord tumors
Pseudogout	Reflex sympathetic dystrophy
Pigmented villonodular synovitis	Causalgia
Sprain	**Vascular Abnormalities**
Strain	Vasculitis
Hemarthrosis	Raynaud syndrome
Periarticular Abnormalities	Takayasu arteritis
Tendon sheath disorders	Scleroderma
Trigger finger	**Referred Pain**
Flexor tenosynovitis	Shoulder-hand syndrome
Extensor tenosynovitis	Angina
de Quervain tenosynovitis	
Dupuytren contracture	
Ganglion cyst	
Gouty tophi	
Subcutaneous nodules associated with rheumatoid arthritis	
Glomus tumor	

Cheiralgia paresthetica is an uncommon cause of wrist and hand pain and numbness; it is also known as handcuff neuropathy. The onset of symptoms usually occurs after compression of the sensory branch of the radial nerve at the wrist by tight handcuffs, wristwatch bands, or casts (Fig. 103-1). Cheiralgia paresthetica presents as pain and associated paresthesias and numbness of the radial aspect of the dorsum of the hand to the base of the thumb. Because there is significant interpatient variability in the distribution of the sensory branch of the radial nerve caused by overlap of the lateral antebrachial cutaneous nerve, the signs and symptoms of cheiralgia paresthetica may vary from patient to patient, and localization of the nerve by ultrasound imaging may be useful in difficult cases (Fig. 103-2). Direct trauma to the nerve at this level by radial fracture or surgical trauma during de Quervain tenosynovitis surgery can also result in a similar clinical presentation.

Physical findings of cheiralgia paresthetica include tenderness over the radial nerve at the wrist. A positive Tinel sign over the radial nerve at the distal forearm usually is present (Fig. 103-3). Decreased sensation in the distribution of the sensory branch of the radial nerve often is

present, although, as mentioned earlier, the overlap of the lateral antebrachial cutaneous nerve can result in a confusing clinical presentation. Flexion and pronation of the wrist, as well as adduction, often cause paresthesias in the distribution of the sensory branch of the radial nerve

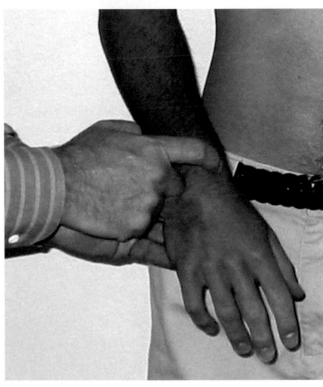

• **Figure 103-2** The positive Tinel sign over the radial nerve in cheiralgia paresthetica.

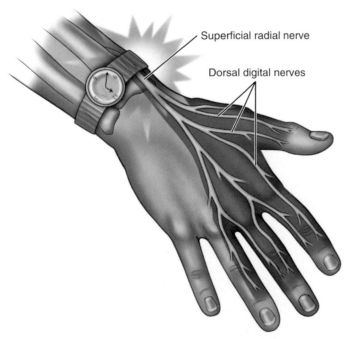

Superficial radial nerve

Dorsal digital nerves

• **Figure 103-1** Cheiralgia paresthetica presents as pain, paresthesia, and numbness of the radial aspect of the dorsum or the hand to the base of the thumb. (From Waldman SD: *Atlas of uncommon pain syndromes*, Philadelphia, 2003, Saunders, p 99.)

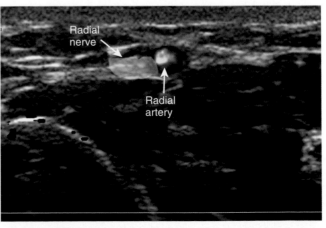

Radial nerve

Radial artery

• **Figure 103-3** Color Doppler image demonstrating the anatomic relationship of the radial artery and nerve at the wrist.

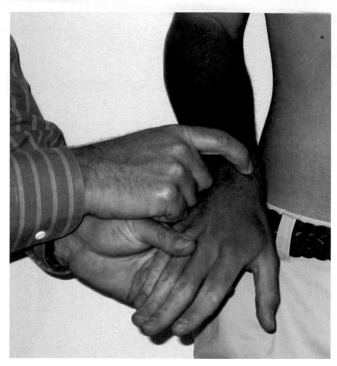

• **Figure 103-4** The wristwatch test for cheiralgia paresthetica.

in patients who suffer from cheiralgia paresthetica. Most patients suffering from cheiralgia paresthetica will also exhibit a positive wristwatch test. To perform the wristwatch test for cheiralgia paresthetica, the examiner has the patient fully pronate the affected extremity. The examiner then exerts firm pressure over the radial nerve at the wrist and then instructs the patient to fully adduct his or her wrist (Fig. 103-4). The wristwatch sign is considered positive if the patient experiences pain, paresthesias, or numbness with this maneuver.

De Quervain tenosynovitis is caused by inflammation and swelling of the tendons of the abductor pollicis longus and extensor pollicis brevis at the level of the radial styloid process. The inflammation and swelling are usually the result of trauma to the tendon from repetitive twisting motions. If the inflammation and swelling become chronic, a thickening of the tendon sheath occurs, with a resulting constriction of the sheath (Figs. 104-1 and 104-2). A triggering phenomenon may result, with the tendon catching within the sheath, causing the thumb to lock or "trigger." Arthritis and gout of the first metacarpal joint also may coexist with and exacerbate the pain and disability of de Quervain tenosynovitis.

De Quervain tenosynovitis occurs in patients who engage in repetitive activities that include hand grasping, such as politicians shaking hands, or high-torque wrist turning, such as scooping ice cream at an ice cream parlor

(Fig. 104-3). De Quervain tenosynovitis also may develop without obvious antecedent trauma in the patient.

The pain of de Quervain tenosynovitis is localized to the region of the radial styloid. It is constant and made worse with active pinching activities of the thumb or ulnar deviation of the wrist. Patients note an inability to hold a coffee cup or turn a screwdriver. Sleep disturbance is common. On physical examination, there are tenderness and swelling over the tendons and tendon sheaths along the distal radius, with point tenderness over the radial styloid (Fig. 104-4). Many patients with de Quervain tenosynovitis exhibit a creaking sensation with flexion and extension of the thumb. Range of motion of the thumb may be decreased because of the pain, and a trigger thumb phenomenon may be noted. Patients with de Quervain tenosynovitis demonstrate a positive Finkelstein test. The Finkelstein test is performed by stabilizing the patient's forearm and having the patient fully

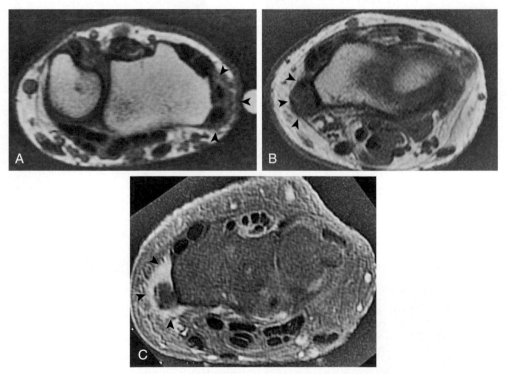

• **Figure 104-1 A,** T1 axial image, wrist. Painful mass over the radial styloid process in this postpartum woman proved to be fibrosis surrounding the extensor pollicis brevis and abductor pollicis longus tendons *(arrowheads),* causing obliteration of the subcutaneous fat that normally surrounds these tendons. **B,** T1 axial image, wrist (different patient than in **A**). The tendons of the first dorsal compartment are not discrete, low-signal structures like other wrist tendons and appear enlarged *(arrowheads).* The subcutaneous fat surrounding the tendons remains normal in this patient. **C,** T1 fat-saturation image, with contrast, axial wrist (different patient than in **A** and **B**). There is increased signal and size of the tendons of the first dorsal compartment and contrast enhancement surrounding the tendons *(arrowheads)* from extensive tenosynovitis. (From Kaplan PA, Helms CA, Dussault R, et al: *Musculoskeletal MRI,* Philadelphia, 2001, Saunders, p 259.)

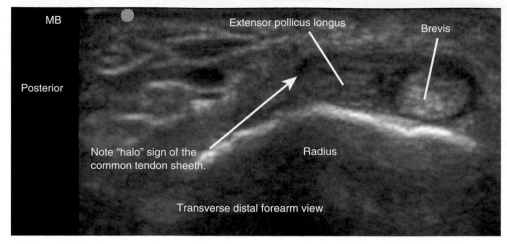

MB

Extensor pollicus longus

Brevis

Posterior

Note "halo" sign of the common tendon sheath.

Radius

Transverse distal forearm view

• **Figure 104-2** Transverse ultrasound image demonstrating de Quervain tenosynovitis. Note the positive halo sign indicating fluid surrounding the inflamed tendons.

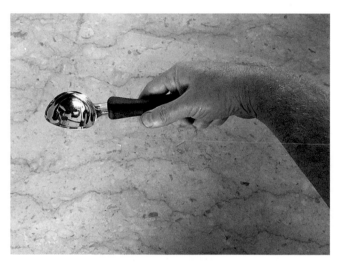

• **Figure 104-3** De Quervain tenosynovitis occurs in patients who engage in repetitive activities that include hand grasping, such as politicians shaking hands, or high-torque wrist turning, such as scooping ice cream at an ice cream parlor.

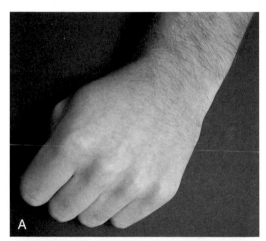

A

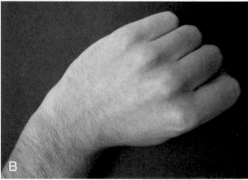

B

• **Figure 104-5 A** and **B,** The Finkelstein test for de Quervain tenosynovitis.

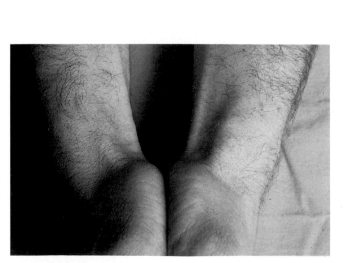

• **Figure 104-4** De Quervain tenosynovitis. (From Fam AG: The wrist and hand. In Klippel JH, Dieppe PA, editors: *Rheumatology,* ed 2, London, 1998, Mosby, pp 4-6.9.)

flex his or her thumb into the palm (Fig. 104-5, *A*). The examiner then actively forces the wrist toward the ulna (Fig. 104-5, *B*). Sudden severe pain is highly suggestive of de Quervain tenosynovitis (Video 104-1).

Entrapment of the lateral antebrachial cutaneous nerve, arthritis of the first metacarpal joint, gout, cheiralgia paresthetica, and, occasionally, C6-C7 radiculopathy can mimic de Quervain tenosynovitis. Cheiralgia paresthetica is an entrapment neuropathy, the result of entrapment of the superficial branch of the radial nerve at the wrist. Electromyography helps to distinguish cervical radiculopathy and cheiralgia paresthetica from de Quervain tenosynovitis.

The Allen test for patency of the radial and ulnar arteries is useful in helping the clinician identify compromise of the superficial and deep palmar arches, which are continuations of the ulnar and radial arteries, respectively. Although trauma to the arteries is the most common cause of compromise of the vasculature of the hand, embolism, thrombosis, aneurysm, and vasculitis are but a few of the other problems that can result in ischemic pain and associated dysfunction of the hand (Fig. 105-1).

To perform the Allen test, the patient is asked to raise his or her hand and to make a fist while the examiner occludes the radial and ulnar arteries at the wrist (Fig. 105-2). The patient is then asked to extend his or her hand, and blanching of the palmar surface should be seen,

indicating occlusion of the radial and ulnar arteries at the wrist by the examiner (Fig. 105-3). The radial artery is then released by the examiner. If the radial artery is patent, the color will immediately return to the patient's hand (Fig. 105-4). If the color does not return to the hand, the Allen test is considered positive for occlusion of the radial artery at the wrist. The test is then repeated, with the examiner this time releasing the ulnar artery first. If the ulnar artery is patent, the color will return to the hand. If the color does not return to the hand, the Allen test is positive for occlusion of the ulnar artery.

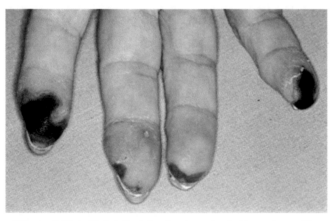

• **Figure 105-1** Digital tip infarction in polyarteritis nodosa. (From Hochberg MC, Silman AJ, Smolen JS, et al, editors: *Rheumatology,* ed 4, vol 2, Philadelphia, 2008, Mosby, p 1515.)

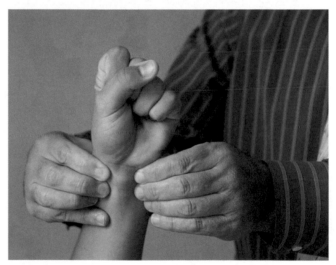

• **Figure 105-2** The Allen test for patency of the radial and ulnar arteries at the wrist: the examiner occludes the radial and ulnar arteries at the wrist.

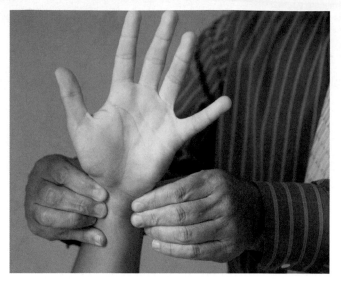

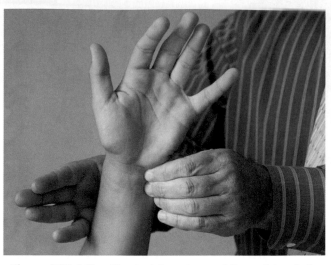

• **Figure 105-3** The Allen test for patency of the radial and ulnar arteries at the wrist: the patient is asked to extend his or her hand, and blanching of the palmar surface should be seen, indicating occlusion of the radial and ulnar arteries at the wrist by the examiner.

• **Figure 105-4** The Allen test for patency of the radial and ulnar arteries at the wrist: if the radial artery is patent, the color will immediately return to the patient's hand.

The carpometacarpal joint of the thumb is susceptible to the development of arthritis from a variety of conditions that have in common the ability to damage the joint cartilage. Osteoarthritis of the joint is the most common form of arthritis that results in pain in the carpometacarpal joint of the thumb (Fig. 106-1). Rheumatoid arthritis, posttraumatic arthritis, and psoriatic arthritis are also common causes of carpometacarpal joint pain secondary to arthritis. Less common causes of arthritis-induced carpometacarpal pain include the collagen vascular diseases, infection, and Lyme disease.

The majority of patients with carpometacarpal pain secondary to osteoarthritis and posttraumatic arthritis pain present with the complaint of pain that is localized to the base of the thumb. Activity, especially with pinching and gripping motions, exacerbates the pain, with rest and heat providing some relief. The pain is constant and is characterized as aching in nature. The pain may interfere with sleep.

Some patients complain of a grating or "popping" sensation with use of the joint, and crepitus may be present on physical examination. The Watson stress test is positive in patients who suffer from inflammation and arthritis of the carpometacarpal joint of the thumb.

The Watson test is performed by having the patient place the dorsum of the hand against a table with the fingers fully extended and then pushing the thumb back toward the table (Fig. 106-2). The test is positive if the patient's pain is reproduced.

In addition to the above-mentioned pain, patients who suffer from arthritis of the carpometacarpal joint often experience a gradual decrease in functional ability, with decreasing pinch and grip strength, thereby making everyday tasks such as using a pencil or opening a jar quite difficult. With continued disuse, muscle wasting may occur, and an adhesive capsulitis with subsequent ankylosis may develop.

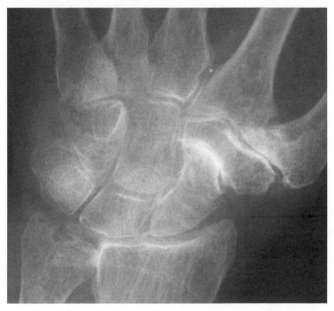

• **Figure 106-1** Plain radiograph demonstrating osteoarthritis of the first carpometacarpal and scaphotrapeziotrapezoid joint in a patient with a positive Watson test. (From Waldman SD, Campbell, RSD: *Imaging of pain,* Philadelphia, 2010, Saunders/Elsevier, p 298, fig 117-1.)

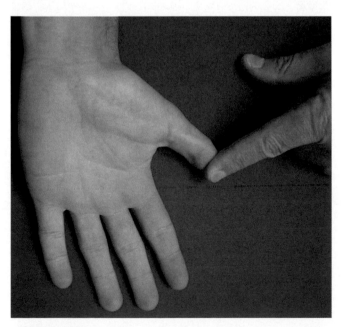

• **Figure 106-2** The Watson stress test for arthritis of the carpometacarpal joint of the thumb.

Ulnar impaction syndrome is an overuse syndrome associated with repetitive activities that have in common the gripping of heavy objects held away from the body. Ulnar impaction syndrome is seen in chefs and candymakers who hold hot, heavy pots or frying pans by the handle away from their bodies. To maximize grip strength, the wrist is forced into a slightly plantar-flexed position with significant ulnar deviation. This results in an excessive load-bearing across the ulnar aspect of the wrist. Over time, chronic impaction of the ulnar head against the triangular fibroelastic cartilage, triquetrum, and lunate results in degenerative changes (Fig. 107-1).

Patients who present with ulnar impaction syndrome will complain of pain across the ulnar aspect of the wrist and an increasing inability to perform the task that caused the syndrome in the first place. On physical examination, the examiner will often identify swelling and diffuse tenderness across the ulnar aspect of the wrist. Decreased grip strength is often present, and the patient's pain is made worse with ulnar loading. Most patients with ulnar impaction syndrome will also exhibit a positive click test with ulnar loading.

To perform the ulnar click test for ulnar impaction syndrome, the examiner has the patient flex the elbow of the affected extremity to 90 degrees and then has the patient maximally clench the fist on the affected side (Fig. 107-2, *A*). The examiner then exerts increasingly heavy loading onto the ulnar aspect of the wrist (Fig. 107-2, *B*). If ulnar impaction syndrome is present, a palpable and occasionally audible click will be appreciated as the ulnar load-bearing components of the wrist fail.

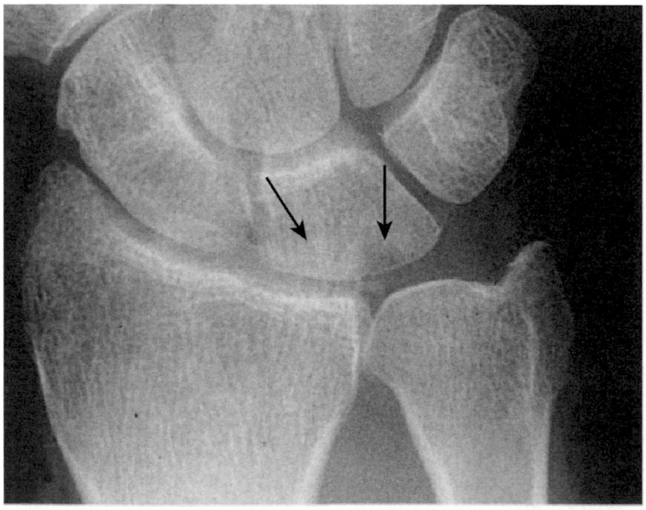

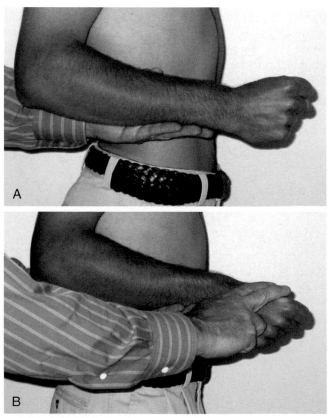

• **Figure 107-1** Plain radiography of the ulnar impaction syndrome. Note cysts and sclerosis *(arrows)* in the lunate bone. (From Resnick D, Kang HS: *Internal derangement of the joints: emphasis on MR imaging*, Philadelphia, 1997, Saunders.)

• **Figure 107-2 A** and **B,** The ulnar click test for ulnar impaction syndrome.

Carpal tunnel syndrome is caused by compression of the median nerve as it passes through the carpal canal at the wrist. The median nerve is made up of fibers from the C5-T1 spinal roots. The nerve lies anterior and superior to the axillary artery in the 12 o'clock to 3 o'clock quadrant. Exiting the axilla, the median nerve descends into the upper arm along with the brachial artery. At the level of the elbow, the brachial artery is just medial to the biceps muscle. At this level, the median nerve lies just medial to the brachial artery. As the median nerve proceeds downward into the forearm, it gives off numerous branches that provide motor innervation to the flexor muscles of the forearm. These branches are susceptible to nerve entrapment by aberrant ligaments, muscle hypertrophy, and direct trauma. The nerve approaches the wrist overlying the radius. It lies deep within and between the tendons of the palmaris longus muscle and the flexor carpi radialis muscle at the wrist.

The median nerve then passes beneath the flexor retinaculum and through the carpal tunnel, with the nerve's terminal branches providing sensory innervation to a portion of the palmar surface of the hand as well as the palmar surface of the thumb, index and middle fingers, and radial portion of the ring finger (Figs. 108-1 and 108-2). The median nerve also provides sensory innervation to the distal dorsal surface of the index and middle fingers and the radial portion of the ring finger (see Fig. 108-2). The carpal tunnel is bounded on three sides by the carpal bones and is covered by the transverse carpal ligament. In addition to the median nerve, it contains a number of flexor tendon sheaths, blood vessels, and lymphatics.

The most common causes of compression of the median nerve at this anatomic location include flexor tenosynovitis, rheumatoid arthritis, pregnancy, amyloidosis, and space-occupying lesions including abnormalities of the median nerve and artery, for example, persistent median artery, that compromise the median nerve as it passes though this closed space (Fig. 108-3). This entrapment neuropathy presents as pain, numbness, paresthesias, and associated weakness in the hand and wrist that radiates to the thumb, index and

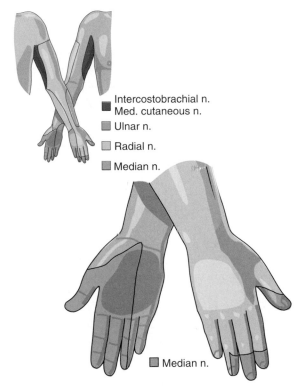

Intercostobrachial n.
Med. cutaneous n.
Ulnar n.
Radial n.
Median n.

Median n.

• **Figure 108-2** The sensory distribution of the median nerve. (From Waldman S: *Atlas of interventional pain management,* ed 4, Philadelphia, 2015, Elsevier, p 267, fig 59-7.)

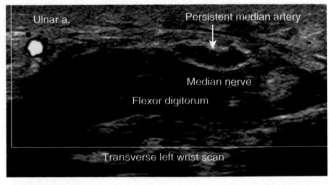

• **Figure 108-3** Transverse ultrasound image demonstrating a persistent median artery compressing the median nerve within the carpal tunnel.

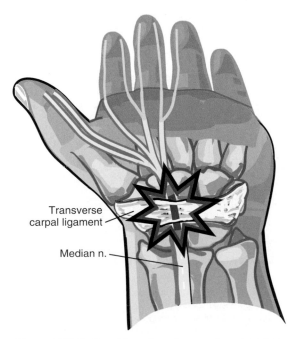

Transverse carpal ligament

Median n.

• **Figure 108-1** Carpal tunnel syndrome: relevant anatomy.

middle fingers, and radial half of the ring finger. These symptoms also may radiate proximal to the entrapment into the forearm. Untreated, progressive motor deficit and ultimately flexion contracture of the affected fingers can result. The onset of symptoms is usually after repetitive wrist motions or from repeated pressure on the wrist, such as resting the wrists on the edge of a computer keyboard. Direct trauma to the median nerve as it enters the carpal tunnel also may result in a similar clinical presentation. The pain of carpal tunnel syndrome is often worse at night, with the patient awakened from a sound sleep to find his or her hand numb and a need to shake the affected hands to get the "circulation going."

Physical findings include tenderness over the median nerve at the wrist. A positive Tinel sign over the median nerve as it passes beneath the flexor retinaculum usually is present (see Chapter 109). A positive Phalen test is also highly suggestive of carpal tunnel syndrome (see Chapter 110). Weakness of thumb opposition and wasting of the thenar eminence often are seen in advanced carpal tunnel syndrome, although because of the complex motion of the thumb, subtle motor deficits easily may be missed (Fig. 108-4; see also Chapters 111 and 112). Early in the course of the evolution of carpal tunnel syndrome, the only physical finding other than tenderness over the nerve may be the loss of sensation in the above-mentioned fingers, which can be most easily identified with the two-point discrimination test (see Chapter 113). Later in the disease, the examiner may appreciate a hotdog-shaped swelling along the ulnar side of the palmaris longus tendon extending proximally from the wrist crease (see Chapter 114).

Carpal tunnel syndrome is often misdiagnosed as arthritis of the carpometacarpal joint of the thumb, cervical radiculopathy, or diabetic polyneuropathy. Patients with arthritis of the carpometacarpal joint of the thumb have a positive Watson test and radiographic evidence of arthritis. Most patients who suffer from a cervical radiculopathy have reflex, motor, and sensory changes associated with neck pain, whereas patients with carpal tunnel syndrome have no

reflex changes, and motor and sensory changes are limited to the distal median nerve. Diabetic polyneuropathy generally presents as symmetric sensory deficit involving the entire hand, rather than limited just to the distribution of the median nerve. Because carpal tunnel syndrome is commonly seen in patients with diabetes, it is not surprising that diabetic polyneuropathy is usually present in diabetic patients with carpal tunnel syndrome.

Electromyography helps distinguish cervical radiculopathy and diabetic polyneuropathy from carpal tunnel syndrome. Plain radiographs are indicated in all patients who present with carpal tunnel syndrome to rule out occult bony pathology. On the basis of the patient's clinical presentation, additional testing might be indicated, including complete blood count, uric acid, sedimentation rate, and antinuclear antibody testing. Magnetic resonance and ultrasound imaging of the wrist might also help identify not only the presence of median nerve entrapment at the wrist but also the anatomic structures that are responsible for the entrapment (Fig. 108-5). Ultrasound imaging with measurement

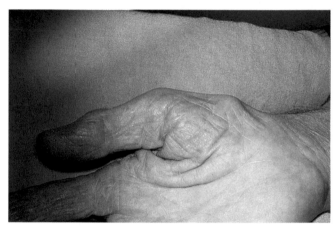

• **Figure 108-4** Thenar muscle atrophy. Chronic entrapment of the median nerve in the carpal tunnel or more proximally can produce thenar atrophy as seen in the patient. (From Nahsel DJ: Soft tissue. In: Klippel JH, Dieppe PA, editors: *Rheumatology,* ed 2, London, 1998, Mosby, pp 4–16.7.)

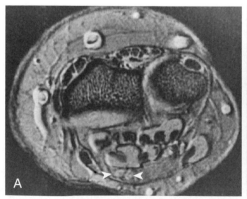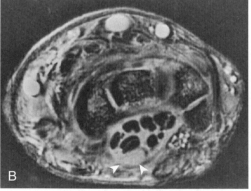

• **Figure 108-5 A,** T2* axial image, wrist at the distal radioulnar joint. The median nerve *(arrowheads)* has a normal size and signal prior to entering the carpal tunnel. **B,** T2* axial magnetic resonance (MR) image, wrist at the pisiform. The median nerve *(arrowheads)* is enlarged and has a high signal. The flexor retinaculum is bowed volarly, and there is increased signal and space between flexor tendons from tenosynovitis. (From Kaplan PA, Helms CA, Dussault R, et al: *Musculoskeletal MRI,* Philadelphia, 2001, Saunders, p 263.)

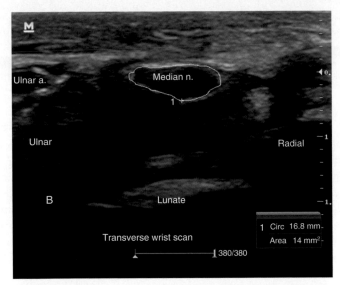

• **Figure 108-6** Transverse ultrasound image demonstrating an enlarged median nerve at the level of the proximal wrist crease with a cross-sectional area 14 mm². Cross-sectional measurement of the median nerve at this level of greater than 11 mm² strongly suggests a diagnosis of carpal tunnel syndrome.

of the cross-sectional area of the median nerve at the level of the proximal wrist crease has been shown to be highly accurate in helping diagnose carpal tunnel syndrome, with nerves with a cross-sectional area greater than 11 mm² highly suggestive of the diagnosis of carpal tunnel syndrome (Fig. 108-6).

Carpal tunnel syndrome also should be differentiated from cervical radiculopathy involving the cervical nerve roots, which at times mimics median nerve compression. Furthermore, it should be remembered that cervical radiculopathy and median nerve entrapment may coexist in the so-called double crush syndrome. The double crush syndrome is seen most commonly with median nerve entrapment at the wrist or carpal tunnel syndrome.

109 The Tinel Sign for Carpal Tunnel Syndrome

There are a number of clinical tests and signs to aid the clinician in the physical diagnosis of carpal tunnel syndrome. Perhaps the most famous is the Tinel sign.

To elicit the Tinel sign for carpal tunnel syndrome, the patient is asked to relax the affected extremity. The patient is then asked to place the palm upward, and the examiner brings the affected hand into a full but not forced dorsiflexed position to compress the carpal tunnel with the overlying flexor retinaculum and flexor tendons (Fig. 109-1). The examiner then percusses the median nerve using the broad side of a neurologic hammer, which is more effective at compressing the entire transverse carpal ligament over the nerve. The Tinel sign is positive if the patient perceives paresthesias that radiate distally into the thumb and index and middle fingers (Video 109-1).

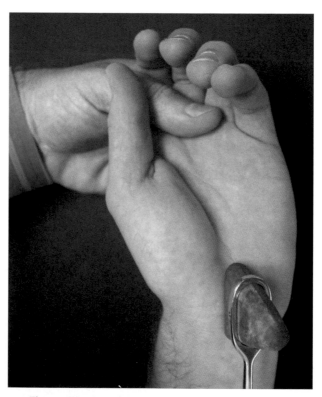

• **Figure 109-1** The Tinel sign for carpal tunnel syndrome.

To perform the Phalen test for carpal tunnel syndrome, the patient is asked to relax both upper extremities with the arms held at the patient's sides. The patient is then asked to allow the wrists to hang downward in a fully, but not forced, palmar-flexed position for a minimum of 30 seconds (Fig. 110-1). The Phalen test is positive for a presumptive diagnosis of carpal tunnel syndrome if the patient's symptoms are reproduced or worsened (Video 110-1).

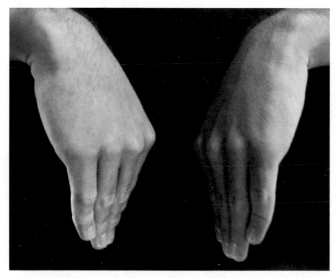

• **Figure 110-1** The Phalen test for carpal tunnel syndrome.

The opponens weakness test, which tests the strength of the adductor pollicis brevis muscle, is another of the many tests that aid in diagnosis of carpal tunnel syndrome.

To perform the opponens weakness test for carpal tunnel syndrome, the patient is asked to relax the affected upper extremity, with the dorsal surface of the affected hand resting comfortably on the examination table. The patient is then asked to adduct the thumb toward the little finger (Fig. 111-1, *A*) and then to abduct the thumb against the examiner's resistance against the distal phalanx (Fig. 111-1, *B*). The opponens weakness test is positive for a presumptive diagnosis of carpal tunnel syndrome if the patient demonstrates weakness of adduction indicating compromise of the adductor pollicis brevis muscle (Video 111-1).

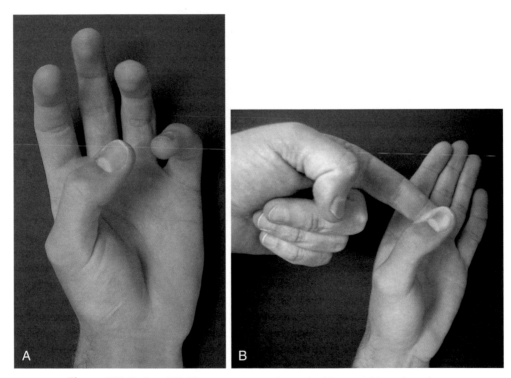

• **Figure 111-1 A** and **B,** The opponens weakness test for carpal tunnel syndrome.

The opponens pinch test evaluates the strength of the adductor pollicis muscle. To perform the opponens pinch test for carpal tunnel syndrome, the patient is asked to relax the affected upper extremity, with the dorsal surface of the affected hand resting comfortably on the examination table. The patient is then asked to pinch the thumb against the little finger. The patient is asked to hold the pinch as tightly as possible. The examiner then tries to break the pinch against the patient's resistance (Fig. 112-1). The opponens pinch test is positive for a presumptive diagnosis of carpal tunnel syndrome if the patient demonstrates an inability to hold the pinch, which indicates compromise of the adductor pollicis muscle (Video 112-1).

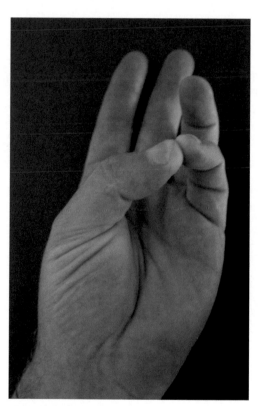

• **Figure 112-1** The opponens pinch test for carpal tunnel syndrome.

Among the number of clinical tests and signs to aid in physical diagnosis is the two-point discrimination test, which tests the sensory fibers of the median nerve. To perform the two-point discrimination test for carpal tunnel syndrome, the patient is asked to relax the affected upper extremity, with the dorsal surface of the affected hand resting comfortably on the examination table. The examiner then uses an electrocardiograph caliper to test the ability of the patient to distinguish whether there are 1 or 2 points touching the tip of the index finger. The points of the calipers are initially placed 1 cm apart and are gradually brought together (Fig. 113-1). The two-point discrimination test is positive for a presumptive diagnosis of carpal tunnel syndrome if the patient demonstrates an inability to distinguish whether the tip of the index finger is being touched by 1 or 2 points as the calipers are brought closer than 0.5 cm together, which indicates compromise of the sensory fibers of the median nerve.

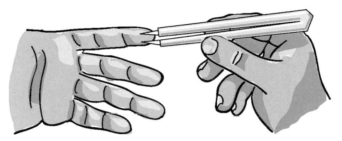

• **Figure 113-1** The two-point discrimination test for carpal tunnel syndrome.

The Dowart hotdog sign is thought to be caused by the bowing out of the flexor retinaculum and flexor tendons because of pressure from an enlarged median nerve (Fig. 114-1).

The Dowart hotdog sign is identified by having the patient relax the affected upper extremity and rest the dorsum of the hand comfortably on the examination table.

The palmaris longus tendon is then identified by asking the patient to flex his or her wrist against resistance. After the tendon is identified, the patient is asked to again relax the affected hand and wrist. The Dowart hotdog sign is considered positive if the examiner observes a hotdog-shaped swelling along the ulnar side of the palmaris longus tendon that extends proximally from the wrist crease (Fig. 114-2).

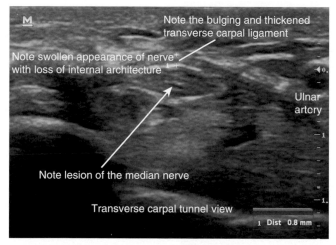

• **Figure 114-1** Transverse ultrasound image demonstrating a bulging and thickened transverse carpal ligament.

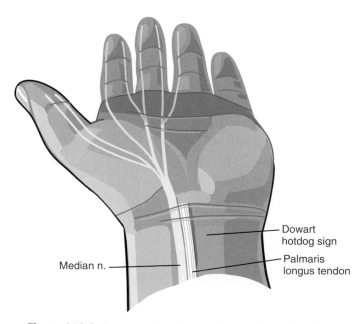

• **Figure 114-2** The Dowart hotdog sign for carpal tunnel syndrome.

Ulnar tunnel syndrome is caused by compression of the ulnar nerve as it passes through Guyon canal at the wrist. The most common causes of compression of the ulnar nerve at this anatomic location are space-occupying lesions, including ganglion cysts and ulnar artery aneurysms; fractures of the distal ulna and carpals; and repetitive motion injuries that compromise the ulnar nerve as it passes though this closed space (Figs. 115-1 and 115-2). This entrapment neuropathy presents most commonly as a pure motor neuropathy without pain, which is caused by compression of the deep palmar branch of the ulnar nerve as it passes through Guyon canal (see Figs. 115-1 and 115-2). This pure motor neuropathy presents as painless paralysis of the intrinsic muscles of the hand.

Ulnar tunnel syndrome may also present as a mixed sensory and motor neuropathy. Clinically this mixed neuropathy presents as pain, numbness, and paresthesias of the wrist that radiate into the ulnar aspect of the palm and dorsum of the hand and the little finger, as well as the ulnar half of the ring finger. These symptoms also may radiate proximal to the nerve entrapment into the forearm. Like carpal tunnel syndrome, the pain of ulnar tunnel syndrome is frequently worse at night and made worse by vigorous flexion and extension of the wrist. If it is left untreated, progressive motor deficit and ultimately flexion contracture of the affected fingers can result. The onset of symptoms is usually after repetitive wrist motions or from direct trauma to the wrist, such as wrist fractures or direct trauma to the proximal hypothenar eminence, which may occur when the hand is used to hammer on hubcaps or from handlebar compression during long-distance cycling (Fig. 115-3).

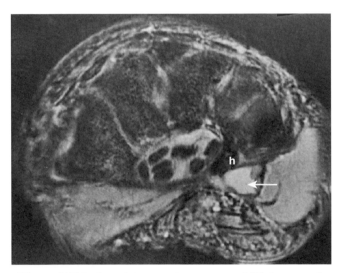

• **Figure 115-1** T2* axial magnetic resonance (MR) image, wrist. There is a ganglion cyst *(arrow)* in the ulnar tunnel adjacent to the hook of the hamate *(h)*, causing a compressive neuropathy of the ulnar nerve. (From Kaplan PA, Helms CA, Dussault R, et al: *Musculoskeletal MRI,* Philadelphia, 2001, Saunders, p 265.)

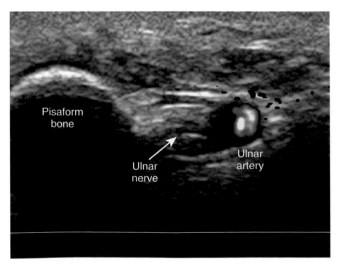

• **Figure 115-2** Transverse color Doppler image demonstrating the anatomic relationship of the ulnar artery and nerve as they pass through Guyon canal.

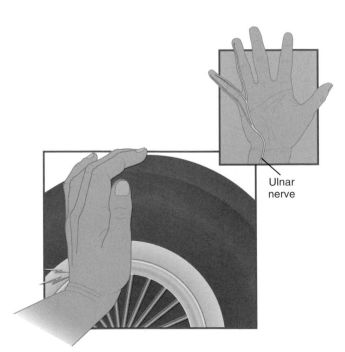

• **Figure 115-3** The onset of ulnar tunnel syndrome is usually after repetitive wrist motions. (From Waldman SD: *Atlas of pain management injection techniques,* Philadelphia, 2000, Saunders, p 151.)

Physical findings include tenderness over the ulnar nerve at the wrist. A positive Tinel sign over the ulnar nerve as it passes beneath the transverse carpal ligament is usually present. If the sensory branches are involved, there is decreased sensation into the ulnar aspect of the hand and the little finger as well as the ulnar half of the ring finger. Depending on the location of neural compromise, the patient might have weakness of the intrinsic muscles of the hand, as evidenced by the inability to spread the fingers, or weakness of the hypothenar eminence. This weakness of the intrinsic hand muscles is called a positive spread sign.

To perform the spread sign, the patient is asked to relax the affected extremity and comfortably rest the wrist on the examination table. The patient is then asked to spread his or her fingers apart as far as possible. A positive spread sign is observed if the patient is unable to spread 2 or more fingers apart (Fig. 115-4). The examiner should be aware that the little finger is often spared while at the same time the patient is unable to spread apart the other fingers because the compromise is limited to the deep palmar branch of the ulnar nerve (Video 115-1).

Ulnar tunnel syndrome is often misdiagnosed as arthritis of the carpometacarpal joints, cervical radiculopathy, or diabetic polyneuropathy. Patients with arthritis of the carpometacarpal joint usually have radiographic evidence and physical findings that might be suggestive of arthritis. Most patients who suffer from a cervical radiculopathy have reflex, motor, and sensory changes associated with neck pain, whereas patients with ulnar tunnel syndrome have no reflex changes, and motor and sensory changes are limited to the distal ulnar nerve. Diabetic polyneuropathy generally presents as symmetric sensory deficit involving the entire hand, rather than being limited just to the distribution of the ulnar nerve. It should be remembered that cervical radiculopathy and ulnar nerve entrapment may coexist as the so-called double crush syndrome. Furthermore, because ulnar tunnel syndrome is commonly seen in patients with diabetes, it is not surprising that diabetic polyneuropathy is usually present in diabetic patients with ulnar tunnel syndrome. Pancoast tumor invading the medial cord of the brachial plexus also may mimic an isolated ulnar nerve

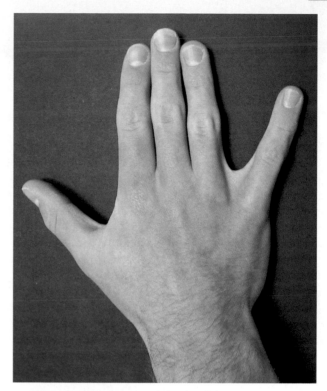

• **Figure 115-4** The spread sign for ulnar tunnel syndrome.

entrapment and should be ruled out by apical lordotic chest radiograph.

Electromyography helps distinguish cervical radiculopathy, diabetic polyneuropathy, and Pancoast tumor from ulnar tunnel syndrome. Plain radiographs are indicated in all patients who present with ulnar tunnel syndrome to rule out occult bony pathology. On the basis of the patient's clinical presentation, additional testing including complete blood count, uric acid, sedimentation rate, and antinuclear antibody testing might be indicated. Magnetic resonance and ultrasound imaging of the wrist is indicated if joint instability or a space-occupying lesion is suspected and to help confirm the diagnosis.

The dorsal and volar aspect of the wrist is especially susceptible to the development of ganglion cysts. These cysts are thought to form as the result of herniation of synovial fluid–containing tissues from joint capsules or tendon sheaths. This tissue may then become irritated and begin to produce increased amounts of synovial fluid, which can pool in cystlike cavities overlying the tendons and joint space. A one-way valve phenomenon may cause these cystlike cavities to expand, because the fluid cannot flow freely back into the synovial cavity.

Activity, especially extreme flexion and extension, makes the pain worse, with rest and heat providing some relief. The pain is constant and is characterized as aching in nature. It is often the unsightly nature of the ganglion cyst, rather than the pain, that causes the patient to seek medical attention (Fig. 116-1). The ganglion is smooth to palpation and transilluminates with a penlight, in contradistinction to solid tumors, which do not transilluminate. Palpation of the ganglion may increase the pain. Patients with ganglion cysts of the dorsal and volar aspect of the wrist will exhibit a positive extreme flexion/extension test.

To perform the extreme flexion/extension test for ganglion cyst of the wrist, the examiner first localizes the ganglion cyst to the dorsal or volar aspect of the wrist (Fig. 116-2). If the ganglion is on the dorsal aspect, the examiner forcefully flexes the patient's affected wrist. If the ganglion cyst is located on the volar aspect of the wrist, the examiner forcefully extends the patient's affected wrist. The extreme flexion/extension test is positive if the forceful flexion or extension of the wrist causes a marked increase in the patient's pain.

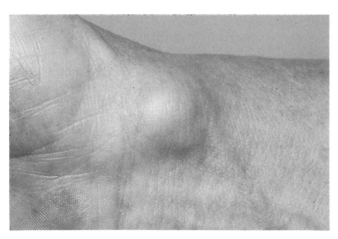

• **Figure 116-1** A ganglion on the volar aspect of the wrist. (From Fam AG: The wrist and hand. In Klippel JH, Dieppe PA, editors: *Rheumatology*, ed 2, London, 1998, Mosby, pp 4-9.3.)

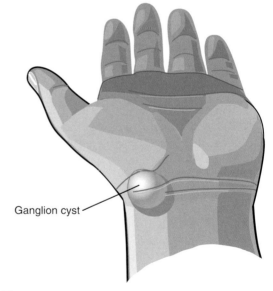

Ganglion cyst

• **Figure 116-2** Localization of the ganglion cyst of the wrist.

Carpal boss, which is also known as os styloideum, is the term used to described a painful exostosis that arises along the dorsal surface of the second or third carpometacarpal joints. The carpal boss is thought to be the result of repetitive microtrauma or fusion of an accessory ossicle that results in this development of bony exostosis. The patient with carpal boss presents with aching across the dorsal surface of the wrist in the area of the second and third carpometacarpal joints that is made worse with strenuous activity that requires repetitive finger or wrist extension. This bony excrescence is often mistaken for a dorsal ganglion cyst (Fig. 117-1). Palpation of this area reveals point tenderness, and the examiner may appreciate a dorsal bony prominence known as the hunchback carpal sign (Fig. 117-2). Extreme flexion will often make identification easier (Fig. 117-3). Plain radiographs or magnetic resonance and/or ultrasound imaging will confirm the clinical diagnosis of carpal boss and guide treatment, which consists of local injections of corticosteroid and surgical removal (Fig. 117-4).

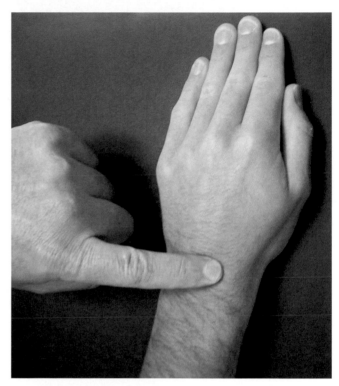

• **Figure 117-2** The hunchback carpal sign for carpal boss.

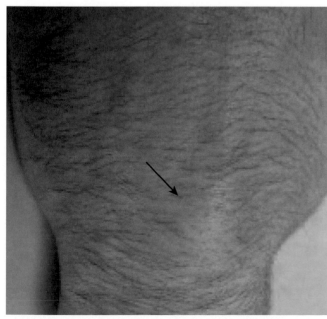

• **Figure 117-1** Appearance of a carpal boss *(arrow)*. (From Park MJ, Namdari S, Weiss A-P: The carpal boss: review of diagnosis and treatment. *J Hand Surg* 33(3):446–449, 2008, fig 1.)

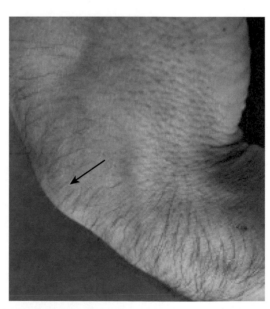

• **Figure 117-3** Extreme flexion of the wrist may simplify the identification of a carpal boss *(arrow)*. (From Park MJ, Namdari S, Weiss A-P: The carpal boss: review of diagnosis and treatment. *J Hand Surg* 33(3):446–449, 2008, fig 2.)

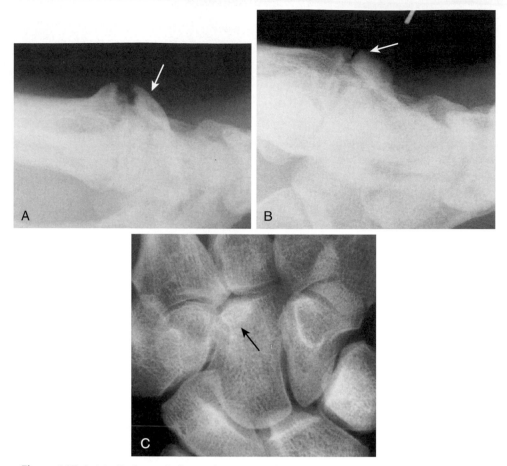

• **Figure 117-4 A** to **C,** *Arrows* indicate a bony exostosis consistent with a carpal boss. (From Resnick D: *Diagnosis of bone and joint disorders,* Philadelphia, 2002, Saunders, p 1312.)

The extensor tendons of the wrist pass beneath the extensor retinaculum via six tendon sheaths. These tendon sheaths are susceptible to inflammation and scarring, which can cause pain and functional disability. As this process becomes chronic, a thickening of the extensor tendon sheaths results in an ovoid swelling on the dorsum of the hand. On physical examination, this swollen area is warm and tender. On palpation, the examiner may appreciate a creaking sensation as the fingers move through the inflamed and narrowed tendon sheaths. In addition, many patients with active extensor tenosynovitis of the wrist will exhibit a positive tuck sign. To elicit a tuck sign, the examiner has the patient lightly clench his or her fist for 30 seconds. The examiner observes the dorsum of the clenched fist for swelling that is consistent with extensor tenosynovitis (Fig. 118-1). If it is present, the examiner has the patient gradually fully extend the fingers of the clenched fist. The tuck sign for extensor tenosynovitis of the wrist is considered positive if as the patient extends his or her hand, the area of swelling moves proximally and folds under the flexor retinaculum like a sheet being tucked under a mattress (Fig. 118-2).

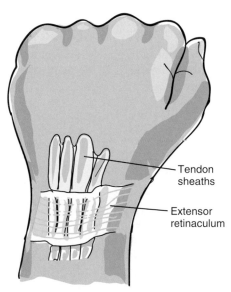

• **Figure 118-1** The examiner should observe the dorsum of the clenched fist for swelling consistent with extensor tenosynovitis.

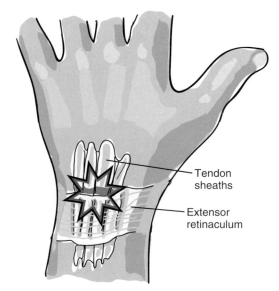

• **Figure 118-2** The tuck sign for extensor tenosynovitis of the wrist.

119 The Palmar Band Sign for Dupuytren Contracture

Dupuytren contracture is caused by a progressive fibrosis of the palmar fascia. Initially, the patient might notice fibrotic nodules that are tender to palpation along the course of the flexor tendons of the hand. These nodules arise from the palmar fascia and initially do not involve the flexor tendons (Fig. 119-1). As the disease advances, these fibrous nodules coalesce and form fibrous bands that gradually thicken and contract around the flexor tendons, a process that has the effect of drawing the affected fingers into flexion. Although all fingers can develop Dupuytren contracture, the ring and little fingers are most commonly affected. If untreated, the fingers will develop permanent flexion contractures. The pain of Dupuytren contracture seems to burn itself out as the disease progresses.

Dupuytren contracture is thought to have a genetic basis and occurs most frequently in males of northern Scandinavian descent. The disease also may be associated with trauma to the palm, diabetes, alcoholism, and chronic barbiturate use. The disease rarely occurs before the fourth decade. The plantar fascia also may be concurrently affected.

In the early stages of the disease, hard, fibrotic nodules may be palpated along the path of the flexor tendons. These nodules often are misdiagnosed as calluses or warts. At this early stage, pain is invariably present. As the disease progresses, the clinician notes taut, fibrous bands that may cross the metacarpophalangeal joint and ultimately the proximal interphalangeal joint, which constitutes a positive palmar band sign that is pathognomonic for Dupuytren contracture (Fig. 119-2). As the disease progresses, these bands become less painful to palpation, and although they limit finger extension, finger flexion remains relatively normal. It is at this point that patients often seek medical advice, as they begin having difficulty putting on gloves and reaching into their pockets to retrieve keys. In the final stages of the disease, the flexion contracture develops with its attendant negative impact on function. Arthritis and gout involving the metacarpal and interphalangeal joints and trigger finger may coexist with and exacerbate the pain and disability of Dupuytren contracture.

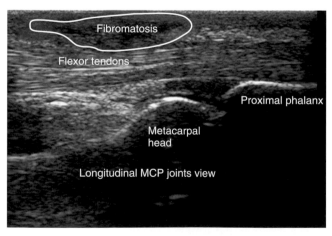

• **Figure 119-1** Longitudinal ultrasound image demonstrating the classic palmar fibrosis associated with Dupuytren contracture. Note that there is no involvement of the flexor tendon. *MCP,* Metacarpophalangeal.

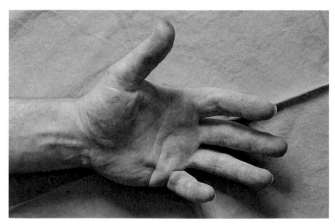

• **Figure 119-2** Dupuytren contracture of the palmar fascia. (From Fam AG: The wrist and hand. In Klippel JH, Dieppe PA, editors: *Rheumatology,* ed 2, London, 1998, Mosby, p 4-9.7.)

The Allen test for patency of the digital arteries is useful in helping the clinician identify compromise of the digital arteries. Although trauma to the arteries is the most common cause of compromise of the vasculature of the fingers, embolism, thrombosis, aneurysm, and vasculitis are but a few of the other problems that can result in ischemic pain and associated dysfunction of the fingers (see Fig. 105-1).

To perform the Allen test, the patient is asked to raise his or her hand and to tightly flex the affected digit while the examiner occludes the digital arteries on each side of the digit (Fig. 120-1). The patient is then asked to extend the affected finger, and blanching of the finger should be seen, indicating occlusion of digital arteries by the examiner (Fig. 120-2). The digital artery on the radial side of the finger is then released by the examiner. If the artery is patent, the color will immediately return to the patient's finger (Fig. 120-3). If the color does not return to the finger, the Allen test is considered positive for occlusion of the digital artery on the radial side of the finger. The test is then repeated, with the examiner this time releasing the artery on the ulnar side of the artery first. If that digital artery is patent, the color will return to the finger. If the color does not return to the finger, the Allen test is positive for occlusion of the digital artery on the ulnar side of the affected finger.

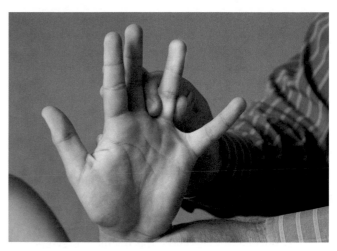

• **Figure 120-2** The Allen test for patency of the digital arteries of the fingers: the patient is asked to extend the affected finger; blanching of the finger should be seen, indicating occlusion of digital arteries by the examiner.

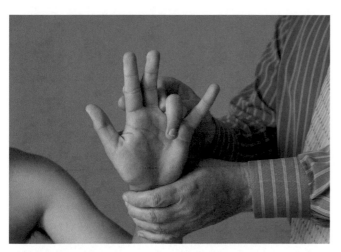

• **Figure 120-1** The Allen test for patency of the digital arteries of the fingers: the patient is asked to raise his or her hand and to tightly flex the affected digit while the examiner occludes the digital arteries on each side of the digit.

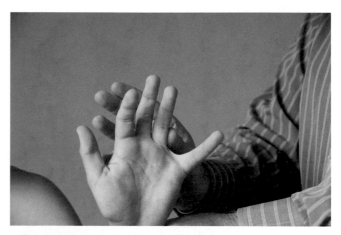

• **Figure 120-3** The Allen test for patency of the digital arteries of the fingers: the digital artery on the radial side of the finger is released by the examiner. If the artery is patent, the color will immediately return to the patient's finger. If the color does not return to the finger, the Allen test is considered positive for occlusion of the digital artery on the radial side of the finger.

121 The Catching Tendon Sign for Trigger Finger Syndrome

Trigger finger is caused by inflammation and swelling of the tendons of the flexor digitorum superficialis muscle caused by compression and irritation of the tendons by the heads of the metacarpal bones (Fig. 121-1). Sesamoid bones in this region also may cause compression and trauma to the tendons. The inflammation and swelling of the tendon are usually the result of trauma to the tendon from repetitive motion or pressure overlying the tendon as it passes over these bony prominences. If the inflammation and swelling become chronic, a thickening of the tendon sheath occurs, with a resulting constriction of the sheath. Frequently, a nodule develops on the tendon due to chronic pressure and irritation. These nodules often can be palpated when the patient flexes and extends the fingers. Such nodules may catch in the tendon sheath as the nodule passes under a restraining tendon pulley and cause a triggering phenomenon, causing the finger to catch or lock as the nodule catches on the pulley (Fig. 121-2).

Coexistent arthritis and gout of the metacarpal and interphalangeal joints may also exacerbate the pain and disability of trigger finger. Trigger finger occurs in patients who engage in repetitive activities that include hand clenching, such as gripping a steering wheel or holding a horse's reins too tightly.

The pain of trigger finger is localized to the distal palm, with tender tendon nodules often palpated. The pain of trigger finger is constant and is made worse with active gripping activities of the hand. Patients note significant stiffness when flexing the fingers. Sleep disturbance is common, and the patient often awakens to find that the finger has become locked in a flexed position during sleep. On physical examination, there are tenderness and swelling over the tendon with maximal point tenderness over the heads of the metacarpals. Many patients with trigger finger exhibit a "creaking" sensation with flexion and extension of the fingers. Range of motion of the fingers may be decreased because of the pain, and a trigger finger phenomenon may be noted. Patients with trigger finger often have palpable nodules on the tendons of the flexor digitorum superficialis muscle as well as a positive catching tendon sign on passive extension of the tendon.

To identify the catching tendon sign for trigger finger, the examiner has the patient hold his or her fist in a tightly clenched position for 30 seconds. The examiner then instructs the patient to relax but not open his or her fist. The examiner then passively extends the affected finger. The catching tendon sign is positive if the examiner appreciates a locking, popping, or catching of the tendon as the finger is straightened (Fig. 121-3 and Video 121-1).

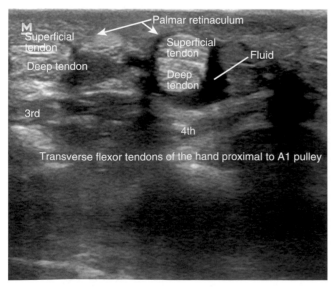

• **Figure 121-1** Transverse ultrasound image demonstrating inflammation of the flexor tendon sheaths in a patient with triggering of the ring finger. Note the effusion surrounding the tendon of the ring finger.

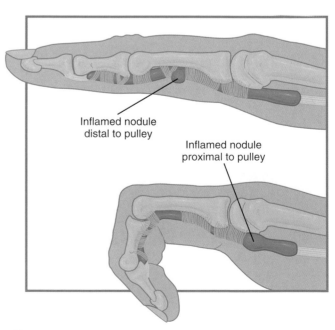

• **Figure 121-2** Inflamed nodules on the tendon distal and proximal to the pulley. (From Waldman SD: *Atlas of pain management injection techniques,* Philadelphia, 2000, Saunders, p 135.)

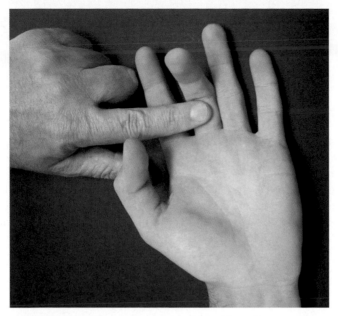

• **Figure 121-3** The catching tendon sign for trigger finger syndrome.

122 The Sausage Finger Sign for Psoriatic Arthritis

Physical examination of the joints of the fingers can provide important diagnostic information if the clinician understands the patterns of joint disease and their relationship to specific pathologic processes. Inflammation, pain, or swelling of a single joint of the hand points to an infectious or localized process, such as septic joint, gouty arthritis, and foreign body arthritis, as opposed to a more symmetric pattern of inflammation, pain, or swelling, which is more indicative of a systemic arthritis, such as rheumatoid arthritis, psoriatic arthritis, or the collagen vascular diseases.

When the inflammatory process extends beyond the joint proper and involves the surrounding structures, including tendons and ligaments, it is called an enthesopathy. If this inflammatory process involves a digit and progresses unchecked, inflammation of the entire digit can result. This generalized inflammation and swelling are called dactylitis. Dactylitis occurs commonly in patients who suffer from psoriatic arthritis, resulting in a classic appearing digit called a sausage finger (Fig. 122-1). A positive sausage finger sign is considered pathognomonic for psoriatic arthritis.

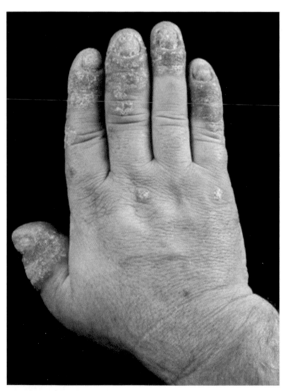

• **Figure 122-1** Sausage fingers in psoriatic arthropathy; note dorsal and volar aspects of dactylitis at the third finger. (From Hubscher O: Pattern recognition. In Klippel JH, Dieppe PA editors: *Rheumatology*, ed 2, London, 1998, Mosby, p 2-3.4.)

The swan neck deformity consists of hyperextension of the proximal interphalangeal joint, flexion of the distal interphalangeal joint, and sometimes flexion of the meta-carpophalangeal joint (Fig. 123-1). It is most commonly associated with rheumatoid arthritis that has been inade-quately treated (Fig. 123-2). Other causes of swan neck deformity include rupture of the flexor tendon of the proximal interphalangeal (PIP) joint, untreated mallet finger, laxity of the ligaments of the volar aspect of the PIP joint, spasticity of intrinsic hand muscles, and malunion of a fracture of the middle or proximal phalanx. Swan neck deformity results in the inability to compensate for hyper-extension of the proximal interphalangeal joint; it makes finger closure impossible and can cause severe disability.

Normal joint

Swan neck deformity

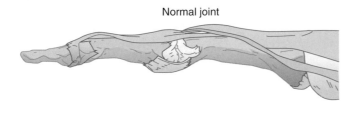

• **Figure 123-1** The swan neck deformity consists of hyperextension of the proximal interphalangeal joint, flexion of the distal interphalangeal joint, and sometimes flexion of the metacarpophalangeal joint.

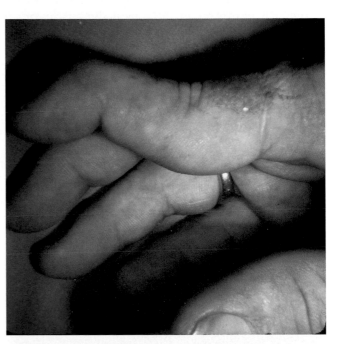

• **Figure 123-2** Fixed rheumatoid swan neck deformity, with proximal interphalangeal joint hyperextension and distal interphalangeal joint flexion. (From Canale ST, Beaty J, editors: *Campbell's operative ortho-paedics,* ed 11, vol 4, Philadelphia, 2007, Mosby, p 4204.)

Commonly associated with rheumatoid arthritis, the boutonnière deformity consists of flexion of the proximal interphalangeal joint accompanied by hyperextension of the distal interphalangeal joint (Fig. 124-1). Other causes of the boutonnière deformity include extensor tendon lacerations, fractures of the phalanges, dislocations, and severe osteoarthritis. What these pathologic processes have in common is disruption of the central slip attachment of the extensor tendon to the base of the middle phalanx, allowing the proximal phalanx to protrude between the lateral bands of the extensor tendon in a manner analogous to a button passing through a buttonhole. Frequently, other deformities such as the swan neck deformity can be seen in conjunction with the boutonnière deformity (Fig. 124-2) (see Chapter 123).

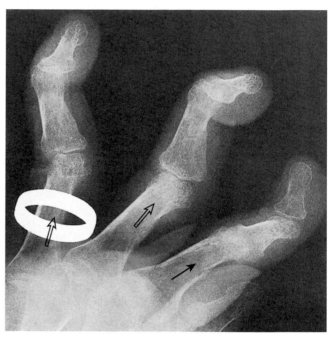

• **Figure 124-2** Boutonnière and swan neck deformities of the digits. A typical swan neck deformity of the third and fourth digits *(open arrows)* and boutonnière deformity of the second digit *(closed arrow)* are evident in this patient with rheumatoid arthritis. (From Resnick D, Kransdorf MJ, editors: *Bone and joint imaging*, ed 3, Philadelphia, 2005, Saunders, p 230.)

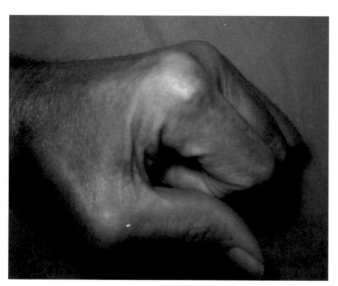

• **Figure 124-1** Thumb with fixed rheumatoid boutonnière deformity (type 1). Note tight metacarpophalangeal flexion and interphalangeal hyperextension. (From Canale ST, Beaty J, editors: *Campbell's operative orthopaedics*, vol 4, ed 11, Philadelphia, 2007, Mosby, p 4197.)

125 The Heberden Node Sign for Osteoarthritis of the Distal Interphalangeal Joints

Although William Heberden is most famous for his classic description of angina pectoris, he is also credited with the first description of the classic finger deformity associated with osteoarthritis that bears his name. The Heberden node is the name given to the deformity of a distal interphalangeal joint when it is damaged by osteoarthritis (Fig. 125-1). The exact cause of this deformity is not known, but there are several known risk factors, including overuse of the joints, especially by excessive precision gripping; being of female gender; previous trauma to the distal interphalangeal joints; and having a genetic predisposition. A positive Heberden node sign is pathognomonic for osteoarthritis of the distal interphalangeal joint.

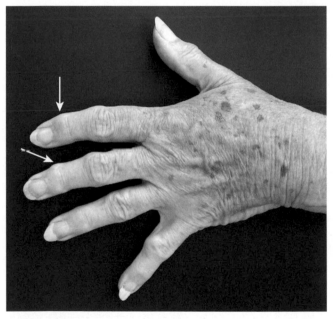

• **Figure 125-1** The Heberden node sign *(arrows)* for osteoarthritis of the distal interphalangeal joints.

The nineteenth-century French physician Charles Jacques Bouchard is credited with the first description of the classic finger deformity associated with osteoarthritis that bears his name. The Bouchard node is the name given to the deformity of a proximal interphalangeal joint when it is damaged by osteoarthritis (Fig. 126-1). Although the exact cause of this deformity is not known, there are several risk factors, including overuse of the joints, especially by excessive precision gripping; being of the female gender; previous trauma to the proximal interphalangeal joints; and having a genetic predisposition. A positive Bouchard node sign is pathognomonic for osteoarthritis of the proximal interphalangeal joint.

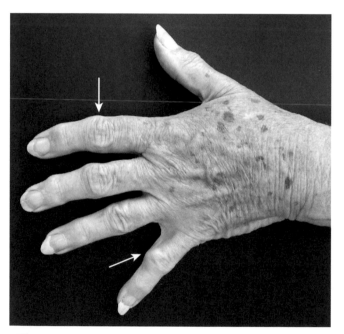

• **Figure 126-1** The Bouchard node sign *(arrows)* for osteoarthritis of the proximal interphalangeal joints.

127 The Ice Water Test for Glomus Tumor of the Finger

Glomus tumor of the hand is an uncommon cause of distal finger pain. It is the result of tumor formation of the glomus body, which is a neuromyoarterial apparatus whose function is to regulate peripheral blood flow in the digits. The majority of patients who suffer from glomus tumor are females between the ages of 30 and 50 years. The pain is very severe and is lancinating and boring in nature. The tumor frequently involves the nail bed and may invade the distal phalanx. Patients suffering from glomus tumor of the hand will exhibit the classic triad of excruciating distal finger pain, cold intolerance, and tenderness to palpation of the affected digit. Multiple glomus tumors are present in approximately 25% of patients who are diagnosed with this disease. Glomus tumors can also occur in the foot and occasionally in other parts of the body.

The diagnosis of glomus tumor of the hand is based primarily on 3 points in the patient's clinical history: (1) excruciating pain that is localized to a distal digit, (2) the ability to trigger the pain by palpating the area, and (3) marked intolerance to cold. Patients who suffer from glomus tumor of the digit will exhibit a positive ice water test. The pain of glomus tumor can be reproduced by placing the affected digit in a glass of ice water. If glomus tumor is present, the characteristic lancinating, boring pain will occur within 30 to 60 seconds, constituting a positive ice water test. Placing other unaffected fingers of the same hand in ice water will not trigger the pain in the affected finger. Nail bed ridging is present in many patients with glomus tumor of the hand, and a small blue or dark red spot at the base of the nail is visible in 10% to 15% of patients suffering from the disease (Fig. 127-1). The patient with glomus tumor of the hand will frequently wear a finger protector on the affected digit and will guard against hitting the digit on anything to avoid triggering the pain.

Magnetic resonance image scanning of the affected digit will often reveal the actual glomus tumor and may also reveal erosion or a perforating lesion of the phalanx beneath the tumor. The tumor will appear as a very high and homogeneous signal on T2-weighted images (Fig. 127-2). Ultrasound and color Doppler imaging may also reveal the size and exact localization of the tumor (Fig. 127-3). The bony changes associated with glomus tumor of the hand may also appear on plain radiographs if a careful comparison of the corresponding contralateral digit is made. Radionuclide bone scan may also reveal localized bony destruction.

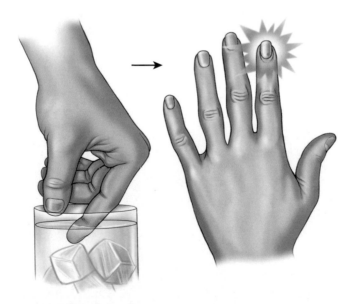

• **Figure 127-1** Glomus tumor is characterized by (1) excruciating distal digit pain, (2) ability to trigger the pain by palpation, and (3) marked intolerance to cold. It is easily diagnosed by the ice water test. (From Waldman SD: *Atlas of uncommon pain syndromes,* Philadelphia, 2003, Saunders, p 108.)

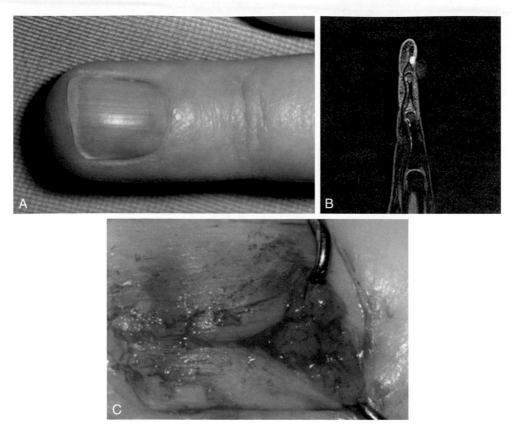

• **Figure 127-2** Glomus tumor of the finger. **A,** Classic clinical appearance of the tumor as demonstrated by bluish discoloration at the base of the nail. **B,** MRI slice confirming location of the tumor. **C,** Intraoperative appearance of the subungual glomus tumor. (From Joory K, Mikalef P, Rajive MJ: Smoking and glomus tumours, *J Plast Reconstr Aesthet Surg* 67(11):1600–1601, 2014, fig 1.)

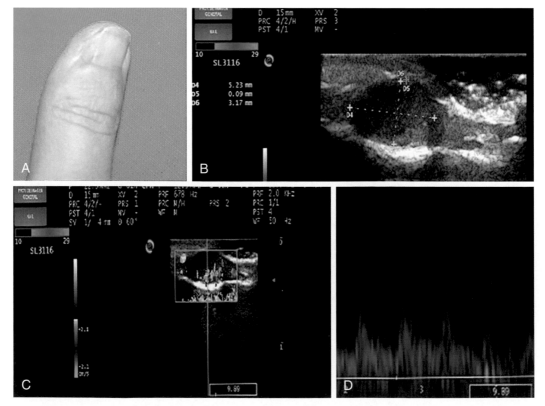

• **Figure 127-3 A,** Characteristic nail ridging dystrophy on the medial face of the first finger of the right hand in a patient with glomus tumor. **B,** B mode Doppler image showing a well-defined, solid hypoechoic lesion with an oval form and regular borders. **C,** In color Doppler mode, extensive vascularization can be seen in the nail bed. **D,** Spectral analysis shows low-grade systolic arterial flow within the lesion. (From Gómez-Sánchez ME, Alfageme-Roldán F, Roustán-Gullón G, et al: The usefulness of ultrasound imaging in digital and extradigital glomus tumors, *Actas Dermosifiliogr* 105(7):e45–e49, 2014, fig 2.)

SECTION 6

The Chest Wall, Thorax, and Thoracic Spine

128 The Winged Scapula Sign for Entrapment of the Long Thoracic Nerve of Bell

Long thoracic nerve entrapment syndrome is caused by compression or stretching of the long thoracic nerve as it passes beneath the subscapularis muscle to innervate the serratus anterior muscle (Fig. 128-1). The most common causes of compression of the long thoracic nerve at this anatomic location include direct trauma to the nerve during surgical procedures, such as radical mastectomy and surgery for thoracic outlet syndrome. Direct blunt trauma from heavy items falling from shelves also can cause long thoracic nerve entrapment syndrome. Damage to the long thoracic nerve following first rib fracture also has been reported. Stretch injuries to the long thoracic nerve often occur from prolonged heavy labor or wearing improperly fitting heavy backpacks.

Clinically the patient presents with painless paralysis of the serratus anterior muscle that results in the classic finding of winged scapula sign. The winged scapula sign is the result of the inability of the serratus anterior muscle to hold the scapula firmly against the posterior chest wall. The winged scapula sign can be identified by having the patient place both hands against the wall and press outward. The clinician, by observing the patient from behind, identifies the affected scapula projecting posteriorly or winging away from the posterior chest wall (Fig. 128-2). The patient with long thoracic nerve syndrome also is unable to fully extend the upper extremity overhead on the affected side, the last 25 to 30 degrees of extension being lost.

Electromyography helps to diagnose long thoracic nerve entrapment syndrome. Plain radiographs are indicated in all patients who present with long thoracic nerve entrapment syndrome to rule out occult bony pathology, including scapular and first rib fractures.

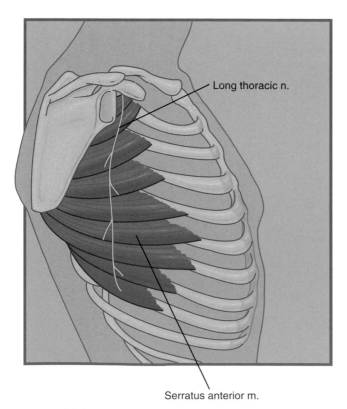

Long thoracic n.

Serratus anterior m.

• **Figure 128-1** Long thoracic nerve entrapment syndrome: relevant anatomy. (From Waldman SD: *Atlas of pain management injection techniques*, Philadelphia, 2000, Saunders, p 167.)

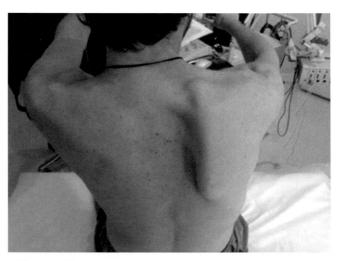

• **Figure 128-2** Winged scapula. Note how the scapula projects posteriorly and wings away from the posterior chest wall. (Fig. 1 from Deroux JP, Brion L, Hyerle A, et al: Association between hepatitis E and neurological disorders: two case studies and literature review, *J Clin Virol* 60(1):60–62, 2014.)

The Suprascapular Notch Sign for Suprascapular Nerve Entrapment Syndrome

Suprascapular nerve entrapment syndrome is caused by compression of the suprascapular nerve as it passes through the suprascapular notch (Fig. 129-1). The most common causes of compression of the suprascapular nerve at this anatomic location include the prolonged wearing of heavy backpacks and direct blows to the nerve such as occur in

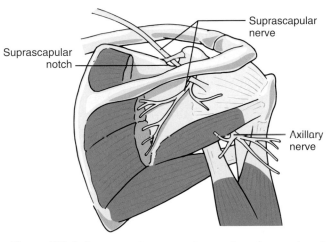

• **Figure 129-1** Suprascapular nerve entrapment syndrome: relevant anatomy.

football injuries and in falls from trampolines (see Fig. 129-1). This entrapment neuropathy presents most commonly as a severe, deep, aching pain that radiates from the top of the scapula to the ipsilateral shoulder. On physical examination, patients who are suffering from suprascapular nerve entrapment will exhibit a positive suprascapular notch sign. Tenderness over the suprascapular notch is usually present. Shoulder movement, especially reaching across the chest, may increase the pain. If suprascapular nerve entrapment remains untreated, weakness and atrophy of the supraspinatus and infraspinatus muscles will occur.

To elicit the suprascapular notch sign for suprascapular nerve entrapment, the patient is asked to face away from the examiner with the arms hanging loosely at the sides. The examiner then identifies the patient's suprascapular notch and exerts a sudden, firm pressure on the notch (Fig. 129-2, *A*). Patients who are suffering from suprascapular nerve entrapment will note that this pressure reproduces their pain, and they will reflexively withdraw away from the palpating finger (Fig. 129-2, *B*).

Suprascapular nerve entrapment syndrome is often misdiagnosed as bursitis, tendinitis, or arthritis of the shoulder. Cervical radiculopathy of the C5 nerve root also can mimic the clinical presentation of suprascapular nerve entrapment syndrome. Parsonage-Turner syndrome (idiopathic brachial neuritis) also may present as a sudden onset of shoulder pain

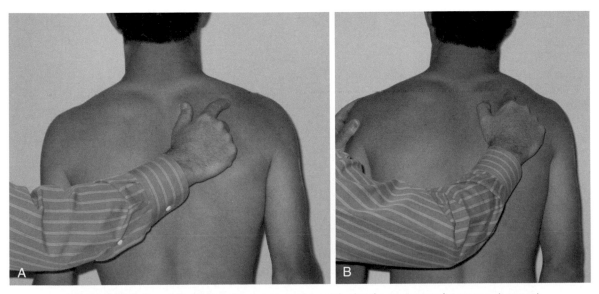

• **Figure 129-2 A** and **B,** Eliciting the suprascapular notch sign for suprascapular nerve entrapment syndrome.

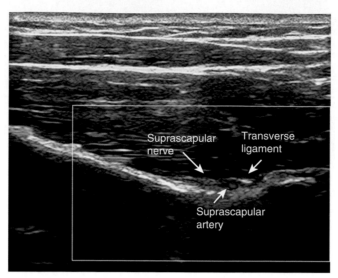

• **Figure 129-3** Color Doppler image demonstrating the relationship of the suprascapular artery and nerve as they pass beneath the transverse suprascapular ligament.

and can be confused with suprascapular nerve entrapment. A tumor that involves the superior scapular region or shoulder also should be considered in the differential diagnosis of suprascapular nerve entrapment syndrome.

Electromyography helps to distinguish cervical radiculopathy and Parsonage-Turner syndrome from suprascapular nerve entrapment syndrome. Plain radiographs are indicated in all patients who present with suprascapular nerve entrapment syndrome to rule out occult bony pathology. Ultrasound and color Doppler imaging can also aid in identification of the cause of suprascapular nerve entrapment (Fig. 129-3).

The costosternal joints can serve as a source of pain that can often mimic the pain of cardiac origin. The costosternal joints are susceptible to the development of arthritis, including osteoarthritis, rheumatoid arthritis, ankylosing spondylitis, Reiter syndrome, and psoriatic arthritis. The joints often are traumatized during acceleration/deceleration injuries and blunt trauma to the chest. With severe trauma, the joints may sublux or dislocate. Overuse or misuse also can result in acute inflammation of the costosternal joint, which can be quite debilitating. The joints also are subject to invasion by tumor from primary malignancies, including thymoma, as well as by metastatic disease.

Physical examination of patients who suffer from costosternal syndrome reveals that the patient will vigorously attempt to splint the joints by keeping the shoulders stiffly in neutral position. Such patients will also exhibit a positive shoulder retraction test.

To elicit a shoulder retraction test in patients who are suspected of suffering from costosternal syndrome, the patient is placed in the standing position with the shoulders in neutral position, facing the examiner. The patient is then asked to retract the shoulder vigorously (Fig. 130-1). The shoulder retraction test is considered positive if the retraction maneuver reproduces the patient's anterior chest wall pain.

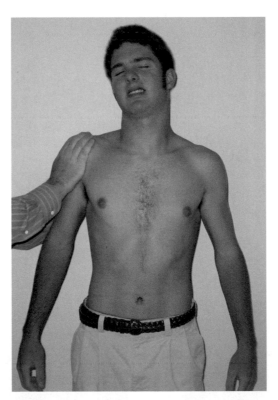

• **Figure 130-1** The shoulder retraction test for costosternal syndrome.

Tietze syndrome is distinct from costosternal syndrome (see Chapter 130). First described in 1921, Tietze syndrome is characterized by acute painful swelling of the costal cartilages. The second and third costal cartilages are most commonly involved. In contradistinction to costosternal syndrome, which usually occurs no earlier than the fourth decade of life, Tietze syndrome is a disease of the second and third decades of life. The onset is acute and often associated with a concurrent viral respiratory tract infection (Fig. 131-1). It has been postulated that microtrauma to the costosternal joints from severe coughing or heavy labor might also cause Tietze syndrome. Painful swelling of the second and third costochondral joints is the sine qua non of Tietze syndrome, and this swelling forms the basis for the swollen costosternal joint sign for Tietze syndrome (Fig. 131-2). Such swelling is absent in costosternal syndrome, which occurs much more frequently than Tietze syndrome.

Physical examination reveals that the patient who suffers from Tietze syndrome will vigorously attempt to splint the joints by keeping the shoulders stiffly in neutral position. Pain is reproduced with active protraction or retraction of the shoulder, deep inspiration, and full elevation of the arm. Shrugging of the shoulder also can reproduce the pain. Coughing may be difficult, and this can lead to inadequate pulmonary toilet in patients who suffer from Tietze

syndrome. The costosternal joints, especially the second and third, are swollen and exquisitely tender to palpation. This swelling constitutes a positive swollen costosternal joint sign, which is pathognomonic for Tietze syndrome. Magnetic resonance and ultrasound imaging can help confirm the diagnosis (Fig. 131-3).

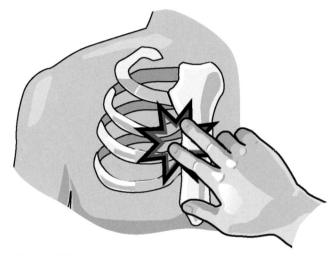

• **Figure 131-2** Inspection of the costosternal joint for swelling indicative of Tietze syndrome.

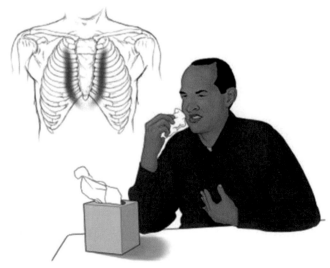

• **Figure 131-1** Acute pain and swelling of the second and third costochondral joints associated with an upper respiratory tract infection is the hallmark sign of Tietze syndrome. (From Waldman SD: Tietze's syndrome. In: *Atlas of common pain syndromes,* Philadelphia, 2002, WB Saunders, p 159.)

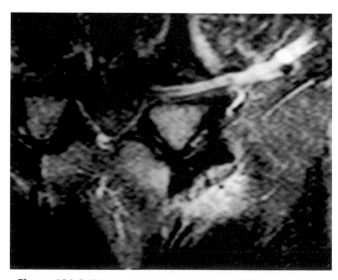

• **Figure 131-3** Tietze syndrome: a coronal short TI inversion recovery magnetic resonance image of the thorax, showing high-intensity signal at the costosternal joint. (From Resnick D, editor: *Diagnosis of bone and joint disorders,* ed 4, Philadelphia, 2002, WB Saunders, p 2605.)

132 The Shrug Test for Sternoclavicular Joint Dysfunction

The sternoclavicular joint can serve as a source of pain that often mimics pain of cardiac origin. The sternoclavicular joint is a double gliding joint with an actual synovial cavity. Articulation occurs between the sternal end of the clavicle, the sternal manubrium, and the cartilage of the first rib. The clavicle and sternal manubrium are separated by an articular disc. The joint is reinforced in front and back by the sternoclavicular ligaments. Additional support is provided by the costoclavicular ligament, which runs from the junction of the first rib and its costal cartilage to the inferior surface of the clavicle.

The sternoclavicular joint is susceptible to the development of arthritis, including osteoarthritis, rheumatoid arthritis, ankylosing spondylitis, Reiter syndrome, and psoriatic arthritis. The joint is often traumatized during acceleration/deceleration injuries and blunt trauma to the chest. With severe trauma, the joint may sublux or dislocate. Overuse or misuse can also result in acute inflammation of the sternoclavicular joint, which can be quite debilitating. The joint is also subject to invasion by tumor from primary malignancies, including thymoma, as well as from metastatic disease. Rarely, the sternoclavicular joint can become infected (Fig. 132-1).

Physical examination reveals that the patient will vigorously attempt to splint the joint by keeping the shoulders stiffly in neutral position. The sternoclavicular joint may be tender to palpation and feel hot and swollen if acutely inflamed. Pain is reproduced by active protraction or retraction of the shoulder as well as full elevation of the arm. Patients who are suffering from sternoclavicular joint dysfunction will also exhibit a positive shrug test.

To perform the shrug test for sternoclavicular joint dysfunction, the patient is asked to stand facing the examiner with the shoulders and upper extremities in a relaxed, neutral position. The examiner places his or her hand over the affected sternoclavicular joint (Fig. 132-2, *A*) and then has the patient rapidly shrug the affected shoulder (Fig. 132-2, *B*). The shrug test is positive if the examiner appreciates a click with maximum shoulder shrug (Video 132-1).

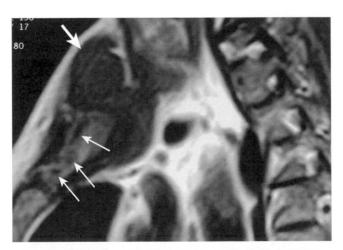

• **Figure 132-1** Sternoclavicular joint infection and osteomyelitis in a 48-year-old man with an infected subclavian venous catheter. Sagittal T1-weighted (repetition time [TR] = 400 ms, echo time [TE] = 12 ms) magnetic resonance image shows abnormal areas of low signal intensity *(smaller arrows)* in the sternal marrow, consistent with osteomyelitis. Surrounding low signal intensity *(thick arrow)* in the soft tissues is consistent with abscess. (From Knisely BL, Broderick LS, Kuhlman JE: MR imaging of the pleura and chest wall, *MRI Clin North Am* 8:125, 2000.)

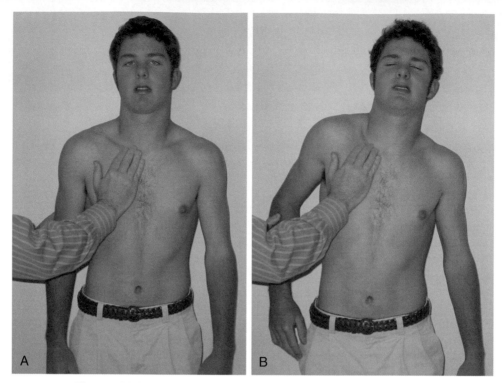

• **Figure 132-2 A** and **B,** The shrug test for sternoclavicular joint dysfunction.

133 The Hooking Maneuver Test for Slipping Rib Syndrome

Slipping rib syndrome is a constellation of symptoms, including severe knife-like pain emanating from the lower costal cartilages associated with hypermobility of the anterior end of the lower costal cartilages. The tenth rib is most commonly involved, but the eight and ninth ribs also can be affected. This syndrome is also known as rib-tip syndrome. Slipping rib syndrome is almost always associated with trauma to the costal cartilage of the lower ribs. These cartilages often are traumatized during acceleration/deceleration injuries and blunt trauma to the chest. With severe trauma, the cartilage may sublux or dislocate from the ribs. Patients with slipping rib syndrome also may complain of a "clicking" sensation with movement of the affected ribs and associated cartilage and may exhibit a positive hooking maneuver test.

Physical examination reveals that the patient will vigorously attempt to splint the affected costal cartilage joints by keeping the thoracolumbar spine slightly flexed. Pain is reproduced with pressure on the affected costal cartilage. Patients with slipping rib syndrome exhibit a positive hooking maneuver test. The hooking maneuver test is performed by having the patient lie in the supine position with the abdominal muscles relaxed while the clinician hooks his or her fingers under the lower rib cage and pulls gently outward (Fig. 133-1). Pain and a clicking or snapping sensation of the affected ribs and cartilage indicate a positive test.

Plain radiographs are indicated for all patients who present with pain that is thought to be emanating from the lower costal cartilage and ribs to rule out occult bony pathology, including rib fracture and tumor. On the basis of the patient's clinical presentation, additional testing may be indicated, including complete blood count, prostate-specific antigen, sedimentation rate, and antinuclear antibody testing. Magnetic resonance and ultrasound imaging of the affected ribs and cartilage is indicated if joint instability or occult mass is suspected.

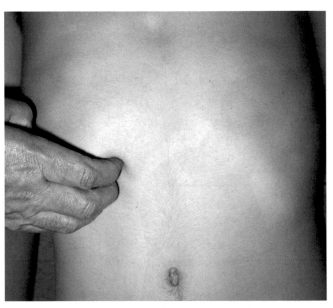

• **Figure 133-1** The hooking maneuver test for slipping rib syndrome.

SECTION 7

The Lumbar Spine

135 Functional Anatomy of the Lumbar Spine

THE BONY ELEMENTS

The lumbar spine comprises 5 vertebrae numbered from cephalad to caudad L1 to L5. The primary function of the lumbar vertebrae is to bear the weight of the upper body and to allow for coordinated movement of the lower back and pelvis in flexion, extension, and lateral bending. Like the rest of the spine, the lumbar vertebrae serve a secondary protective role by enclosing the cauda equina and related structures in a bony canal. Unlike the specialized cervical and thoracic vertebrae, which are dissimilar from their lower counterparts, the lumbar vertebrae are structurally similar.

Each vertebra is made up of an anterior weight-bearing vertebral body and a posterior neural arch. The posterior neural arch has 3 specialized processes that allow attachment of the muscles of posture and a variety of ligaments (Fig. 135-1). These processes are the spinous process, which lies in the midline posteriorly, and the 2 transverse processes, which lie laterally. The area of the neural arch between the spinous process and the transverse process is called the lamina. The area between the transverse process and the vertebral body is called the pedicle.

MOVEMENT

Movement of adjacent lumbar vertebrae is allowed by 3 joints. The first comprises the inferior and superior end plates of the vertebral bodies and their interposed intervertebral disc (Fig. 135-2). The second and third are the 2 facet joints, also known as zygapophyseal joints, which are made up of the inferior articular process of the superior adjacent vertebra and the ipsilateral superior articular process of the inferior adjacent vertebra (Fig. 135-3). This configuration allows flexion, extension, and a limited degree of lateral bending while at the same time contributing significantly to the lateral stability of the lumbar spine.

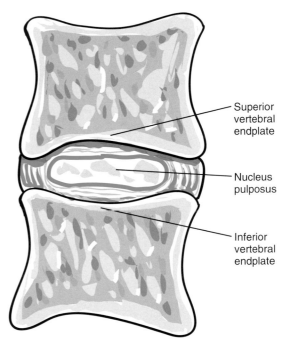

• **Figure 135-2** Movement of adjacent lumbar vertebrae is allowed by 3 joints. The first comprises the inferior and superior endplates of the vertebral bodies and their interposed intervertebral disc.

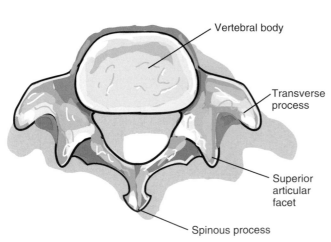

• **Figure 135-1** The processes of the posterior neural arch.

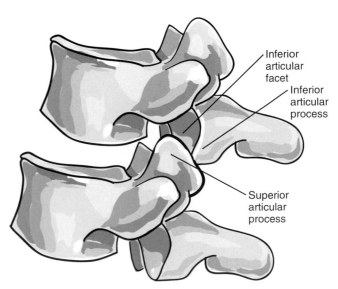

• **Figure 135-3** The zygapophyseal joints are made up of the inferior articular process of the superior adjacent vertebra and the ipsilateral superior articular process of the inferior adjacent vertebra.

THE INTERVERTEBRAL DISC

The lumbar intervertebral disc has 2 major functions: (1) to serve as the major shock-absorbing structure of the lumbar spine and (2) to facilitate the synchronized movement of the lumbar spine while helping to prevent impingement of the neural structures and associated structures that traverse the lumbar spine. Both the shock-absorbing function and the movement/protective function of the lumbar intervertebral disc are functions of the disc's structure as well as the laws of physics that affect it (see later discussion).

To understand how the lumbar intervertebral disc functions in health and becomes dysfunctional in disease, it is useful to think of the disc as a closed, fluid-filled container. The outside of the container is made up of a top and bottom called the endplates, which are composed of relatively inflexible hyaline cartilage. The sides of the lumbar intervertebral disc are made up of a woven criss-crossing matrix of fibroelastic fibers that tightly attaches to the top and bottom endplates. This woven matrix of fibers is called the annulus, and it completely surrounds the sides of the disc (see Fig. 135-2). The interlaced structure of the annulus results in an enclosing mesh that is extremely strong yet very flexible, which facilitates the compression of the disc during the wide range of motion of the lumbar spine.

Inside this container made of the top and bottom endplates and the surrounding annulus is the water-containing mucopolysaccharide gel-like substance called the nucleus pulposus (see Fig. 135-2). The nucleus pulposus is incompressible, and any pressure that is placed on one portion of the disc is transmitted throughout the entire nucleus pulposus. In health, the water-filled gel creates a positive intradiscal pressure that forces the adjacent vertebrae apart and helps to protect the spinal cord and exiting nerve roots. When the lumbar spine moves, the incompressible nature of the nucleus pulposus maintains a constant intradiscal pressure while some fibers of the disc relax and others contract.

As the lumbar intervertebral disc ages, it becomes less vascular and loses its ability to absorb water into the disc. This results in a degradation of the disc's shock-absorbing and motion-facilitating functions. This problem is made worse by degeneration of the annulus, which allows portions of the disc wall to bulge, distorting the ability of the nucleus pulposus to evenly distribute the forces that are placed on it throughout the entire disc. This exacerbates the disc dysfunction and can contribute to further disc deterioration, which can ultimately lead to complete disruption of the annulus and extrusion of the nucleus. The deterioration of the disc is responsible for many of the painful conditions that emanate from the lumbar spine and are encountered in clinical practice.

Much confusion surrounds the nomenclature that is used to describe the diseased lumbar disc. Such confusion exists in part because of a system of nomenclature that was devised before the advent of computed tomography and magnetic resonance imaging (MRI) and in part because of the focus by radiologists and clinicians alike on the impingement of the intervertebral disc on neural structures as the sole source of pain emanating from the spine.

This second viewpoint ignores the disc and facet joint as an independent source of spine pain and leads to misdiagnosis, treatment plans with little chance of success, and needless suffering of the patient. By standardizing the nomenclature of the diseased lumbar disc, the radiologist and clinician can do much to avoid these pitfalls when caring for the patient with spinal pain.

The following classification system will allow the radiologist and clinician to communicate with each other in the same language. It also takes into account the fact that the intervertebral disc might be the sole source of spinal pain and that certain findings on MRI should point the clinician to a discogenic source of pain and an early consideration of discography as a diagnostic maneuver prior to surgical interventions. More than 90% of clinically significant disc abnormalities of the lumbar spine occur at L4-L5 or L5-S1.

THE NORMAL DISC

As discussed in Chapter 137, the normal disc consists of the central gel-like nucleus pulposus, which is surrounded concentrically by a dense fibroelastic ring called the annulus. The top and bottom of the disc are contained by a cartilaginous endplate that is adjacent to the vertebral body. On MRI, the normal lumbar disc appears symmetrical with low signal intensity on T1-weighted images and high signal intensity throughout the disc on T2-weighted images. In health, the margins of the lumbar disc do not extend beyond the margins of the adjacent vertebral bodies (Fig. 136-1).

THE DEGENERATED DISC

As the disc ages, both the nucleus pulposus and the annulus undergo structural and biochemical changes that affect both the disc's appearance on MRI and the disc's ability to function properly. This degenerative process is a normal part of aging, and it can be accelerated by trauma to the lumbar spine, infection, and smoking. If the degenerative process is severe enough, many but not all patients will experience clinical symptoms.

As the degenerative process occurs, the nucleus pulposus begins to lose its ability to maintain an adequate level of

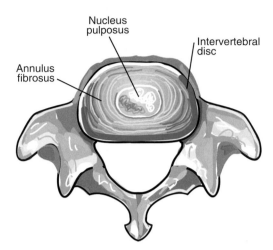

• **Figure 136-1** Normal lumbar disc.

hydration as well as its ability to maintain a proper mixture of proteoglycans necessary to keep the gel-like consistency of the nuclear material (Fig. 136-2). Degenerative clefts develop within the nuclear matrix, and portions of the nucleus become replaced with collagen, which leads to a further degradation of the shock-absorbing abilities and flexibility of the disc. As this process continues, the disc's ability to maintain an adequate intradiscal pressure to push the adjacent vertebrae apart begins to deteriorate, leading to a further deterioration of function with the onset of clinical symptoms.

In addition to changes that affect the nucleus pulposus, the degenerative process affects the annulus as well. As the annulus ages, the complex interwoven mesh of fibroelastic fibers begins to break down, and small tears occur within the mesh. As these tears occur, the exposed collagen fibers stimulate the ingrowth of richly innervated granulation tissue that can account for discogenic pain. These tears can be easily demonstrated on MRI as linear structures of high signal intensity on T2-weighted images, which correlate with positive results when provocative discography is performed on the affected disc (Figs. 136-2 and 136-3). When identified as the source of pain on discography, these annular tears can be treated with intradiscal electrothermal annuloplasty with good results (Fig. 136-4).

THE DIFFUSELY BULGING DISC

As the degenerative process continues, further breakdown and tearing of the annular fibers and continued loss of hydration of the nucleus pulposus lead to a loss of intradiscal pressure with resultant disc space narrowing, which can lead to an exacerbation of clinical symptoms. As the disc

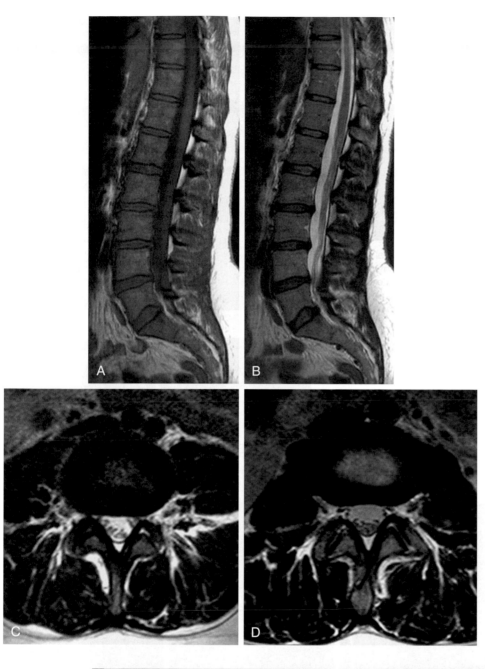

• **Figure 136-2** Sagittal T1W **(A)** and T2W **(B)** magnetic resonance (MR) images of the lumbar spine. The SI of the intervertebral discs is normal on the T1W MR images, but there is disc space narrowing at L2-L3 and L3-L4. The T2W MR image shows early loss of disc hydration with low–signal intensity changes at L2-L3, L3-L4, and L4-L5. In addition, there is bulging of the posterior discs beyond the posterior margin vertebral body wall at these 3 levels, which is most marked at L3-L4. **C,** An axial T2W MR image shows that the posterior margin of the disc is flat, but without significant narrowing of the lateral recesses and with no compression of the thecal sac. **D,** An axial T2W MR image of a normal L3-L4 disc shows that the posterior margin of the disc should be slightly concave. (From Waldman SD, Campbell, RSD: *Imaging of pain,* Philadelphia, 2010, Saunders/ Elsevier, p 120, fig 47-1.)

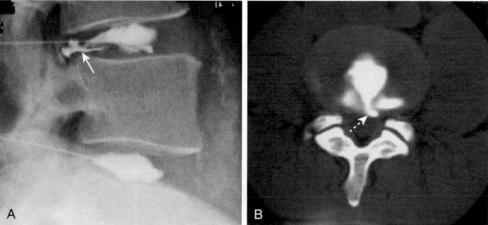

• **Figure 136-3 A,** Fluoroscopic discogram demonstrating an annular fissure extending from the nucleus pulposus to the posterior disc margin *(arrow)*. **B,** The same appearance is seen on a computed tomography discogram, with high-density contrast medium extending into a posterior annular fissure *(broken arrow)*. (From Waldman SD, Campbell, RSD: *Imaging of pain,* Philadelphia, 2010, Saunders/Elsevier, p 124, fig 49-2.)

THE FOCAL DISC PROTRUSION

As the disc annulus and nucleus pulposus continue to degenerate, the ability of the annulus to completely contain and compress the nucleus pulposus is lost and with it the incompressible nature of the nucleus pulposus. This leads to focal areas of annular wall weakness, which allow the nucleus pulposus to protrude into the spinal canal or against pain-sensitive structures (Fig. 136-5, C). Such protrusions are focal in nature and are easily seen on both T1- and T2-weighted MRI (Fig. 136-7). These focal disc protrusions can be either relatively asymptomatic if the focal bulge does not impinge on any pain-sensitive structures or highly symptomatic, presenting clinically as pure discogenic pain or as radicular pain if the focal protrusion extends into a neural foramen or the spinal canal.

THE FOCAL DISC EXTRUSION

Focal disc extrusion is frequently symptomatic because the disc material frequently migrates cranially or caudally, resulting in impingement of exiting nerve roots and the creation of an intense inflammatory reaction as the nuclear material irritates the nerve root. This chemical irritation is thought to be responsible for the intense pain that is experienced by many patients with focal disc extrusion and can be seen on MRI as high-intensity signals on T2-weighted images (Fig. 136-8). Although more pronounced than a focal disc protrusion, focal disc extrusion is similar in that the extruded disc material remains contiguous with the parent disc material (Fig. 136-5, D).

THE SEQUESTERED DISC

When a portion of the nuclear material detaches itself from its parent disc material and migrates, the disc fragment is called a sequestered disc (Fig. 136-5, E). Sequestered disc fragments frequently migrate in a cranial or caudal direction

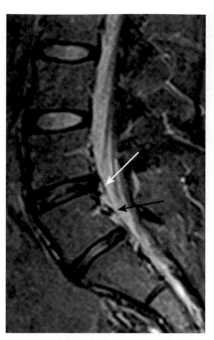

• **Figure 136-9** Axial T2-weighted MR image of the lumbar spine. *Arrows* point to an annular fissure associated with a focal disc protrusion. (From Chou R, Deyo RA, Jarvik JG: Appropriate use of lumbar imaging for evaluation of low back pain. *Radiol Clin North Am* 50(4):569–585, 2012, fig 4.)

and become impacted beneath a nerve root or between the posterior longitudinal ligament and the bony spine. Sequestered disc fragments can cause significant clinical pain and often require surgical intervention. Sequestered disc fragments will often enhance on contrast-enhanced T1-weighted images and demonstrate a peripheral rim of high-intensity signal caused by the inflammatory reaction that the nuclear material elicits on T2-weighted images (Fig. 136-9). Failure to identify and remove sequestered disc fragments often leads to a poor surgical result.

137 An Overview of Painful Conditions Emanating from the Lumbar Spine

The initial general physical examination of the lumbar spine and lumbar dermatomes guides the clinician in narrowing his or her differential diagnosis and helps to suggest which specialized physical examination maneuvers and laboratory and radiographic testing will aid in confirming the cause of the patient's low back pain and dysfunction. For the clinician to make best use of the initial information gleaned from the general physical examination of the lumbar spine and lumbar dermatomes, a grouping of the common causes of pain and dysfunction emanating from the lumbar spine is exceedingly helpful. Although no classification of lumbar spine pain and dysfunction can be all inclusive or all exclusive, because of the frequently overlapping and multifactorial nature of lumbar spine pathology, Table 137-1 should help to improve the diagnostic accuracy of the clinician who is confronted with the patient complaining of low back or lower extremity pain and dysfunction and help the clinician avoid overlooking less common diagnoses.

The list in Table 137-1 is by no means comprehensive, but it does aid the clinician in organizing the potential sources of pathology presenting as pain and dysfunction emanating from the lumbar spine. It should be noted that the most commonly missed categories of low back and lower extremity pain and the categories that most often result in misadventures in diagnosis and treatment are the last 3 categories. The knowledge of this potential pitfall should help clinicians keep these sometimes overlooked causes of low back and lower extremity pain and dysfunction in their differential diagnosis.

TABLE 137-1 Overview of Causes of Low Back and/or Lower Extremity Pain

Localized Bony, Disc Space, or Joint Space Pathology	Primary Hip Pathology	Systemic Disease	Sympathetically Mediated Pain	Pain Referred from Other Body Areas
Vertebral fracture	Bursitis	Rheumatoid arthritis	Causalgia	Pancreatitis
Primary bone tumor	Tendinitis	Collagen vascular disease	Reflex sympathetic dystrophy	Malignancy of the retroperitoneal space
Facet joint disease	Aseptic necrosis	Reiter syndrome	Postthrombophlebitis pain (milk leg)	Lumbar Plexopathy
Localized or generalized degenerative arthritis	Osteoarthritis	Gout		Fibromyalgia
Osteophyte formation	Joint instability	Other crystal arthropathies		Myofascial pain syndromes
Disc space infection	Muscle strain	Charcot neuropathic arthritis		Entrapment neuropathies
Herniated lumbar disc	Muscle sprain	Multiple sclerosis		Intraabdominal tumors
Degenerative disc disease	Periarticular infection not involving joint space	Ischemic pain secondary to peripheral vascular insufficiency		
Primary spinal cord and/or cauda equina pathology		Ankylosing spondylitis		
Osteomyelitis				
Epidural abcess				
Epidural hematoma				

The lumbar spine has movement among all 5 of its structural elements, with the major movements of flexion and limited extension and lateral bending facilitated by the facet joints, which are paired diarthrodial planar joints. In health, movement of the lumbar spine requires synchronized movement of all the elements of the spine. In disease, problems at one level can cause functional disability at other levels.

FLEXION AND EXTENSION

To assess the range of motion of the lumbar spine, the clinician has the patient place the spine in a neutral position. The patient is then asked to flex his or her lumbar spine forward while the clinician observes for any limitation in range of motion and a lack of a smooth, synchronized flexion that might be indicative of pain or spinal segment dysfunction (Fig. 140-1). The patient is then asked to return the lumbar spine to neutral position and then to extend the lumbar spine while the clinician observes for any limitation in range of motion or a lack of a smooth, synchronized extension that might indicate pain or spinal segment dysfunction (Fig. 140-2). With both of these maneuvers, the clinician should be sure that movement occurs only at the level of the lumbar spine and that the patient is not using the thoracic or cervical spine to compensate for a limitation of range of motion of the lumbar segments.

ROTATION AND LATERAL BENDING

To assess the range of motion of rotation of the lumbar spine, the clinician has the patient place the spine in neutral position. The patient is then asked to fully rotate his or her lumbar spine in both the left and right directions while the clinician observes for any limitation in range of motion or a lack of a smooth, synchronized rotation that might indicate pain or spinal segment dysfunction (Fig. 140-3). The facet joints allow relatively limited rotation, although some rotation does occur at the L5-S1 joint because of its more coronal orientation.

The patient is then asked to return the lumbar spine to neutral position and to laterally bend the lumbar spine while the clinician observes for any limitation in range of motion or a lack of smooth, synchronized lateral bending that might indicate pain or spinal segment dysfunction (Fig. 140-4). With both of these maneuvers, the clinician should be sure that movement occurs only at the level of the lumbar spine and that the patient is not using the thoracic or cervical spine to compensate for a limitation of range of motion of the lumbar segments.

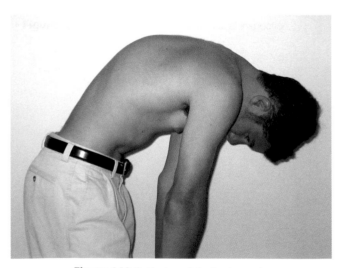

• **Figure 140-1** Flexion of the lumbar spine.

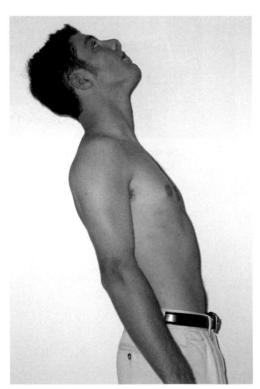

• **Figure 140-2** Extension of the lumbar spine.

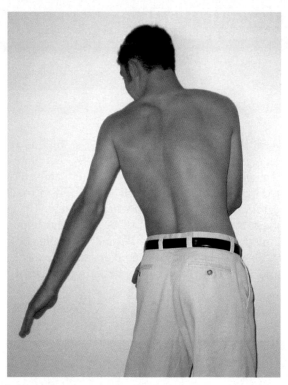

• **Figure 140-3** Rotation of the lumbar spine.

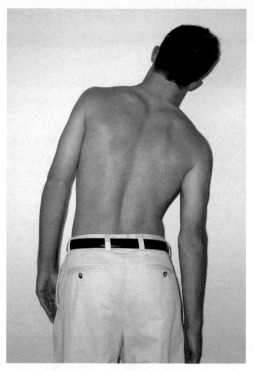

• **Figure 140-4** Lateral bending of the lumbar spine.

First described in 1937, the Schober test for lumbar spine flexion is useful in helping the clinician to quantify the actual degree of lumbar spine flexion by isolating the movement for the lumbar spine from that of flexion of the hips, which the patient may be utilizing to compensate for decreased flexion of the lumbar spine. The test is especially useful in identifying patients with undiagnosed ankylosing spondylitis.

To perform the Schober test for lumbar flexion, with the patient in the standing position, the examiner first identifies the sacral dimples and then identifies the midline at that level and places a mark (Fig. 141-1). The examiner then marks a point 10 cm above that point and 5 cm below that point (Fig. 141-2). The patient is then asked to touch his or her toes to maximally flex the lumbar spine. The examiner then measures the distance between the upper and lower marks while the patient's spine is maximally flexed (Fig. 141-3). The distance should increase to more than 21 cm if the patient's lumbar spine flexion is normal.

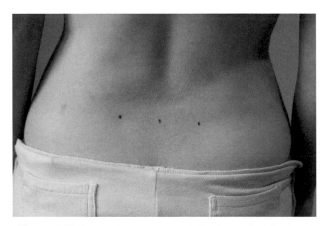

• **Figure 141-1** Identification of sacral dimples and midline mark.

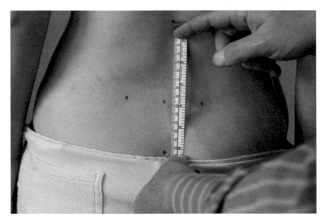

• **Figure 141-2** Markings at 10 cm above and 5 cm below the midline mark.

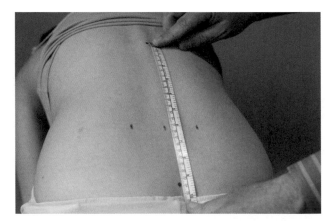

• **Figure 141-3** Measurement between upper and lower marks as patient's back is maximally flexed. A distance of 21 cm or more indicates normal lumbar spine flexion.

The Kemp test for lumbar facet joint pain is useful in helping the clinician to identify if the facet joint is the nidus of the patient's low back pain as well as to determine if there is a radicular component to the patient's pain.

To perform the Kemp test to identify lumbar facet joint pain, with the patient in the standing position, the examiner first identifies the side that the pain is on. The examiner then has the patient extend the spine (Fig. 142-1). The patient is then asked to laterally bend the spine away from the most painful side. The patient is then asked to rotate the shoulder on the less painful side posteriorly while the examiner exerts firm downward pressure on the shoulder (Fig. 142-2). The test is positive if it reproduces and/or exacerbates the patient's back pain. If the patient also experiences pain that radiates from the low back to below the knee in either lower extremity, a radicular component is also present.

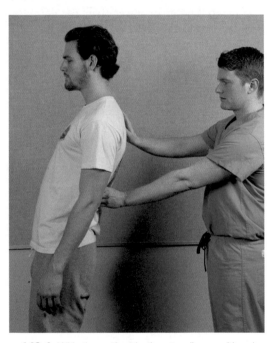

• **Figure 142-1** With the patient in the standing position, he or she is asked to extend the lumbar spine.

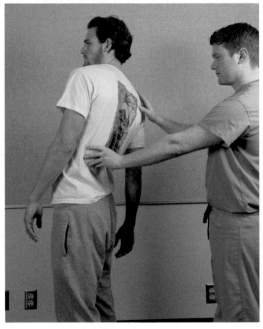

• **Figure 142-2** The patient is then asked to rotate the shoulder on the less painful side backward while the examiner exerts firm downward pressure on the shoulder.

143 The Lumbar Dermatomes

In humans, the innervation of the skin, muscles, and deep structures is determined embryologically at an early stage of fetal development, and there is amazingly little intersubject variability. Each segment of the spinal cord and its corresponding spinal nerve has a consistent segmental relationship that allows the clinician to ascertain the probable spinal level of dysfunction based on the pattern of pain, muscle weakness, and deep tendon reflex changes.

Figure 143-1 is a dermatome chart that the clinician will find useful in determining the specific spinal level subserving a patient's pain. In general, in humans, the more proximal the muscle, the more cephalad the spinal segment, with the ventral muscles innervated by higher spinal segments than the corresponding dorsal muscles.

Figure 143-2 is a myotome chart that the clinician will find useful when trying to correlate clinical weakness with a specific spinal segment. It should be remembered that pain that is perceived in the region of a given muscle or joint might not be coming from that muscle or joint but might simply be referred pain, caused by problems at the same lumbar spinal segment that innervated the muscles.

Furthermore, the clinician needs to be aware that the relatively consistent pattern of dermatomal and myotomal distribution breaks down when the pain is perceived in the deep structures of the upper extremity, such as the joints and tendinous insertions. With pain in these regions, the clinician should refer to the sclerotomal chart in Figure 143-3. This is particularly important if a neurodestructive procedure at the spinal cord level is being considered, as the sclerotomal level of the nerves subserving the pain may be several segments higher or lower than the dermatomal or myotomal levels that the clinician would expect.

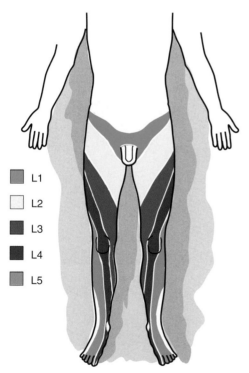

• **Figure 143-1** Lumbar dermatomes.

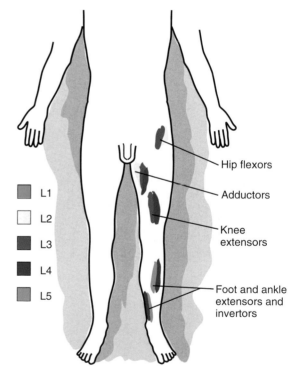

• **Figure 143-2** Lumbar myotomes.

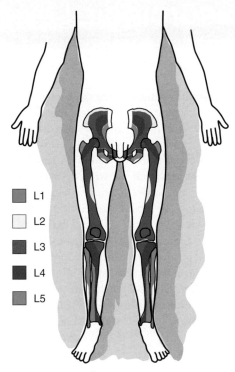

L1
L2
L3
L4
L5

• **Figure 143-3** Lumbar sclerotomes.

The concept of diagnosing a problem at a specific neurologic level via physical examination has its basis in the fact that pathology at the lumbar spinal cord or lumbar nerve root level manifests itself in a relatively consistent manner by dysfunction, numbness, and pain of the upper extremity that occurs in a dermatomal distribution. Although not foolproof, a careful physical examination of the lower extremity with an eye to the neurologic level that is affected can frequently guide the clinician in designing a more targeted workup and treatment plan. By overlapping the information gleaned from physical examination with the neuroanatomic information gained from magnetic resonance imaging and the neurophysiologic information gleaned from electromyography, a highly accurate diagnosis as to which level of the lumbar spine is responsible for the patient's symptoms can be made (Video 144-1).

Testing for the L4 dermatome is best carried out by a careful sensory evaluation of the medial side of the great toe (Fig. 144-1). Decreased sensation in this anatomic region can be ascribed to proximal lesions of the spinal cord and cauda equina, such as a syrinx or spinal cord tumor; to more distal lesions of the L4 nerve root, such as impingement by herniated disc; or to a lesion of a more peripheral nerve, such as the deep peroneal nerve. For this reason, correlation with manual muscle testing and evaluation of the deep tendon reflex combined with radiographic and electromyographic testing can help to determine the exact site of pathology.

Testing for the L4 myotome is best carried out by manual muscle testing of the tibialis anterior muscle. The tibialis anterior muscle is innervated primarily by the L4 nerve, with a small contribution in most patients from the L5 nerve. Because in most patients foot inversion by the tibialis anterior muscle is primarily an L4 function, the muscle should be tested as follows. The patient is placed in the sitting position with the knee flexed at 90 degrees and the affected extremity hanging comfortably off the examination table. The patient is asked to forcefully invert the foot of the affected extremity against the examiner's resistance (Fig. 144-2). If the manual muscle testing is normal, the examiner should not be able to resist the foot inversion or to force the foot back toward neutral position.

The patellar deep tendon reflex is mediated via the L4 spinal segment. To test the patellar reflex, the patient is placed in the sitting position with the knee flexed at 90 degrees and the affected extremity hanging comfortably off the examination table. The clinician then strikes the inferior patellar tendon at the elbow with a neurologic hammer and grades the response (Fig. 144-3). A diminished or absent reflex may point to compromise of the L4 segment, whereas a hyperactive response may suggest an upper motor neuron lesion, such as myelopathy.

SENSORY

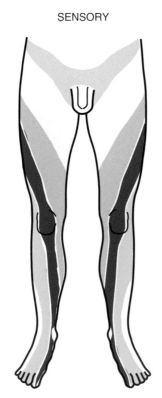

• **Figure 144-1** Sensory distribution of the L4 dermatome.

MOTOR

L4

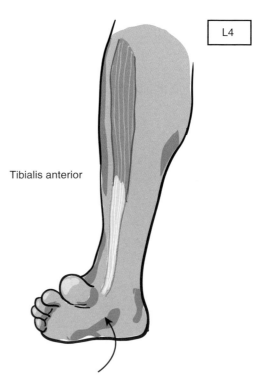

Tibialis anterior

• **Figure 144-2** L4 myotome integrity testing.

REFLEX

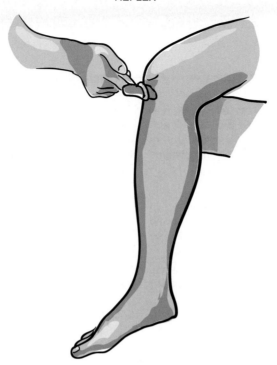

• **Figure 144-3** Patellar deep tendon reflex.

Testing for the L5 dermatome is best carried out by a careful sensory evaluation of the dorsum of the foot (Fig. 145-1). Decreased sensation in this anatomic region can be ascribed to proximal lesions of the spinal cord and cauda equina, such as a syrinx or spinal cord tumor; to more distal lesions of the L5 nerve root, such as impingement by herniated disc; or to a lesion of a more peripheral nerve, such as the deep peroneal nerve. For this reason, correlation with manual muscle testing and evaluation of the deep tendon reflex combined with radiographic and electromyographic testing can help to determine the exact site of pathology.

Testing for the L5 myotome is best carried out by manual muscle testing of the extensor digitorum longus muscle. The extensor digitorum longus muscle is primarily innervated by the L5 nerve. Because in most patients extension of the great toe by the extensor digitorum longus muscle is primarily an L5 function, the muscle should be tested as follows. The patient is placed in the sitting position with the knee flexed at 90 degrees and the affected extremity hanging comfortably off the examination table. The patient is asked to forcefully extend the middle toes of the affected extremity against the examiner's resistance (Fig. 145-2). If the manual muscle testing is normal, the examiner should not be able to resist the extension of the toes or to force the toe back toward neutral position (Video 145-1). There is no deep tendon reflex that can allow clinically useful testing of the L5 spinal segment.

SENSORY

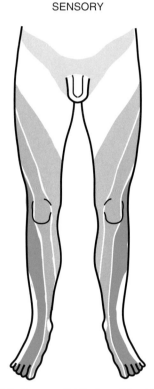

• **Figure 145-1** Sensory distribution of the L5 dermatome.

MOTOR

L5

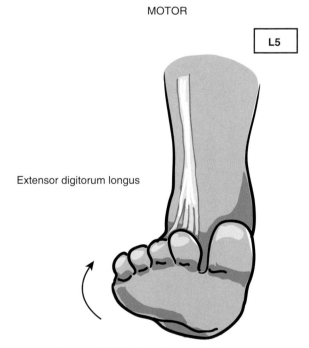

Extensor digitorum longus

• **Figure 145-2** L5 myotome integrity testing.

Testing for the S1 dermatome is best carried out by a careful sensory evaluation of the lateral side of the little toe (Fig. 146-1). Decreased sensation in this anatomic region can be ascribed to proximal lesions of the spinal cord and cauda equina, such as a syrinx or spinal cord tumor; to more distal lesions of the S1 nerve root, such as impingement by herniated disc; or to a lesion of a more peripheral nerve, such as the tibial nerve. For this reason, correlation with manual muscle testing and evaluation of the deep tendon reflex combined with radiographic and electromyographic testing can help to determine the exact site of pathology.

Testing for the S1 myotome is best carried out by manual muscle testing of the peroneus brevis and longus muscles. The peroneal brevis muscle is innervated primarily by the S1 nerve, with a small contribution in some patients from the L5 nerve. The peroneal longus muscle has contribution from both S1 and L5. Because in most patients foot eversion by these muscles is primarily an S1 function, the muscle should be tested as follows. The patient is placed in the sitting position with the knee flexed at 90 degrees and the affected extremity hanging comfortably off the examination table. The patient is asked to forcefully evert the foot of the affected extremity against the examiner's resistance (Fig. 146-2). If the manual muscle testing is normal, the examiner should not be able to resist the foot eversion or to force the foot back toward neutral position (Video 146-1).

The Achilles deep tendon reflex is mediated via the S1 spinal segment. To test the Achilles reflex, the patient is placed in the sitting position with the knee flexed at 90 degrees and the affected extremity hanging comfortably off the examination table. The clinician then strikes the Achilles tendon at the ankle with a neurologic hammer and grades the response (Fig. 146-3). A diminished or absent reflex may point to compromise of the S1 segment, whereas a hyperactive response may suggest an upper motor neuron lesion, such as myelopathy.

SENSORY

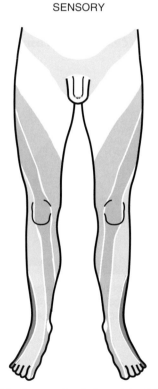

• **Figure 146-1** Sensory distribution of the S1 dermatome.

MOTOR

Peroneus longus
Peroneus brevis

S1
myotome

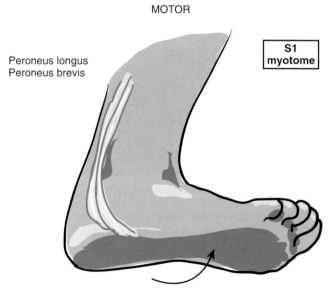

• **Figure 146-2** S1 myotome integrity testing.

Some investigators believe that performing the straight leg raising test in the sitting position provides the examiner with more accurate test results when compared with the classic Lasegue straight leg raising test (see Chapter 147).

To perform the sitting straight leg raising test, the patient is placed in the sitting position. The examiner then has the patient lean slightly forward to increase tension on the lumbar nerve roots (Fig. 148-1). With the ankle of the affected leg placed at 90 degrees of flexion, the examiner slowly raises the affected leg toward the ceiling while keeping the knee fully extended (Fig. 148-2). The test is positive if the patient complains of pain and paresthesias into the affected extremity that are similar to the pain that the patient has been experiencing.

Tight hamstring muscles might confuse the examination and lead to false positive results. If the results are in question, the examiner should note the amount of elevation necessary to elicit the patient's symptoms. Then, after lowering the patient's affected extremity back to the table, the examiner reelevates the leg to a level just below the degree of elevation necessary to reproduce the patient pain. The examiner holds the leg at that level for 10 seconds and then dorsiflexes the foot. If this maneuver reproduces the patient's pain, the test may be considered positive, and additional investigation, including magnetic resonance imaging of the lumbar spine and electromyography, is indicated. Other confirmatory tests include the Lasegue straight leg raising test (see Chapter 147) and the Naffziger test (see Chapter 149).

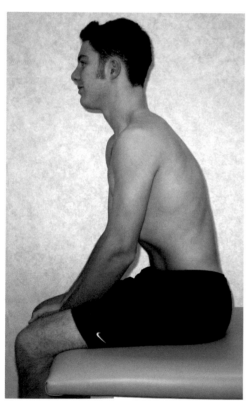

• **Figure 148-1** Sitting straight leg raising test: the patient is in the sitting position. The patient should lean forward slightly to increase tension on the lumbar nerve roots.

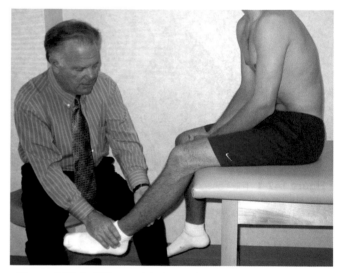

• **Figure 148-2** Sitting straight leg raising test: with the ankle of the affected leg at 90 degrees of flexion, the leg is slowly raised toward the ceiling while the knee is kept fully extended.

149 The Naffziger Jugular Compression Test for an Equivocal Lasegue Straight Leg Raising Test

The Lasegue straight leg raising test remains a mainstay in the physical diagnosis of lower lumber nerve irritation. It has good correlation with positive findings on magnetic resonance imaging of the lumbar spine and lumbar plexus as well as electromyography. The ease of performance of this test combined with excellent intraobserver consistency makes it a good starting point in the physical examination of patients who present with low back pain that radiates into the lower extremity. Unfortunately, the results of this test are sometimes equivocal. When this occurs, the test may be repeated in the sitting position (see Chapter 148) or the Naffziger jugular compression test can be added to improve the diagnostic accuracy of the physical examination.

To perform the Naffziger jugular compression test, the examiner first performs the classic Lasegue straight leg raising test as follows. The patient is placed in the supine position on the examination table with the unaffected leg flexed to 45 degrees at the knee and the affected leg placed flat against the table (see Fig. 147-1). With the ankle of the affected leg placed at 90 degrees of flexion, the examiner slowly raises the affected leg toward the ceiling while the knee is kept fully extended (see Fig. 147-2). At this point, if the results of the straight leg raising test are equivocal, the examiner has his or her assistant compress the patient's jugular veins bilaterally, which will increase the intraspinal pressure by distending the spinal venous plexus (Fig. 149-1). The Naffziger test is considered positive if the patient's pain and paresthesias are reproduced within 15 seconds.

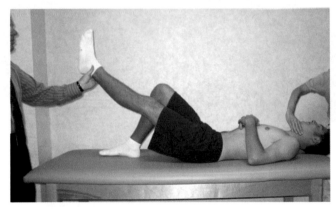

• **Figure 149-1** The Naffziger jugular compression test.

The flip test for lumbar nerve root irritation is an additional test that is available to the clinician who is faced with a patient suffering from low back pain that radiates into the lower extremities. It can be used as a confirmatory test to the straight leg raising tests described in Chapters 147 to 149.

To perform the flip test, the examiner has the patient sit on the side of the examining table with his or her legs dangling comfortably and the hands resting on the edge of the table. The examiner then diverts the patient by asking whether he or she is having any trouble with the knee of the affected leg (Fig. 150-1). The examiner then lifts the foot and extends the knee. If the patient is suffering from significant lumbar nerve root irritation or entrapment, the patient will "flip" backward to relieve the tension on the affected lumbar nerve root (Fig. 150-2). The examiner should take care that the patient does not hit his or her head against the wall when he or she flips backward.

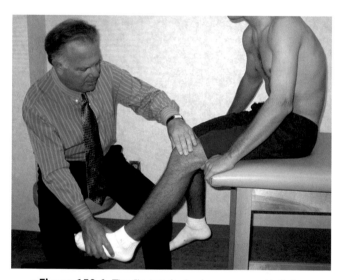

• **Figure 150-1** The flip test for lumbar nerve root irritation.

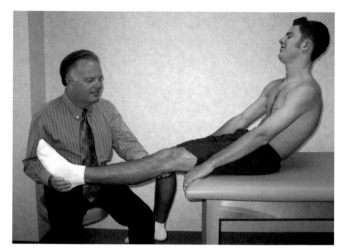

• **Figure 150-2** The patient suffering from significant lumbar nerve root irritation or entrapment will "flip" backward to relieve the tension on the affected lumbar nerve root.

To perform the buckling knee test, the patient is placed in the supine position on the examination table with the unaffected leg flexed to 45 degrees at the knee and the foot of the unaffected leg placed flat against the table (see Fig. 147-1). With the ankle of the affected leg placed at 90 degrees of flexion, the examiner slowly raises the affected leg toward the ceiling while keeping the knee fully extended (Fig. 151-1). The test is positive if the patient complains of pain and paresthesias into the affected extremity that are similar to those that he or she has been experiencing and involuntarily withdraws the affected knee to reduce pressure on the irritated or entrapped lumbar nerve roots (Fig. 151-2).

If this maneuver reproduces the patient's pain, the buckling knee test for lumbar nerve root irritation may be considered positive, and additional investigation, including magnetic resonance imaging of the lumbar spine and electromyography, is indicated.

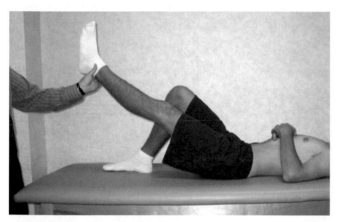

• **Figure 151-1** The buckling knee test for lumbar nerve root irritation.

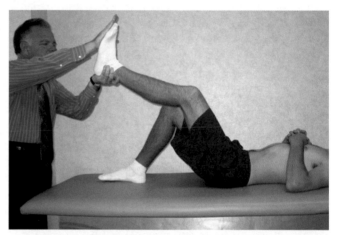

• **Figure 151-2** The buckling knee test is considered positive if it reproduces the patient's pain and paresthesias and the patient involuntarily withdraws the affected knee to reduce pressure on the lumbar nerve root.

To perform the Spurling test, the patient is placed in the supine position on the examination table with the unaffected leg flexed to 45 degrees at the knee and the foot of the unaffected leg placed flat against the table (see Fig. 147-1). With the ankle of the unaffected leg placed at 90 degrees of flexion, the examiner slowly raises the affected leg toward the ceiling while keeping the knee fully extended. The test is positive if the patient complains of pain and paresthesias into the affected extremity that are similar to those that the patient has been experiencing. The examiner notes the degree of elevation that begins to elicit the patient's pain and then returns the affected leg to the table. After allowing the patient's pain to subside for a few moments,

the examiner carefully elevates the leg to a point just below the one at which the patient began to experience the pain. At this point, the examiner forcefully dorsiflexes the patient's foot (Fig. 152-1). The Spurling test is considered positive if this maneuver reproduces the patient's pain (Video 152-1). Modifications of this test abound and include the Sicard test, which involves forced dorsiflexion of the great toe on the affected extremity (Fig. 152-2).

If this maneuver reproduces the patient's pain, the Spurling test for lumbar nerve root irritation may be considered positive, and additional investigation, including magnetic resonance imaging of the lumbar spine and electromyography, is indicated.

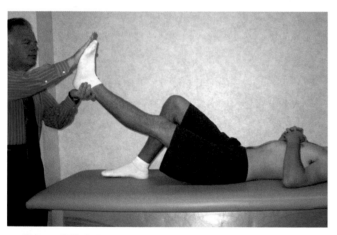

• **Figure 152-1** The Spurling test for lumbar nerve root irritation.

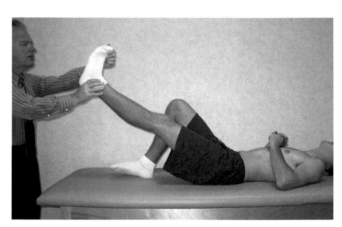

• **Figure 152-2** Sicard test for lumbar nerve root irritation.

To perform the Bragard test, the patient is placed in the supine position on the examination table with the unaffected leg flexed to 45 degrees at the knee and the foot of the unaffected leg placed flat against the table (see Fig. 137-1). The knee of the patient's affected leg is then flexed toward his or her abdomen (Fig. 153-1). The examiner then gradually extends the knee until the leg is straight or the patient's pain and paresthesias are reproduced (Fig. 153-2).

At this point, the examiner forcefully dorsiflexes the foot of the affected leg (Fig. 153-3).

The Bragard test is considered positive if this maneuver exacerbates the patient's pain. If this maneuver reproduces the patient's pain, additional investigation, including magnetic resonance imaging of the lumbar spine and electromyography, is indicated.

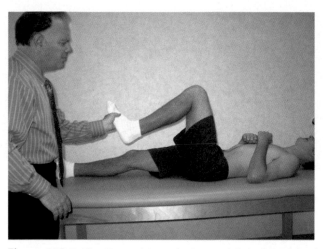

• **Figure 153-1** The Bragard test: the knee of the affected leg is flexed toward the abdomen.

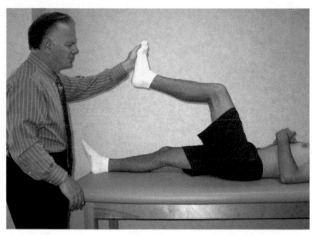

• **Figure 153-2** The Bragard test: the knee is then gradually extended until the leg is straight or the patient's pain and paresthesias are reproduced.

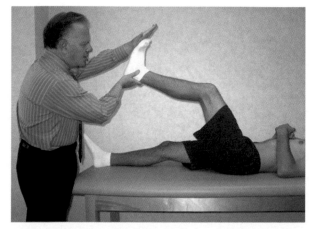

• **Figure 153-3** The Bragard test: the foot of the affected leg is then forcefully dorsiflexed.

To perform the Ely test for lumbar nerve root irritation, the patient is placed in the prone position. The examiner then has the patient flex the affected leg back toward the buttocks (Fig. 154-1) and then has him or her lift the chest off the examining table to extend the back (Fig. 154-2). If this maneuver reproduces the patient's pain, the test may be considered positive, and additional investigation, including magnetic resonance imaging of the lumbar spine and electromyography, is indicated (Video 154-1).

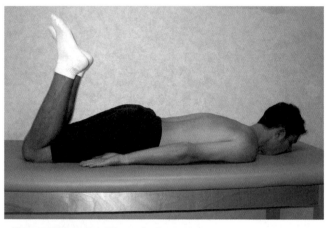

• **Figure 154-1** The Ely test for lumbar nerve root irritation: with the patient in prone position, the affected leg is flexed back toward the buttocks.

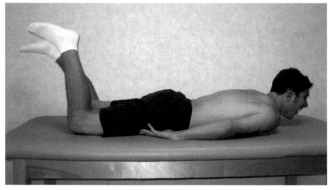

• **Figure 154-2** The Ely test for lumbar nerve root irritation: next, the patient lifts the chest off the examining table to extend the back.

155 The Fajersztajn Test for Lumbar Nerve Root Irritation

To perform the Fajersztajn test, the patient is placed in the supine position on the examination table with the affected leg flexed to 45 degrees at the knee and the foot of the affected leg placed flat against the table (Fig. 155-1). With the ankle of the unaffected leg placed at 90 degrees of flexion, the examiner slowly raises the unaffected leg toward the ceiling while keeping the knee fully extended (Fig. 155-2). The Fajersztajn test is positive if the patient complains of pain and paresthesias into the affected extremity that are similar to the pain that the patient has been experiencing. A positive test suggests that additional investigation, including magnetic resonance imaging of the lumbar spine and electromyography, is indicated.

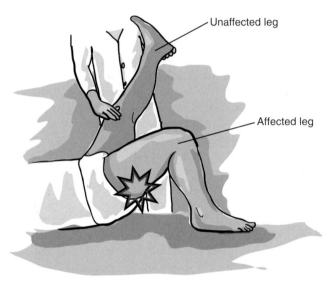

• **Figure 155-2** The examiner slowly raises the unaffected leg toward the ceiling while keeping the knee fully extended.

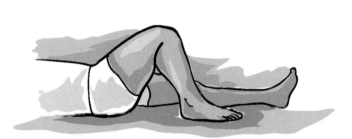

• **Figure 155-1** Patient position for the Fajersztajn test for lumbar nerve root irritation.

Patients suffering from spinal stenosis often experience a constellation of symptoms consisting of cramping, tiredness, weakness, and numbness with walking or running known as pseudoclaudication or neurogenic claudication. These symptoms are generally absent until the patient reaches a maximum distance known as the threshold distance. Once the patient exceeds the threshold distance, the symptoms continue to worsen until the patient is forced to stoop. As the patient begins to experience the symptoms of pseudoclaudication, he or she may assume a simian posture with a forward-flexed trunk and slightly bent knees (Fig. 156-1). This posture is thought to increase the capacity of the spinal canal and improve blood flow to the nerve roots that have become ischemic and unable to keep up with the increased metabolic demands of ambulation. The stoop test has its basis in this hypothesis, and this construct is further reinforced by the fact that a given patient's threshold distance will often be longer when walking up a hill because of the forward-flexed posture that is assumed and, conversely, shortened on the trip back down the hill because of the extended posture that is assumed when walking down a hill.

To perform the stoop test, the patient is asked to walk briskly for 2 or 3 minutes until the threshold distance is identified. The patient is then asked to continue walking for 30 seconds and then to sit upright in a straight-back chair (Fig. 156-2, A). The patient is then asked to lean forward in the chair (Fig. 156-2, B). The stoop test is positive if the patient's pain is relieved by leaning forward and presents the examiner with a presumptive diagnosis of spinal stenosis.

Patients with a positive stoop test should undergo magnetic resonance scanning, computed tomographic scanning, and electromyography with nerve conduction velocities as an initial workup. Myelography of the suspected area of stenosis may also be indicated.

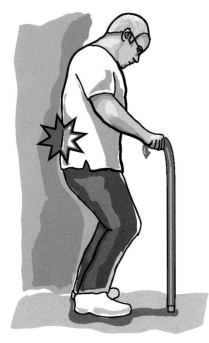

• **Figure 156-1** The simian posture with a forward-flexed trunk and slightly bent knees.

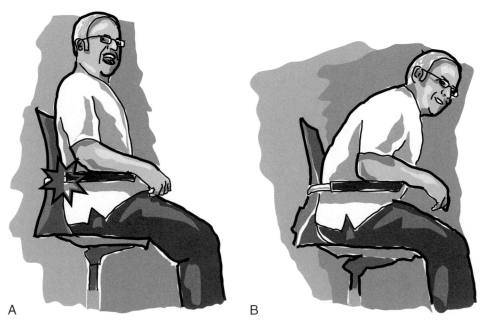

A   B

• **Figure 156-2 A** and **B,** Stoop test for spinal stenosis.

In health, stimulation of the plantar surface of the foot will elicit the consistent response of flexion of the toes with the flexion of the little toe greater than that of the great toe. With disease of the corticospinal system, this normal response is reversed: stimulation of the plantar surface of the foot elicits dorsiflexion of the toes with the dorsiflexion of the great toe greater than that of the little toe. Babinski described this pathologic reflex as *phenomene des orteils,* or dorsiflexion of the toes. He also described another consistent finding in patients with disease of the corticospinal system that he called *signe de l'eventail,* or fanning of the toes. This classic constellation of symptoms has become known as the *Babinski sign* and has become synonymous with diseases of the corticospinal system.

To elicit the Babinski sign, the patient is placed in a comfortable position with the plantar surface of the foot exposed. The lateral plantar surface is then lightly stroked from the heel forward with a blunt object such as a broken tongue depressor (Fig. 157-1, *A*). The stimulus should be light, as more pressure can elicit a nociceptive withdrawal response and produce a false negative test. A positive Babinski sign is produced when light stroking of the plantar surface produces rapid dorsiflexion of the toes with concomitant fanning of the toes, which is strongly suggestive of disease of the corticospinal tract (Fig. 157-1, *B*). As was mentioned previously, plantar flexion of the toes is considered a normal reflex. A positive Babinski sign is a significant physical finding and should prompt the clinician to immediately begin evaluation of the corticospinal system.

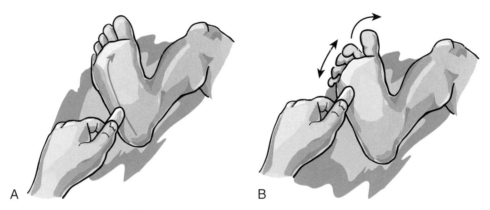

• **Figure 157-1 A** and **B,** Eliciting the Babinski sign.

To perform the Piedallu seated flexion test to determine if the nidus of the patient's pain is the sacroiliac joint, the patient is placed in the sitting position with his or her feet flat on the floor and the examiner seated behind the patient. The pelvis is examined for any asymmetry. The examiner then places his or her thumbs on the patient's posterior superior iliac spines (Fig. 165-1). The patient is then asked to tuck his or her chin and then slowly bend forward at the waist (Fig. 165-2). If there is sacroiliac dysfunction, the side with the painful sacroiliac joint will elevate to reduce the stress on the affected sacroiliac joint. This will cause the examiner's thumb on the painful side to rise (Fig. 165-3).

If this maneuver reproduces the patient's pain, the test may be considered positive, and additional investigation, including plain radiographs, computed tomography, and magnetic resonance imaging of the sacroiliac joint, is indicated.

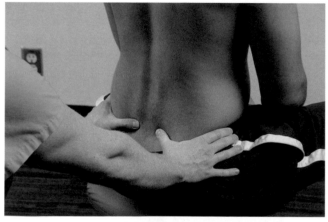

• **Figure 165-1** The Piedallu seated flexion test: the patient is placed in the seated position with the examiner seated behind the patient. The examiner places his or her thumbs over the patient's posterior superior iliac spines.

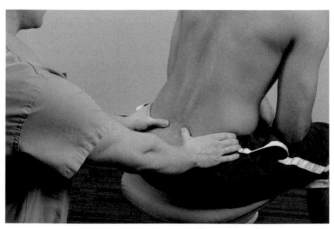

• **Figure 165-2** The Piedallu seated flexion test: the patient is then asked to tuck his or her chin and slowly bend forward at the waist.

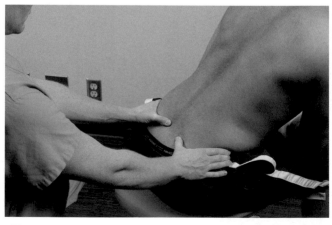

• **Figure 165-3** The Piedallu seated flexion test: as the patient bends forward, it places stress on the sacroiliac joints. The patient will elevate the sacroiliac joint on the affected side in an effort to relieve the stress and resulting pain emanating from the painful joint. This will cause the examiner's thumb to rise.

To perform the Stork test to determine if there is dysfunction of the sacroiliac joint, the patient is placed in the standing position with examiner seated behind the patient. The pelvis is examined for any asymmetry. The examiner then places one thumb on the patient's posterior superior iliac spine and the other thumb on the base of the sacrum (Fig. 166-1). The patient is then asked to flex his or her hip and knee on the nonpainful side to at least 90 degrees while standing on the contralateral leg (Fig. 166-2). If there is no sacroiliac dysfunction, as the patient flexes his or her hip and knee, the thumb on the patient's posterior superior iliac spine of the flexed leg will drop as the ilium rotates in a dorsocaudal direction to brace the pelvis to aid the other leg in receiving the full weight of the upper body (Fig. 166-3). If there is hypomobility of the sacroiliac joint on the painful side, the posterior superior iliac spine of the flexed leg will not drop, as the ilium is unable to rotate in a dorsocaudal direction to brace the pelvis.

If this maneuver reproduces the patient's pain, the test may be considered positive, and additional investigation, including plain radiographs, computed tomography, and magnetic resonance imaging of the sacroiliac joint, is indicated.

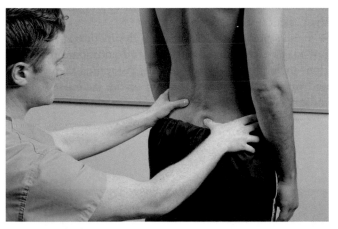

• **Figure 166-1** The Stork test: the patient is placed in the standing position with the examiner seated behind the patient. The examiner places one thumb on the patient's posterior superior iliac spine and the other thumb on the base of the sacrum.

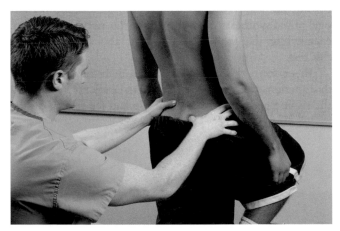

• **Figure 166-2** The Stork test: the patient is then asked to flex his or her hip and knee on the nonpainful side to at least 90 degrees while standing on the contralateral leg.

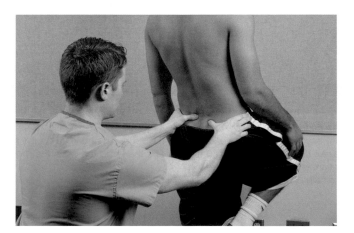

• **Figure 166-3** The Stork test: if there is no sacroiliac dysfunction, as the patient flexes his or her hip and knee, the thumb on the patient's posterior superior iliac spine of the flexed leg will drop as the ilium rotates in a dorsocaudal direction to brace the pelvis to aid the other leg in receiving the full weight of the upper body.

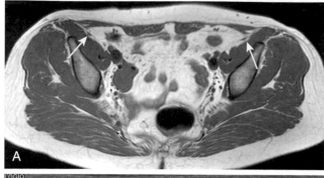

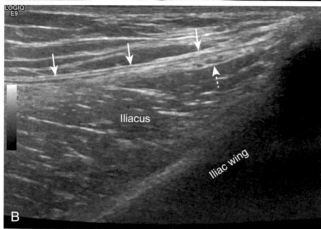

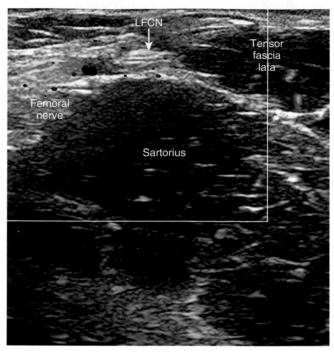

• Figure 171-4 Ultrasound imaging can also aid in the diagnosis and provide accurate guidance for blockade of the lateral femoral cutaneous nerve with local anesthetic, which can also serve as a diagnostic and therapeutic maneuver.

• Figure 171-3 A, Axial T1-weighted magnetic resonance image demonstrating the lateral cutaneous nerve of the thigh on both sides *(arrows),* lying on the surface of the iliacus muscle just proximal to the level of the inguinal ligament. **B,** An oblique ultrasound image in a different subject shows the round nerve *(broken arrow)* lying on the surface of the iliacus muscle immediately deep to the echo-bright inguinal ligament *(arrows).*

whereas patients with meralgia paresthetica have no back pain and no motor or reflex changes. The sensory changes of meralgia paresthetica are limited to the distribution of the lateral femoral cutaneous nerve and should not extend below the knee. It should be remembered that lumbar radiculopathy and lateral femoral cutaneous nerve entrapment may coexist as the so-called double crush syndrome. Occasionally, diabetic femoral neuropathy produces anterior thigh pain, which can confuse the diagnosis.

Electromyography helps to distinguish lumbar radiculopathy and diabetic femoral neuropathy from meralgia paresthetica. Plain radiographs of the back, hip, and pelvis are indicated for all patients who present with meralgia paresthetica to rule out occult bony pathology. On the basis of the patient's clinical presentation, additional testing, including complete blood count, uric acid, sedimentation rate, and antinuclear antibody testing, might be indicated. Magnetic resonance imaging of the spine and pelvis is indicated if herniated disc, spinal stenosis, or a space-occupying lesion is suspected and to help identify the cause of entrapment of the lateral femoral cutaneous nerve. Ultrasound imaging can also aid in the diagnosis and provide accurate guidance for blockade of the lateral femoral cutaneous nerve with local anesthetic, which can also serve as a diagnostic and therapeutic maneuver.

SECTION 9

The Hip

The hip is a ball-and-socket joint that comprises the femoral head and the cup-shaped acetabulum (Fig. 172-1). The femoral head is completely covered with hyaline cartilage except for a central area called the fovea, which is the point of attachment for the ligamentum teres. In contradistinction to its homolog, the glenoid fossa of the shoulder, which is very shallow, the acetabulum, which comprises the confluence of the ilium, ischium, and pubic bones, is much deeper. This deeper, cup-shaped configuration of the acetabulum adds much stability to the hip joint when compared with the shoulder, whose stability is primarily from the ligaments and labrum. The cup of the acetabulum is endowed with a horseshoe-shaped articular cartilage with the open portion of the horseshoe allowing passage of the ligamentum teres (Fig. 172-2). Within the ligamentum teres is the central branch of the obturator artery, which

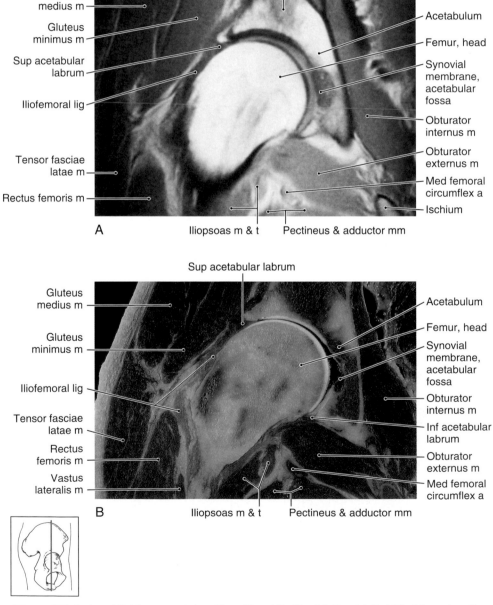

• **Figure 172-1 A** and **B,** Hip, coronal view. (From Kang HS, Ahn JM, Resnick D: *MRI of the extremities,* ed 2, Philadelphia, 2002, Saunders, p 226.)

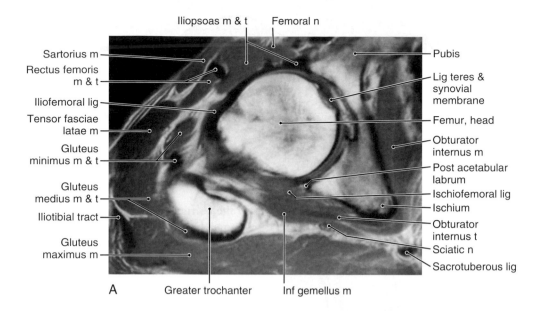

Iliopsoas m & t — Femoral n

Sartorius m —
Rectus femoris m & t —
Iliofemoral lig —
Tensor fasciae latae m —
Gluteus minimus m & t —
Gluteus medius m & t —
Iliotibial tract —
Gluteus maximus m —

Pubis
Lig teres & synovial membrane
Femur, head
Obturator internus m
Post acetabular labrum
Ischiofemoral lig
Ischium
Obturator internus t
Sciatic n
Sacrotuberous lig

A — Greater trochanter — Inf gemellus m

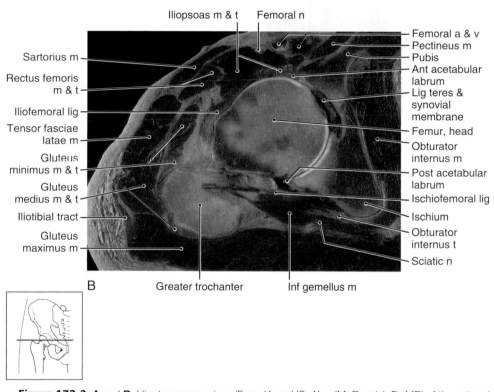

Iliopsoas m & t — Femoral n

Sartorius m —
Rectus femoris m & t —
Iliofemoral lig —
Tensor fasciae latae m —
Gluteus minimus m & t —
Gluteus medius m & t —
Iliotibial tract —
Gluteus maximus m —

Femoral a & v
Pectineus m
Pubis
Ant acetabular labrum
Lig teres & synovial membrane
Femur, head
Obturator internus m
Post acetabular labrum
Ischiofemoral lig
Ischium
Obturator internus t
Sciatic n

B — Greater trochanter — Inf gemellus m

• **Figure 172-2** **A** and **B,** Hip, transverse view. (From Kang HS, Ahn JM, Resnick D: *MRI of the extremities,* ed 2, Philadelphia, 2002, Saunders, p 240.)

provides blood supply to the fovea of the femoral head. This blood supply is very susceptible to disruption from trauma and, if compromised, may cause avascular osteonecrosis of the femoral head (Fig. 172-3).

The femoral head is connected to the femoral shaft by the neck of the femur, which in health forms an angle of 125 to 140 degrees with the femoral shaft and serves to align the femoral head in the coronal plane with the femoral condyles in the standing adult. There are 2 major bony outcroppings at the junction of the femoral neck and shaft of the femur: the greater trochanter and the lesser trochanter. The greater trochanter on the lateral femoral neck serves as the attachment point for the gluteal muscles, and the medially situated lesser trochanter serves as the attachment point for the hip adductors (see Fig. 172-3).

The hip joint is further strengthened by a fibrous articular capsule and a trio of ligaments: the iliofemoral, ischiofemoral, and pubofemoral ligaments. The iliofemoral

Careful palpation of the hip joint and surrounding structures should be the next step after visual inspection of the hip in examining the patient who presents with hip pain and dysfunction. Because of the overlying muscles and soft tissue, direct palpation of the hip joint is difficult, even in thin individuals.

Palpation of the hip must be carried out with the patient undressed to avoid missing physical signs, such as increased temperature, that could be masked by clothing. The anterior, lateral, and posterior aspects of the hip as well as the inguinal region should be palpated for abnormal mass, swelling, increased temperature, joint effusion, and bony abnormalities.

Targeted palpation of the bursae of the hip with particular attention to the ischial and trochanteric bursae will allow the examiner to identify inflamed and painful bursae that may serve as either a primary or contributing cause of the patient's hip pain and dysfunction (Fig. 174-1). Targeted palpation of the inguinal region assists the examiner in identifying inguinal hernia that may also be contributing to the patient's hip pain and dysfunction. The examiner should also assess the hip for the presence of joint instability and crepitus that might be suggestive of tendinitis, adhesive capsulitis, or arthritis.

Positive findings during the palpation of the hip should help guide the examiner in additional physical examination as well as provide a guide as to the ordering of specialized plain radiographic views, ultrasound imaging, and magnetic resonance imaging to further ascertain the cause of the patient's hip pain and dysfunction.

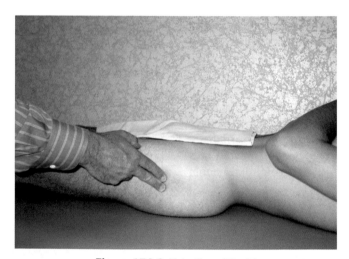

• **Figure 174-1** Palpation of the hip.

175 Flexion of the Hip

To assess hip flexion, the patient is placed in the supine position with the knee flexed to 90 degrees (Fig. 175-1). The patient is then asked to maximally flex his or her hips (Fig. 175-2). The normal hip will flex to approximately 135 degrees with the knee flexed to 90 degrees and the knee fully extended to approximately 90 degrees. Hip flexion deformities are not uncommon findings in patients with chronically painful hips. The Thomas flexion deformity test can help the clinician identify occult hip flexion deformities (see Chapter 182).

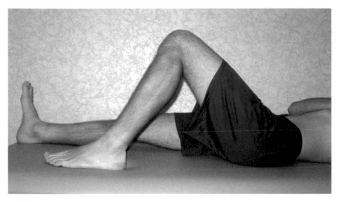

• **Figure 175-1** Patient positioning for assessment of hip flexion.

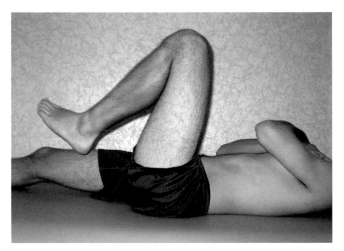

• **Figure 175-2** Maximum flexion of the hip.

Flexion contractures of the hip are not uncommon in patients who suffer from chronic hip pain and dysfunction. The Thomas test for flexion deformity will aid the clinician in identifying these sometimes unrecognized flexion contractures of the hip.

To perform the Thomas test for flexion deformity of the hip, the patient is placed in the supine position on the examination table. The patient is then asked to fully flex the thigh of the leg that is not being tested against the abdomen (Fig. 182-1, A). This position will eliminate any compensatory lumbar hyperlordosis. The patient is then asked to place the leg being tested against the examination table. Failure to fully extend the leg against the table suggests the presence of a flexion contracture of the hip (Figs. 182-1, B, and 182-2). When this occurs, the Thomas test is considered positive.

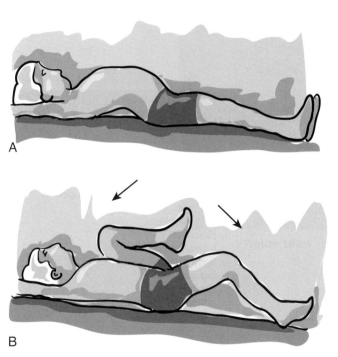

• **Figure 182-1 A** and **B,** Thomas test for flexion deformity of the hip.

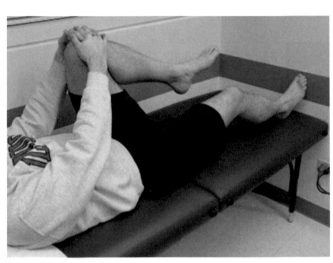

• **Figure 182-2** Positive Thomas test. Note how the lumbar spine is forced flat against the table by the flexion of the hip of the nonpainful side. The patient is unable to fully extend his leg against the table due to flexion contracture of the hip. (From Benjamin A. Hasan: The presenting symptoms, differential diagnosis, and physical examination of patients presenting with hip pain, *Disease-a-Month* 58(9):477–491, 2012, fig 6.)

183 The Trendelenburg Test for Weak Hip Abductors

The Trendelenburg test will allow the clinician to identify patients in whom weak hip abductors are the cause of, or a contributing factor to, the patient's hip pain and hip dysfunction. To perform the Trendelenburg test for weak hip abductors, the patient is asked to assume the standing position and balance on the unaffected leg. The patient is then asked to slowly flex the other knee to 45 degrees while the clinician carefully observes the pelvis. If the pelvis rises on the side with the raised knee, the Trendelenburg test is negative, as the raising of the pelvis indicates adequate hip abductor strength (Fig. 183-1, *A*). If the pelvis drops on the side with the raised knee, then the Trendelenburg test is positive and is indicative of weak hip abductors on that side (Figs. 183-1, *B*, and 183-2).

Patients who exhibit a positive Trendelenburg sign will invariably have an abnormal gait that is manifested clinically as a limp, with the patient swaying the body over the side of the weak abductors to help maintain balance. This abnormal gait is known as a Trendelenburg or abductor gait. If the patient has concomitant pain, the patient might also exhibit an antalgic gait, which can further confuse the clinical picture (see Chapter 184).

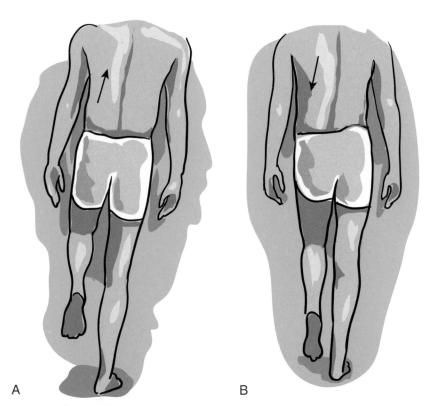

A   B

• **Figure 183-1 A** and **B,** Trendelenburg test for weak hip abductors.

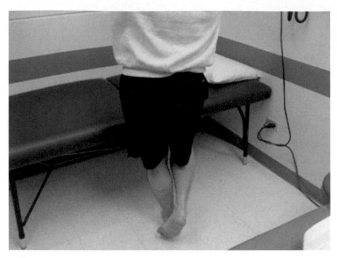

• **Figure 183-2** Positive Trendelenberg test. Note that the right hip drops due to left adductor weakness. (From Benjamin A. Hasan: The presenting symptoms, differential diagnosis, and physical examination of patients presenting with hip pain, *Disease-a-Month* 58(9):477–491, 2012, fig 4.)

184 The Hopalong Cassidy Sign for Antalgic Gait

Assessment of gait abnormalities can provide the clinician with valuable information as to the nature of a patient's hip pain and dysfunction. Although in theory gait assessment is relatively straightforward, in practice, because of the overlapping physical findings, gait assessment can be somewhat more difficult. One of the common confusing factors in assessing abnormal gait is the superimposed sign of an antalgic or painful gait.

To understand gait assessment, the clinician must understand the two components of normal gait: (1) the stance phase and (2) the swing phase. The stance phase begins when the heel strikes the floor and ends with the lift-off of the toes from the floor (Fig. 184-1, *A*). The swing phase begins with toe lift-off from the floor and ends with heel strike (Fig. 184-1, *B*).

Patients with a painful hip will often exhibit a positive Hopalong Cassidy sign, which is synonymous with an antalgic gait. The sign is named after the hero of numerous Western books, movies, and a television show who was named Hopalong due to his antalgic gait after being shot in the leg (Fig. 184-2). To elicit the Hopalong Cassidy sign for antalgic gait, the patient is asked to stand and bear weight on both legs and then to walk away from the examiner. If the patient's hip is painful, the patient will automatically attempt to shorten the stance phase to minimize the amount of time that the painful hip is bearing the weight of the upper body (Fig. 184-3). The attempt by the patient to hurry off the painful hip produces a positive Hopalong Cassidy sign due to the characteristic antalgic gait (Fig. 184-4).

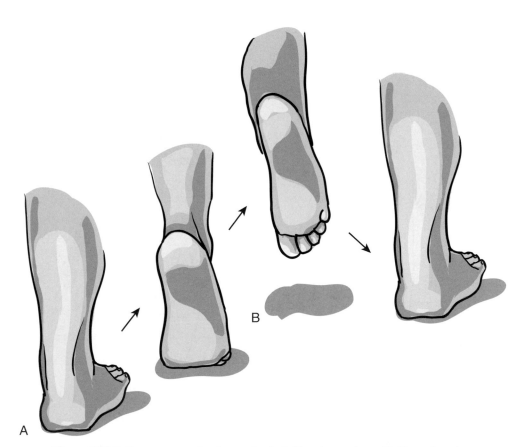

• **Figure 184-1** Two components of normal gait. **A,** The stance phase. **B,** The swing phase.

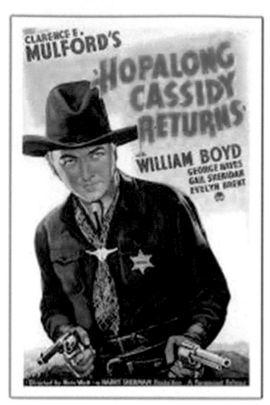

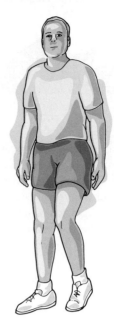

• **Figure 184-3** The Hopalong Cassidy sign. With a painful hip, the stance phase of gait is shortened. Hip extension is avoided by keeping the joint in a slightly flexed position. This slight flexion creates a functional leg length discrepancy with shortening on the involved side and may partially create a lurch.

• **Figure 184-2** Movie poster from 1936 depicting Hopalong Cassidy. Note his antalgic gait as he shortens his stance phase as he stares down an outlaw.

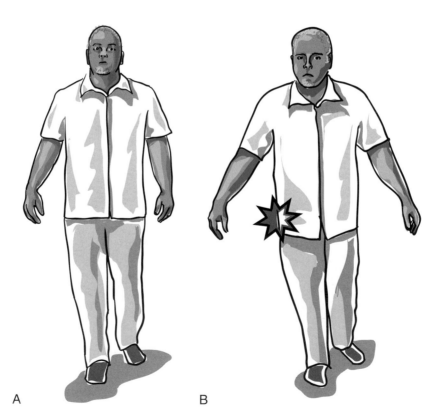

A   B

• **Figure 184-4** **A** and **B,** Eliciting the Hopalong Cassidy sign.

The Patrick/FABER test for internal derangement allows the examiner to quickly identify the presence of hip pathology. FABER is an acronym that helps to remind the examiner that he or she is checking for limitation of pain of **F**lexion, **AB**duction and **E**xternal **R**otation. To perform the Patrick/FABER test, the patient is placed in the supine position and the knee and hip are flexed to 90 degrees (Fig. 185-1, *A*). The examiner then has the patient place the foot of his or her affected extremity on the opposite knee. The thigh is then slowly abducted and externally rotated toward the examination table (Fig. 185-1, *B*). The test is considered positive if the patient complains of groin pain or spasm or the examiner identifies limited range of motion of the hip (Video 185-1).

Plain radiographs of the hip and pelvis are indicated in all patients who exhibit a positive Patrick/FABER test to rule out occult bony pathology. On the basis of the patient's clinical presentation, additional testing, including complete blood count, uric acid, sedimentation rate, and antinuclear antibody testing, might be indicated. Magnetic resonance imaging or ultrasound scanning of the hip and pelvis is indicated if osteonecrosis of the femoral head or a space-occupying lesion is suspected. Blockade of the obturator nerve with local anesthetic can also serve as a diagnostic and therapeutic maneuver.

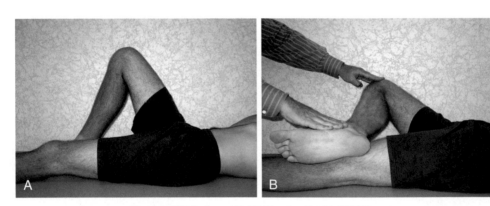

• **Figure 185-1 A** and **B,** Eliciting the Patrick/FABER test.

The musculotendinous unit of the hip joint that is responsible for hip adduction is susceptible to the development of tendinitis due to overuse or trauma from stretch injuries. Inciting factors may include the vigorous use of exercise equipment for lower-extremity strengthening and acute stretching of the musculotendinous units as a result of prolonged horseback riding or from straddle injuries. The pain of adductor tendinitis is sharp, constant, and severe, with sleep disturbance often reported. The patient may attempt to splint the inflamed tendons by adopting an adductor lurch type of gait, that is, shifting the trunk of the body over the affected extremity when walking. The pain of adductor tendinitis is primarily localized to the medial thigh at the groin crease, in contradistinction to the pain of iliopsoas bursitis, which is also made worse with resisted adduction but is localized to the anterior groin just below the groin crease (see Chapter 189).

On physical examination, the patient will report pain on palpation of the origins of the adductor tendons. Active resisted adduction reproduces the pain, as does passive abduction. Patients who suffer from adductor tendinitis will also exhibit a positive Waldman knee squeeze test. To perform the knee squeeze test, the patient is placed in the sitting position with the legs hanging over the edge of the examination table. A tennis ball is then placed between the patient's knees (Fig. 186-1). The patient is then asked to quickly squeeze the ball between the knees as hard as possible. Patients who are suffering from adductor tendinitis will reflexly extend the affected extremity because of the sudden pain from forced adduction, causing the knees to open and the tennis ball to fall (Fig. 186-2). The dropping of the tennis ball is considered a positive Waldman knee squeeze test for adductor tendinitis.

It is important for the clinician to remember that tendinitis of the musculotendinous unit of the hip frequently coexists with bursitis of the associated bursae of the hip joint, creating additional pain and functional disability. In addition to this pain, patients who suffer from adductor

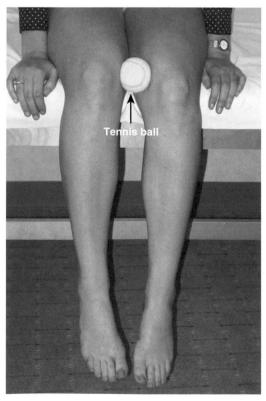

• **Figure 186-1** To perform the Waldman knee squeeze test for adductor tendinitis, the patient quickly squeezes the ball between the legs.

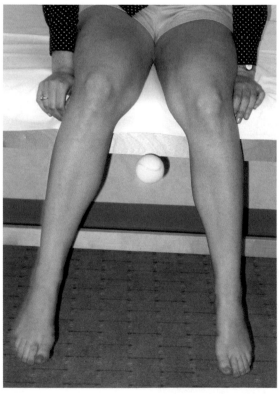

• **Figure 186-2** The Waldman knee squeeze test for adductor tendinitis.

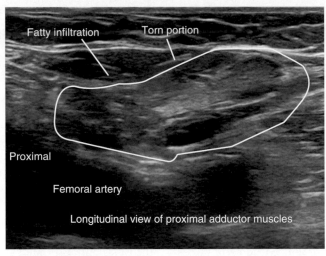

Fatty infiltration   Torn portion

Proximal

Femoral artery

Longitudinal view of proximal adductor muscles

• **Figure 186-3** Longitudinal ultrasound image demonstrating tearing of the proximal adductor muscles.

tendinitis often experience a gradual decrease in functional ability with decreasing hip range of motion, making simple, everyday tasks such as getting into or out of a car quite difficult. With continued disuse, muscle wasting can occur and an adhesive capsulitis of the hip may develop.

Plain radiographs are indicated for all patients who present with hip pain. On the basis of the patient's clinical presentation, additional testing may be indicated, including complete blood count, sedimentation rate, and antinuclear antibody testing. Magnetic resonance imaging and ultrasound scanning of the hip and the proximal adductor muscles is indicated if aseptic necrosis of the hip, occult mass, or tearing of the adductor muscles are suspected (Fig. 186-3).

The ischial bursa lies between the gluteus maximus muscle and the bone of the ischial tuberosity. It may exist as a single bursal sac or, in some patients, as a multisegmented series of sacs that may be loculated in nature. The ischial bursa is vulnerable to injury from both acute trauma and repeated microtrauma. Acute injuries frequently take the form of direct trauma to the bursa from falls directly onto the buttocks and from overuse, such as prolonged riding of horses or bicycles. Running on uneven or soft surfaces such as sand also may cause ischial bursitis. If the inflammation of the ischial bursa becomes chronic, calcification of the bursa may occur.

The patient who is suffering from ischial bursitis frequently complains of pain at the base of the buttock with ambulation. The pain is localized to the area over the ischial tuberosity with referred pain noted into the hamstring muscle, which also may develop coexistent tendinitis. Often the patient is unable to sleep on the affected hip and may complain of a sharp, "catching" sensation when extending and flexing the hip, especially on first awakening. Physical examination may reveal point tenderness over the ischial tuberosity. Passive straight leg raising of the affected lower extremity reproduces the pain. Patients who suffer from ischial bursitis will exhibit a positive resisted hip extension test. To perform the resisted hip extension test for ischial bursitis, the patient is placed in the prone position on the edge of the examination table. The examiner firmly grasps the thigh of the affected extremity and has the patient forcefully extend his or her hip against the examiner's resistance

(Fig. 187-1). The resisted hip extension test for ischial bursitis is considered positive if this maneuver causes a reproduction of the patient's pain that is localized to the base of the buttock. Sudden release of resistance during this maneuver will markedly increase the pain and further strengthen the clinical diagnosis of ischial bursitis (Video 187-1).

Plain radiographs of the hip may reveal calcification of the bursa and associated structures that is consistent with chronic inflammation. Magnetic resonance imaging and ultrasound scanning is indicated if disruption of the hamstring musculotendinous unit is suspected as well as to confirm the diagnosis of ischial bursitis (Fig. 187-2).

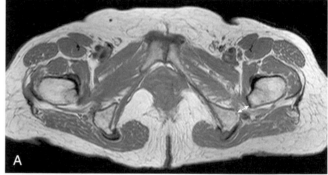
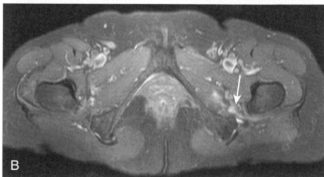

• **Figure 187-2 A,** Axial T1W magnetic resonance image of a middle-aged woman with poorly localized hip pain demonstrates reduced space between the lesser trochanter and the ischium on the left side *(double-headed white arrow)* due to ischiofemoral impingement. **B,** The axial FST2W magnetic resonance image shows high-SI edema within the quadratus femoris muscle and adjacent ischiogluteal bursa *(white arrow).* (From Waldman SD, Campbell, RSD: *Imaging of pain,* Philadelphia, 2010, Saunders/Elsevier, p 350, fig 173-3.)

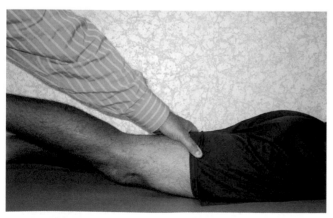

• **Figure 187-1** The resisted hip extension test for ischial bursitis.

The gluteal bursae lie between the gluteal maximus, medius, and minimus muscles as well as between these muscles and the underlying bone. These bursae may exist as a single bursal sac or, in some patients, as a multisegmented series of sacs that may be loculated in nature.

The gluteal bursae are vulnerable to injury from both acute trauma and repeated microtrauma. Acute injuries frequently take the form of direct trauma to the bursae from falls directly onto the buttocks or repeated intramuscular injections, as well as from overuse such as running for long distances, especially on soft or uneven surfaces. If the inflammation of the gluteal bursae becomes chronic, calcification of the bursae may occur.

The patient who suffers from gluteal bursitis frequently complains of pain in the upper outer quadrant of the buttock. The pain is localized to the area over the upper outer quadrant of the buttock with referred pain noted into the sciatic notch. Often the patient is unable to sleep on the affected hip and may complain of a sharp, "catching" sensation when extending and abducting the hip, especially on first awakening. Physical examination may reveal point tenderness in the upper outer quadrant of the buttock. Passive flexion and adduction may reproduce the pain.

Patients who suffer from gluteal bursitis will exhibit a resisted hip abduction test. To perform the resisted hip abduction test, the patient is asked to assume the lateral position with the unaffected leg down. The examiner then firmly grabs the lateral thigh of the affected leg and has the patient forcefully abduct the affected leg against the examiner's resistance (Fig. 188-1). The resisted hip abduction test is considered positive if this maneuver reproduces the patient's gluteal pain. Sudden release of resistance during this maneuver should markedly increase the pain of gluteal bursitis and further strengthens the diagnosis (Video 188-1).

Plain radiographs of the hip may reveal calcification of the bursa and associated structures that is consistent with chronic inflammation. Magnetic resonance imaging and ultrasound scanning is indicated if occult mass or tumor of the hip is suspected as well as to confirm the diagnosis.

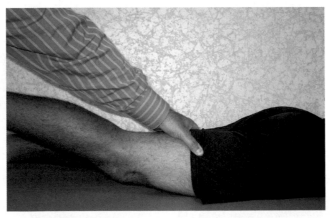

• **Figure 188-1** The resisted hip abduction test for gluteal bursitis.

The iliopsoas bursa lies medially in the femoral triangle between the psoas tendon and the anterior aspect of the neck of the femur (Fig. 189-1). This bursa may exist as a single bursal sac or, in some patients, as a multisegmented series of sacs that may be loculated in nature.

The iliopsoas bursa is vulnerable to injury from both acute trauma and repeated microtrauma. Acute injuries frequently take the form of direct trauma to the bursa from seat-belt injuries as well as from overuse injuries that required repeated hip flexion, such as javelin throwing and ballet dancing. If the inflammation of the iliopsoas bursa becomes chronic, calcification of the bursa may occur.

The patient who suffers from iliopsoas bursitis frequently complains of pain in the groin. The pain is localized to the area just below the crease of the groin anteriorly, with referred pain noted into the hip joint. The anterior location of the pain is in contradistinction to the pain of adductor tendinitis, in which the pain is localized to the medial thigh at the groin crease (see Chapter 186). Often, the patient with iliopsoas bursitis is unable to sleep on the affected hip and may complain of a sharp, "catching" sensation with range of motion of the hip.

Physical examination may reveal point tenderness in the upper thigh just below the crease of the groin. Passive flexion, adduction, and abduction as well as active resisted flexion of the affected lower extremity will reproduce the pain, as will the resisted adduction test for iliopsoas bursitis. To perform the resisted adduction test for iliopsoas bursitis, the patient is asked to assume the sitting position with his or her legs hanging over the edge of the examination table and the knees slightly apart. The examiner then firmly grasps the medial thigh of the affected extremity and instructs the patient to forcefully adduct the hip against the examiner's resistance (Fig. 189-2). The test is considered positive if this maneuver reproduces the patient's anterior groin pain. Sudden release of resistance during this maneuver markedly increases the anterior groin pain, which further strengthens the diagnosis of iliopsoas bursitis. If this maneuver causes the patient to experience medial groin pain, the diagnosis of adductor bursitis should be considered (Video 189-1).

Plain radiographs of the hip may reveal calcification of the bursa and associated structures that is consistent with chronic inflammation. Magnetic resonance imaging and ultrasound scanning is indicated if occult mass or tumor of the hip or groin is suspected as well as to confirm the diagnosis.

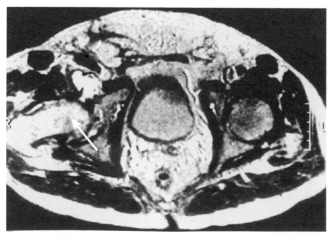

• **Figure 189-1** Iliopsoas bursitis. Axial T2-weighted magnetic resonance image in a 67-year-old woman with rheumatoid arthritis and right hip pain. High-signal mass is noted adjacent to the iliopsoas muscle *(arrow),* consistent with an iliopsoas bursitis. (From Kaplan PA, Helms CA, Dussault R, et al: *Musculoskeletal MRI,* Philadelphia, 2001, Saunders, p 350.)

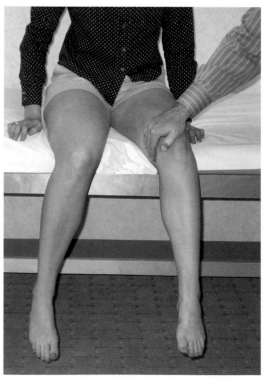

• **Figure 189-2** The resisted hip adduction test for iliopsoas bursitis.

An uncommon cause of sciatica, piriformis syndrome is caused by entrapment and compression of the sciatic nerve by the piriformis muscle at the level of the sciatic notch (Fig. 190-1). Patients suffering from piriformis syndrome complain of pain that begins in the buttocks and radiates into the affected leg all the way to the foot. There is associated numbness and dysesthesias as well as weakness in the distribution of the sciatic nerve. To perform the piriformis test for piriformis syndrome, the patient is placed in the supine position and the symptomatic lower extremity is flexed at the hip to 90 degrees (Fig. 190-2). The examiner then pushes the patient's knee on the symptomatic side upward and inward toward the patient's opposite shoulder (Fig. 190-3). If this maneuver reproduces the patient's pain, the test may be considered positive, and additional investigation, including plain radiographs, computerized tomography, ultrasonography, and magnetic resonance imaging of the sacroiliac joint is indicated.

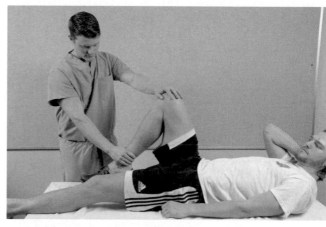

• **Figure 190-2** The patient is placed in the supine position and the symptomatic lower extremity is flexed at the hip to 90 degrees.

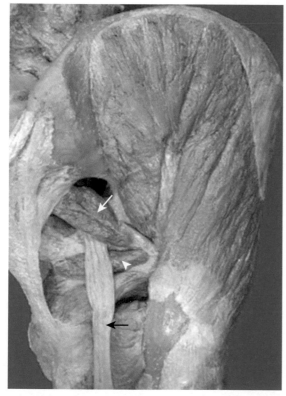

• **Figure 190-1** Posterior view of the right gluteal region. The sciatic nerve *(black arrow)* passes through the infrapiriform foramen, bordered superiorly by the piriformis muscle *(white arrow)* and inferiorly by the portion of the obturator internus muscle that is outside the pelvis *(arrowhead)*.

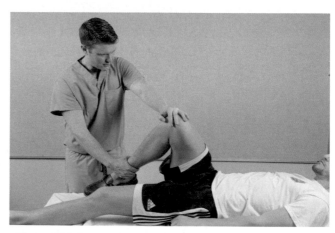

• **Figure 190-3** The examiner then pushes the patient's knee on the symptomatic side upward and inward toward the patient's opposite shoulder.

The trochanteric bursa lies between the greater trochanter and the tendon of the gluteus medius and the iliotibial tract (Fig. 191-1). This bursa may exist as a single bursal sac or, in some patients, as a multisegmented series of sacs that may be loculated in nature.

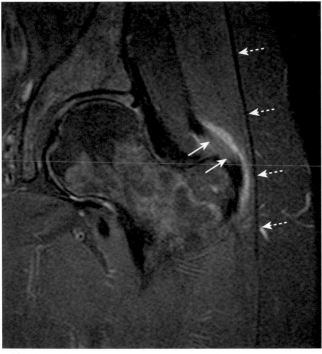

• **Figure 191-1** Coronal T2 magnetic resonance (MR) image of a patient with trochanteric bursitis. Note the high signal intensity fluid lying between the iliotibial tract *(broken arrows)* and the gluteus minimus tendon *(solid arrows)*. (From Waldman SD, Campbell, RSD: *Imaging of pain,* Philadelphia, 2010, Saunders/Elsevier, p 362, fig 142-2.)

The trochanteric bursa is vulnerable to injury from both acute trauma and repeated microtrauma. Acute injuries frequently take the form of direct trauma to the bursa via falls directly onto the greater trochanter or from previous hip surgery, as well as from overuse injuries, including running on soft or uneven surfaces. If the inflammation of the trochanteric bursa becomes chronic, calcification of the bursa may occur.

The patient who suffers from trochanteric bursitis frequently complains of pain in the lateral hip that can radiate down the leg, mimicking sciatica. The pain is localized to the area over the greater trochanter. Often, the patient is unable to sleep on the affected hip and may complain of a sharp, "catching" sensation with range of motion of the hip, especially on first rising. The patient might note that walking upstairs is increasingly difficult. Trochanteric bursitis often coexists with arthritis of the hip joint, back and sacroiliac joint disease, and gait disturbance.

Physical examination may reveal point tenderness in the lateral thigh just over the greater trochanter. Passive adduction and abduction, as well as active resisted abduction of the affected lower extremity, reproduces the pain. Patients suffering from trochanteric bursitis will also exhibit a positive resisted abduction release test. To perform the resisted abduction release test, the examiner has the patient assume the lateral position with the unaffected leg down. The examiner then firmly grasps the lateral thigh and has the patient abduct the hip against the examiner's resistance (Fig. 191-2, *A*). The examiner then suddenly releases the resistance against the patient's active abduction. This sudden release of resistance during this maneuver will markedly increase the pain in the lateral thigh over the greater trochanter if the patient suffers from trochanteric bursitis (Fig. 191-2, *B*). This sudden increase in localized

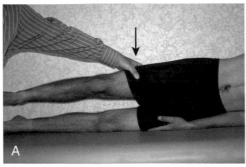
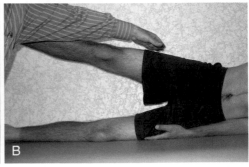

• **Figure 191-2 A** and **B,** The resisted abduction release test.

lateral thigh pain is considered a positive resisted abduction release test.

The clinician should be aware that patients who suffer from trochanteric bursitis should exhibit no sensory deficit in the distribution of the lateral femoral cutaneous nerve, as is seen with meralgia paresthetica, which is often confused with trochanteric bursitis.

Plain radiographs of the hip may reveal calcification of the bursa and associated structures that is consistent with chronic inflammation. Magnetic resonance imaging and ultrasound scanning is indicated if occult mass or tumor of the hip or groin is suspected. Electromyography helps to distinguish trochanteric bursitis from meralgia paresthetica and sciatica.

Stress fractures of the femur are a not uncommon cause of thigh pain in runners, military recruits, and in patients suffering from osteoporosis. These fractures are often initially misdiagnosed, as plain radiographs of the femur are often read as negative (Fig. 192-1). The fulcrum test is highly sensitive in identifying stress fractures of the femur. To perform the fulcrum test, the patient is placed in the sitting position, and the examiner places his or her arm beneath the patient's painful lower extremity and grasps the contralateral thigh (Fig. 192-2). The examiner's arm serves

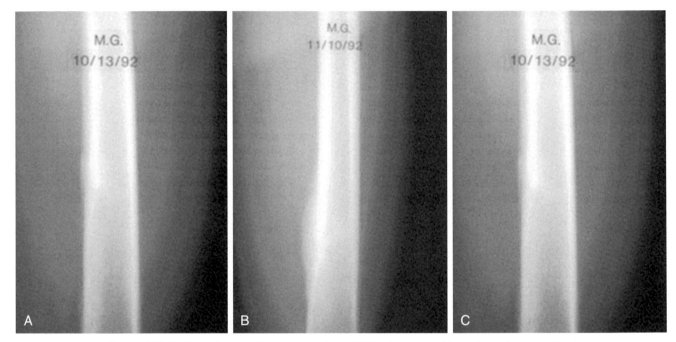

• **Figure 192-1** Femoral stress fractures are often initially missed on plain radiographs, as a classic fracture line may not be evident. **A,** Initial radiograph from an athlete suspected of having a distal femoral stress fracture. **B** and **C,** Radiographs reveal progressive stages of healing in the stress fracture of the distal femoral cortex after initial radiograph was obtained. (From DeFranco MJ, Recht M, Schils J, Parker RD: Stress fractures of the femur in athletes, *Clin Sports Med* 25(1):89–103, 2006, fig 5.)

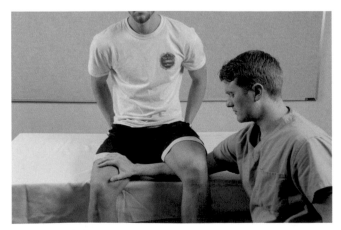

• **Figure 192-2** The patient is placed in the sitting position, and the examiner places his or her arm beneath the patient's painful lower extremity and grasps the contralateral thigh.

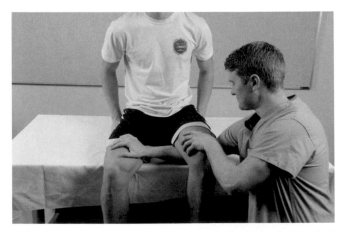

• **Figure 192-3** The examiner then grasps the thigh of the painful lower extremity and exerts a firm downward pressure, which increases stress on the shaft of the femur.

as a fulcrum. The examiner then grasps the thigh of the painful lower extremity and exerts a firm downward pressure, which increases stress on the shaft of the femur (Fig. 192-3). If there is a stress fracture present, the patient will experience a reproduction or exacerbation of their thigh pain and will often exhibit apprehension as the downward pressure is applied. The test can be repeated as the examiner moves his or her arm more proximally to further localize the site of the fracture.

Contracture of the iliotibial band, which is an extension of the deep fascia of the thigh, can occur following trauma of acute inflammation of the iliotibial band (Fig. 193-1). Such contractures can lead to difficulty in hip adduction and can make getting into and out of a car extremely difficult. The Ober test for iliotibial band contracture is performed by having the patient assume the lateral position with the unaffected extremity on the bottom with the hip and the knee flexed to eliminate lumbar lordosis.

The affected leg is then extended and fully abducted (Fig. 193-2, *A*). The examiner then slowly allows the extremity to passively adduct while he or she gently supports the weight of the extremity against gravity. If there is contracture of the iliotibial band, the affected extremity will not completely drop back toward the examination table and will remain partially abducted after the examiner removes his or her supporting hands (Fig. 193-2, *B*).

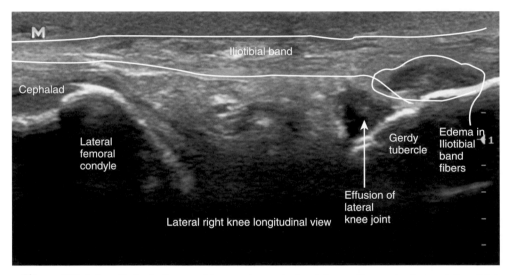

• **Figure 193-1** Longitudinal ultrasound image demonstrating inflammation and edema of the distal iliotibial band.

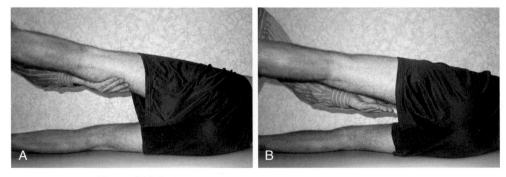

• **Figure 193-2 A** and **B,** The Ober test for iliotibial band contracture.

Snapping hip syndrome is a constellation of symptoms that includes a snapping sensation in the lateral hip associated with sudden, sharp pain in the area of the greater trochanter. The snapping sensation and pain are the result of the iliopsoas tendon subluxing over the greater trochanter or iliopectineal eminence. The symptoms of snapping hip syndrome occur most commonly when the patient rises from a sitting to a standing position or when walking briskly. Often trochanteric bursitis coexists with snapping hip syndrome, further increasing the patient's pain and disability.

Physical examination reveals that the patient can recreate the snapping and pain by moving from a sitting to a standing position and adducting the hip. Point tenderness over the trochanteric bursa that is indicative of trochanteric bursitis also is often present. Patients who suffer from the snapping hip syndrome will exhibit a positive snap test. To perform the snap test for snapping hip syndrome, the patient is asked to assume the squatting position or, if unable to squat, to sit in a straight-backed chair. The examiner then places his or her hand over the greater trochanter and has the patient quickly move from the squatting or sitting position to a standing position (Fig. 194-1, *A*). The snap test for snapping hip syndrome is considered positive if the examiner can appreciate a snapping sensation as the iliopsoas tendon subluxes over the greater trochanter or iliopectineal eminence (Fig. 194-1, *B*). In some severe cases, the examiner will also hear an audible snap.

Plain radiographs are indicated in all patients who present with pain that is thought to be emanating from the hip to rule out occult bony pathology and tumor. On the basis of the patient's clinical presentation, additional testing may be indicated, including complete blood count, prostate-specific antigen, sedimentation rate, and antinuclear antibody testing. Magnetic resonance, fluoroscopy (Fig. 194-2), and ultrasound imaging of the affected hip is indicated if occult mass or aseptic necrosis is suspected and to help confirm the diagnosis.

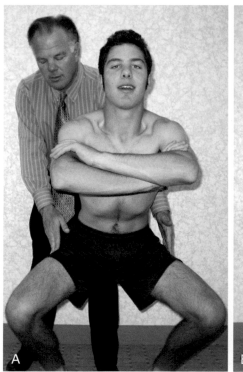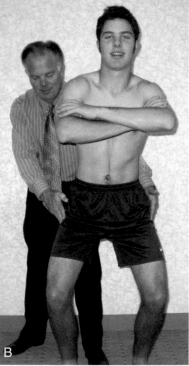

• **Figure 194-1 A** and **B,** Eliciting the snap sign.

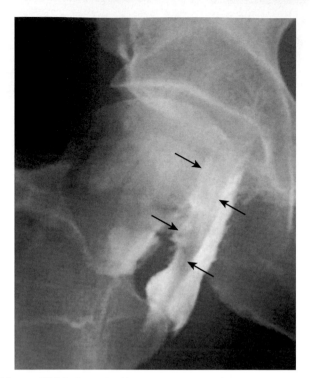

• **Figure 194-2** Snapping hip syndrome. Direct fluoroscopic injection into the tendon sheath outlines the tendon margins *(arrows)* before assessment for abnormal excursion. (From Lazarus ML: Imaging of femoroacetabular impingement and acetabular labral tears of the hip, *Dis Mon* 58(9):495–542, 2012, fig 26.)

SECTION 10

The Knee

Many clinicians approach examination of the knee with the idea that the knee is a relatively straightforward, simple hinge joint that flexes and extends. Nothing could be farther from the truth. The largest joint in the body in terms of articular surface and joint volume, the knee is capable of amazingly complex movements that encompass highly coordinated flexion and extension. The knee joint is best thought of as a cam that is capable of locking in a stable position. Even the simplest movements of the knee involve an elegantly coordinated set of rolling and gliding movements of the femur on the tibia. Because of the complex nature of these movements, the knee is extremely susceptible to functional abnormalities with relatively minor alterations in the anatomy from arthritis or damage to the cartilage or ligaments.

Although both clinicians and laypeople think of the knee joint as a single joint, from the viewpoint of understanding the functional anatomy, it is more helpful to think of the knee as 2 separate but interrelated joints: the femoral-tibial joint and the femoral-patellar joint (Fig. 195-1). The 2 joints share a common synovial cavity, and dysfunction of 1 joint can easily affect the function of the other.

The femoral-tibial joint is made up of the articulation of the femur and the tibia. Interposed between the 2 bones are 2 fibrocartilaginous structures known as the medial and lateral menisci (Fig. 195-2). The menisci help transmit the forces placed on the femur across the joint onto the tibia. The menisci have the property of plasticity in that they are able to change their shape in response to the variable forces placed on the joint through its complex range of motion. The medial and lateral menisci are relatively avascular and receive the bulk of their nourishment from the synovial fluid, which means that there is little potential for healing when these important structures are traumatized.

The primary function of the femoral-patellar joint is to use the patella, which is a large sesamoid bone embedded in the quadriceps tendon, to improve the mechanical advantage of the quadriceps muscle. The medial and lateral articular surfaces of the sesamoid interface with the articular groove of the femur (Fig. 195-3). In extension, only the superior pole of the patella is in contact with the articular surface of the femur. As the knee flexes, the patella is drawn superiorly into the trochlear groove of the femur.

The majority of the knee joint's stability comes from the ligaments and muscles surrounding it with little contribution from the bony elements. The main ligaments of the knee are the anterior and posterior cruciate ligaments, which provide much of the anteroposterior stability of the

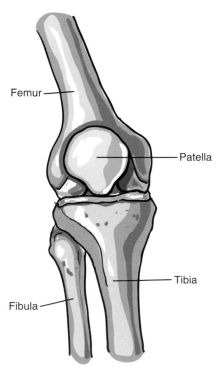

• **Figure 195-1** Functional anatomy of the knee is easier to understand if it is viewed as two separate but interrelated joints: the femoral-tibial and the femoral-patellar joints.

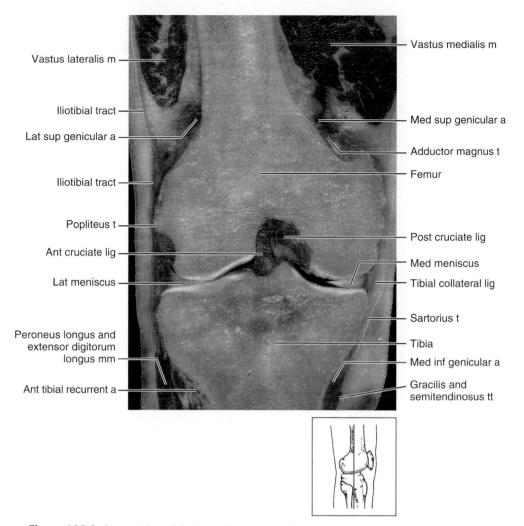

Vastus lateralis m

Iliotibial tract

Lat sup genicular a

Iliotibial tract

Popliteus t

Ant cruciate lig

Lat meniscus

Peroneus longus and
extensor digitorum
longus mm

Ant tibial recurrent a

Vastus medialis m

Med sup genicular a

Adductor magnus t

Femur

Post cruciate lig

Med meniscus

Tibial collateral lig

Sartorius t

Tibia

Med inf genicular a

Gracilis and
semitendinosus tt

• **Figure 195-2** Coronal view of the knee. (From Kang HS, Ahn JM, Resnick D: *MRI of the extremities.* Philadelphia, 2002, Saunders, p 301.)

knee, and the medial and lateral collateral ligaments, which provide much of the valgus and varus stability (Fig. 195-4). All of these ligaments also help prevent excessive rotation of the tibia in either direction. There are also a number of secondary ligaments that add further stability to this inherently unstable joint.

The main extensor of the knee is the quadriceps muscle, which attaches to the patella via the quadriceps tendon. Fibrotendinous expansions of the vastus medialis and vastus lateralis insert into the sides of the patella and are subject to strain and sprain. The hamstrings are the main flexors of the hip, with help from the gastrocnemius, sartorius, and gracilis muscles. Medial rotation of the flexed knee is via the medial hamstring muscle, and lateral rotation of the knee is controlled by the biceps femoris muscle.

The knee is well endowed with a variety of bursae to facilitate movement. Bursae are formed from synovial sacs whose purpose is to allow easy sliding of muscles and tendons across one another at areas of repeated movement (Fig. 195-5). These synovial sacs are lined with a synovial membrane that is invested with a network of blood vessels that secrete synovial fluid. Inflammation of the bursa results in an increase in the production of synovial fluid and swelling of the bursal sac. With overuse or misuse, these bursae may become inflamed, enlarged, and, on rare occasions, infected. Given that the knee shares a common synovial cavity, inflammation of one bursa can cause significant dysfunction and pain of the entire knee.

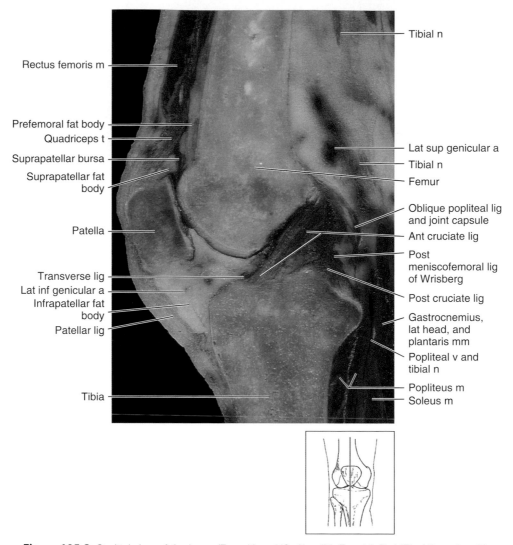

Rectus femoris m

Prefemoral fat body
Quadriceps t
Suprapatellar bursa
Suprapatellar fat body

Patella

Transverse lig
Lat inf genicular a
Infrapatellar fat body
Patellar lig

Tibia

Tibial n

Lat sup genicular a
Tibial n
Femur

Oblique popliteal lig and joint capsule
Ant cruciate lig
Post meniscofemoral lig of Wrisberg
Post cruciate lig
Gastrocnemius, lat head, and plantaris mm
Popliteal v and tibial n
Popliteus m
Soleus m

• **Figure 195-3** Sagittal view of the knee. (From Kang HS, Ahn JM, Resnick D: *MRI of the extremities.* Philadelphia, 2002, Saunders, p 341.)

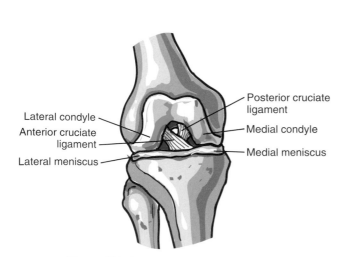

Lateral condyle
Anterior cruciate ligament
Lateral meniscus

Posterior cruciate ligament
Medial condyle
Medial meniscus

• **Figure 195-4** The main ligaments of the knee.

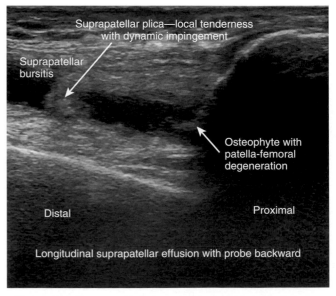

Suprapatellar plica—local tenderness with dynamic impingement
Suprapatellar bursitis
Osteophyte with patella-femoral degeneration
Distal
Proximal
Longitudinal suprapatellar effusion with probe backward

• **Figure 195-5** Longitudinal ultrasound image demonstrating suprapatellar bursitis. Note the suprapatellar plica.

Because of the lack of soft tissue overlying the knee joint, visual inspection can provide the clinician with important clues to the causes of knee pain and dysfunction. The starting point to visual inspection of the knee is an observation of the patient both standing and walking. The degree of valgus or varus of the knee with weight bearing should be noted, as should any other obvious bony deformity (Fig. 196-1). The clinician should then look for evidence of quadriceps wasting, which, if identified, can be quantified

with careful measurement at a point 12 cm above the upper margin of the patella with the knee fully extended. The presence of rubor above, below, or alongside the patella, which might suggest infection, swelling, or an inflammatory process (including bursitis and tendinitis), is also noted. The posterior knee is then inspected for the presence of a popliteal fossa mass that might suggest a Baker cyst (Fig. 196-2).

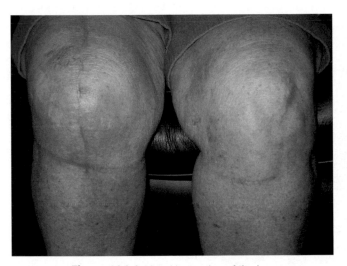

• **Figure 196-1** Visual inspection of the knee.

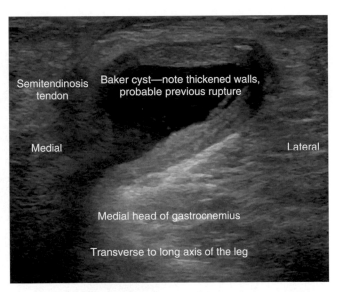

• **Figure 196-2** Transverse ultrasound imaged demonstrating a Baker cyst.

Careful palpation of the knee will often provide the examiner with valuable clues to the cause of the patient's knee pain and dysfunction. The examiner palpates the temperature of both knees, as a localized increase in temperature may indicate inflammation or infection. The presence of swelling in the suprapatellar, prepatellar, or infrapatellar regions that might suggest suprapatellar, prepatellar, or infrapatellar bursitis is then identified. Generalized joint effusion may be identified by performing the bulge test (see Chapter 202).

The bony elements of the knee, including the medial and lateral femoral condyles, the patella, and the tibial tubercle, are then palpated. The patellar tendon is then palpated to identify patellar tendinitis, or jumper's knee (Fig. 197-1). The popliteal fossa is then palpated for evidence of a mass or Baker cyst. The knee joint is then ranged through flexion, extension, and medial and lateral rotation to identify crepitus or limitation of range of motion.

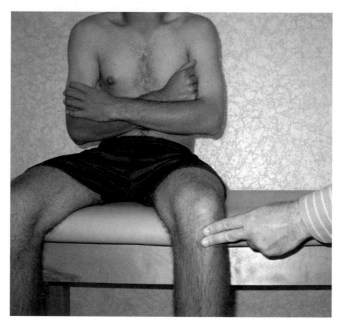

• **Figure 197-1** Palpation of the knee.

The patient is asked to assume the prone position on the examination table. The posterior knee joints are inspected for evidence of mass or swelling. The patient is then asked to actively flex the knee as far as it will flex (Fig. 198-1).

The degree of flexion is then compared with that of the opposite leg. The extent of flexion of the normal knee is limited by the soft tissues of the thigh, calf, and buttocks.

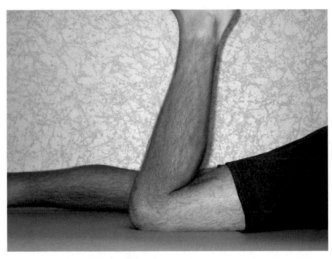

• **Figure 198-1** Flexion of the knee.

The patient is asked to sit on the edge of the examination table. The anterior knee joints are inspected for evidence of mass or swelling. The patient is then asked to actively extend the knee as far as it will extend (Fig. 199-1). The degree of extension is then compared with that of the opposite leg. The patient should be able to extend the knees to 0 degrees of flexion.

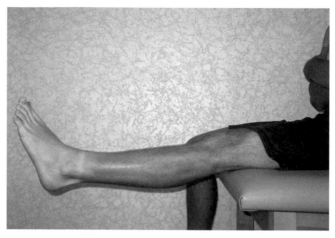

• **Figure 199-1** Extension of the knee.

The patient is asked to sit on the edge of the examination table. The anterior knee joints are inspected for evidence of mass or swelling. The patient is then asked to actively internally rotate the knee as far as possible (Fig. 200-1). The degree of internal rotation is compared with that of the opposite leg. The process is repeated with the patient externally rotating the knee. Pain on rotation is suggestive of medial or collateral ligament strain or sprain, medial meniscal tear, or bursitis of the knee (Fig. 200-2).

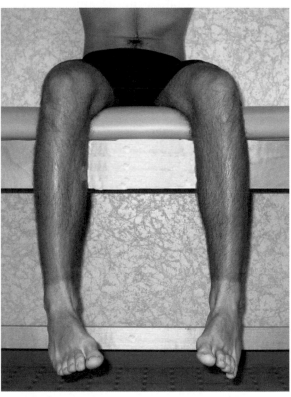

• **Figure 200-1** Internal rotation of the knee.

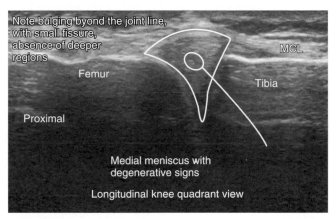

Note bulging byond the joint line, with small fissure, absence of deeper regions

MCL

Femur

Tibia

Proximal

Medial meniscus with degenerative signs

Longitudinal knee quadrant view

• **Figure 200-2** Longitudinal ultrasound image of the knee demonstrating degenerative changes of the medial meniscus. Note the bulging of the meniscus and displacement of the medial collateral ligament (MCL).

201 An Overview of Painful Conditions of the Knee

The initial general physical examination of the knee guides the clinician in narrowing his or her differential diagnosis and helps the clinician determine which specialized physical examination maneuvers, laboratory tests, and radiographic testing will aid in confirming the cause of the patient's knee pain and dysfunction. For the clinician to make the best use of the initial information that is gleaned from the general physical examination of the knee, a grouping of the common causes of knee pain and dysfunction is exceedingly helpful. Although no classification of knee pain and dysfunction can be absolute, because of the frequently overlapping and multifactoral nature of knee pathology, Table 201-1 should help improve the diagnostic accuracy of the clinician who

is confronted with a patient complaining of knee pain and dysfunction and will help the clinician avoid overlooking less common diagnoses.

The list in Table 201-1 is by no means comprehensive, but it does aid the clinician in organizing the potential sources of pathology that present as knee pain and dysfunction. It should be noted that the most commonly missed causes of knee pain that most often result in misadventures in diagnosis and treatment are systemic disease, sympathetically mediated pain, and pain that is referred from other body areas. The knowledge of this potential pitfall should help the clinician keep these sometimes overlooked causes of knee pain and dysfunction in the differential diagnosis.

TABLE 201-1 Most Common Causes of Knee Pain

Localized Bony or Joint Space Pathology	Periarticular Pathology	Systemic Disease	Sympathetically Mediated Pain	Referred from Other Body Areas
Fracture	Bursitis	Rheumatoid arthritis	Causalgia	Lumbar plexopathy
Primary bone tumor	Tendinitis	Collagen vascular disease	Reflex sympathetic dystrophy	Lumbar radiculopathy
Primary synovial tissue tumor	Adhesive capsulitis	Reiter syndrome		Lumbar spondylosis
Joint instability	Joint instability	Gout		Fibromyalgia
Localized arthritis	Muscle strain	Other crystal arthropathies		Myofascial pain syndromes
Osteophyte formation	Muscle sprain	Charcot neuropathic arthritis		Inguinal hernia
Joint space infection	Periarticular infection not involving joint space			Entrapment neuropathies
Hemarthrosis				Intrapelvic tumors
Villonodular synovitis				Retroperitoneal tumors
Intraarticular foreign body				
Osgood-Schlatter disease				
Chronic dislocation of the patella				
Patellofemoral pain syndrome				
Patella alta				

202 The Bulge Sign for Small Joint Effusions

The bulge sign is a useful indicator of joint effusion in the knee. To elicit the bulge sign, the patient is asked to assume the supine position on the examination table and fully extend and relax the affected knees. The examiner milks the effusion up into the suprapatellar area by moving the hand in an upward motion along the medial patellar margin (Fig. 202-1). The examiner then milks the fluid down from the suprapatellar region by milking along the lateral margin of the patella. Clinically significant joint effusions will form a bulge at the medial patellar margin.

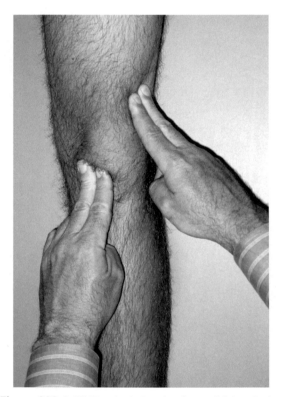

• **Figure 202-1** Eliciting the bulge sign for small joint effusions.

The ballottement test is a useful indicator of joint effusion in the knee. To perform the ballottement test, the patient is asked to assume the supine position on the examination table and fully extend and relax the knees. The examiner then grasps the affected knee just above the joint space and applies pressure, displacing synovial fluid from the suprapatellar pouch into the joint, which elevates the patella (Figs. 203-1, *A,* 203-2, *A,* and Fig. 203-3). The examiner then performs ballottement on the patella (Figs. 203-1, *B* and 203-2, *B*). The test is considered positive if the patella ballottes easily (Video 203-1).

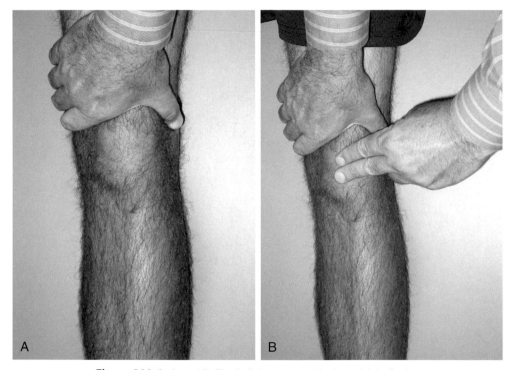

• **Figure 203-1 A** and **B,** The ballottement test for large joint effusions.

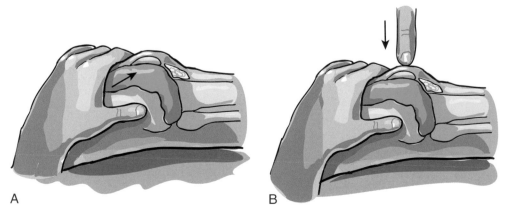

• **Figure 203-2** The ballottement test. **A,** The examiner displaces synovial fluid from the suprapatellar pouch into the joint. **B,** The examiner performs ballottement on the patella.

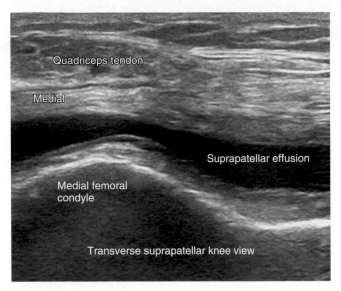

• **Figure 203-3** Longitudinal ultrasound image demonstrating a large suprapatellar effusion.

The valgus stress test provides the clinician with useful information regarding the integrity of the medial collateral ligaments (Fig. 204-1). To perform the valgus stress test, the patient is placed in a supine position on the examination table with the knee flexed 35 degrees and the entire affected extremity relaxed. The examiner places his or her hand above the knee to stabilize the thigh. With the other hand, the examiner forces the lower leg away from the midline while observing for widening of the medial joint compartment and pain (Fig. 204-2). The maneuver is repeated with the other lower extremity, and the results are compared.

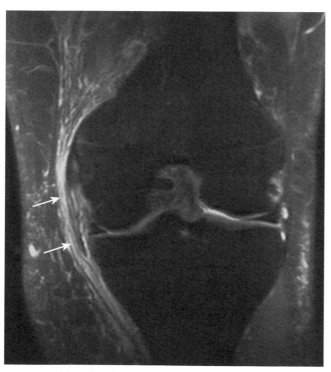

• **Figure 204-1** Coronal sagittal T2-weighted with fat suppression magnetic resonance image of an acute grade 2 tear of the medial collateral ligament with poorly defined ligament fibers and surrounding soft tissue edema. (From Waldman SD, Campbell RSD *Imaging of pain,* Philadelphia, 2010, Saunders/Elsevier, p 382, fig 149-3.)

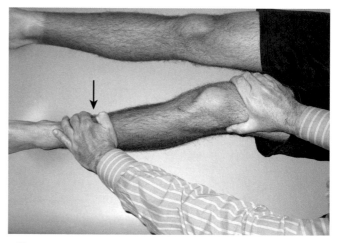

• **Figure 204-2** The valgus stress test for medial collateral ligament integrity. Pull in the direction of the arrow.

205 The Varus Stress Test for Lateral Collateral Ligament Integrity

The varus stress test provides the clinician with useful information regarding the integrity of the lateral collateral ligaments (Fig. 205-1). To perform the varus stress test, the patient is placed in a supine position on the examination table with the knee flexed 35 degrees and the entire affected extremity relaxed. The examiner places his or her hand above the knee to stabilize the thigh. With the other hand, the examiner forces the lower leg toward the midline while observing for widening of the medial joint compartment and pain (Fig. 205-2). The maneuver is repeated with the other lower extremity, and the results are compared.

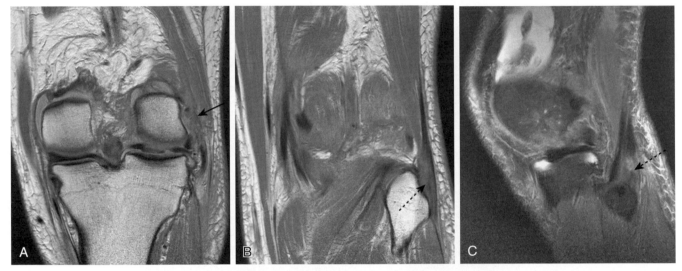

• **Figure 205-1** Magnetic resonance (MR) images of a patient with a combined lateral collateral ligament (LCL) and posterior cruciate ligament injury with lateral meniscal tear. **A,** The coronal protein-density (PD) MR image demonstrates nonvisualization of the proximal LCL due to complete disruption of the ligament *(arrow)*. There are also thickening and increased signal intensity within the conjoint tendon on the coronal PD MR image **(B)** and the sagittal T2-weighted with fat suppression MR image **(C),** due to associated partial tendon tear *(broken arrows)*. Note also the surrounding soft tissue edema and joint effusion. (From Waldman SD, Campbell RSD *Imaging of pain,* Philadelphia, 2010, Saunders/Elsevier, p 386, fig 150-2.)

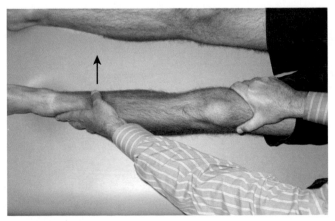

• **Figure 205-2** The varus stress test for lateral collateral ligament integrity. Push in the direction of the arrow.

The anterior drawer test is useful in helping the clinician assess the integrity of the anterior cruciate ligament. To perform the anterior drawer test, the patient is placed in the supine position on the examination table with the patient's head on a pillow to help relax the hamstring muscles. The patient's hip is then flexed to 45 degrees with the patient's foot placed flat on the table. The examiner grasps the affected leg below the knee with both hands and pulls the lower leg forward while stabilizing the foot (Fig. 206-1). The test is considered positive if there is more than 5 mm of anterior motion.

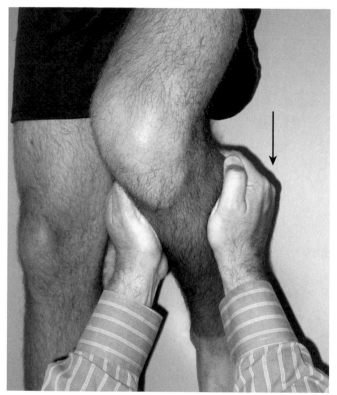

• Figure 206-1 The anterior drawer test for anterior cruciate ligament integrity. Pull in the direction of the arrow.

207 The Flexion-Rotation Anterior Drawer Test for Anterior Cruciate Ligament Instability

By testing the integrity of the anterior cruciate ligament in 2 planes, some investigators believe the flexion-rotation anterior drawer test for anterior cruciate ligament instability is more accurate than the more commonly utilized anterior drawer test. To perform the flexion-rotation anterior drawer test for anterior cruciate ligament instability, the examiner lifts the patient's affected leg upward, taking care not to hyperextend the knee joint (Fig. 207-1). This allows the femur to move posteriorly and rotate externally with antero-lateral tibial subluxation if the anterior cruciate ligament is unstable. The examiner then exerts mild anterior pressure on the patient's calf and valgus stress as the knee is gently flexed to reduce the joint (Fig. 207-2). Reduction of the joint with this mild anterior pressure and valgus stress is considered a positive test, and magnetic resonance imaging of the knee is indicated.

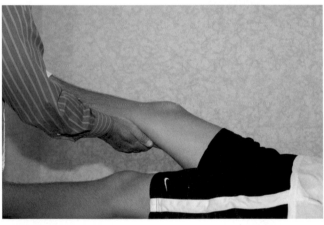

• **Figure 207-1** The flexion-rotation anterior drawer test: the examiner lifts the patient's affected leg upward, taking care not to hyperextend the knee joint.

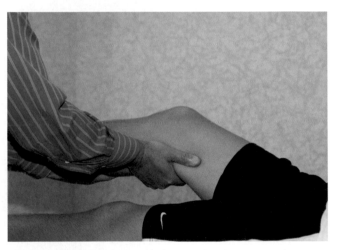

• **Figure 207-2** The flexion-rotation anterior drawer test: the examiner exerts mild anterior pressure on the patient's calf and valgus stress as the knee is gently flexed to reduce the joint.

The Lachman test is useful in helping the clinician assess the integrity of the anterior cruciate ligament. To perform the Lachman test, the patient is placed in the supine position on the examination table with the patient's head on a pillow to help relax the hamstring muscles. The patient's hip is flexed to 30 degrees with the patient's femur supported by the examiner. The examiner flexes the patient's affected knee, grasps the tibia of the affected leg, and applies anterior pressure on the posteromedial portion of the tibia while stabilizing the femur (Fig. 208-1). The test is considered positive if there is more than 5 mm of anterior motion.

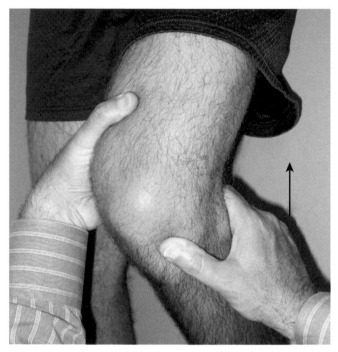

• **Figure 208-1** The Lachman test for anterior cruciate ligament integrity. Push in the direction of the arrow.

The posterior drawer test is useful in helping the clinician assess the integrity of the posterior cruciate ligament (Fig. 209-1). To perform the posterior drawer test, the patient is placed in the supine position on the examination table with his or her head on a pillow to help relax the hamstring muscles. The patient's hip is then flexed to 45 degrees with the patient's foot placed flat on the table. The examiner grasps the affected leg below the knee with both hands and pushes the lower leg backward while stabilizing the foot (Fig. 209-2). The test is considered positive if there is more than 5 mm of posterior motion.

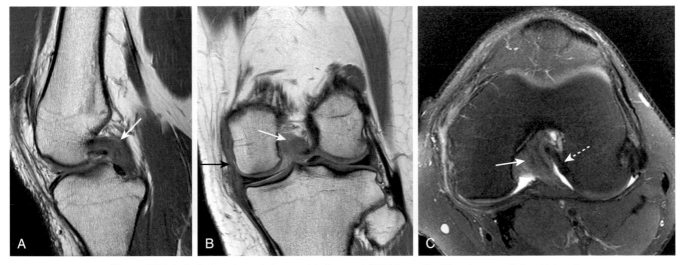

• **Figure 209-1 A,** Subacute posterior cruciate ligament (PCL) tear with diffuse increased signal intensity within the ligament substance *(arrow)* on the sagittal protein-density (PD) magnetic resonance (MR) image. **B,** The coronal PD image also shows the abnormal PCL *(white arrow)*, and there is an associated grade 2 tear of the medial collateral ligament *(black arrow)*. **C,** The axial T2-weighted with fat suppression (FST2W) MR image shows the thickened high-SI PCL *(arrow)* within the intercondylar notch, adjacent to the normal, low-SI anterior cruciate ligament *(broken arrow)*. (From Waldman SD, Campbell RSD: *Imaging of pain,* Philadelphia, 2010, Saunders/Elsevier, p 380, fig 148-2.)

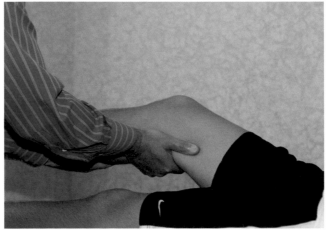

• **Figure 209-2** The posterior drawer test for posterior cruciate ligament integrity.

The pivot shift test is useful in helping the clinician assess the integrity of the anterior cruciate ligament. To perform the pivot shift test, the patient is placed in the supine position on the examination table with the ankle and foot of the patient's affected leg held firmly under the examiner's axilla. The patient's knee is placed in 20 degrees of flexion, and the tibia is rotated internally while the examiner pulls the lower leg outward (Fig. 212-1). The test is considered positive for anterior cruciate ligament insufficiency if the tibia subluxes anteriorly. The examiner can reduce the tibial subluxation by flexing the knee further, to 40 degrees, which will tighten the iliotibial band and pull the anteriorly displaced tibia back into place.

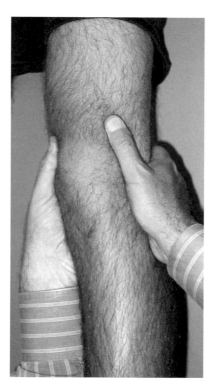

• **Figure 212-1** The pivot shift test for anterolateral rotary instability.

The reverse pivot shift test of Jakob is useful in the identification of posterolateral instability of the knee. To perform the reverse pivot shift test of Jakob, the examiner places the patient's affected lower extremity in full extension and neutral rotation (Fig. 213-1). The examiner then quickly flexes the patient's affected extremity while placing firm continuous valgus stress and allowing the foot to rotate externally (Fig. 213-2). If there is disruption of the posterior cruciate ligament, arcuate complex, and the lateral collateral ligament, at approximately 10 degrees of flexion, the examiner will appreciate a jolt-like shift of the lateral tibial plateau as it moves suddenly from a position of posterior subluxation and external rotation into a position of reduction and neutral rotation.

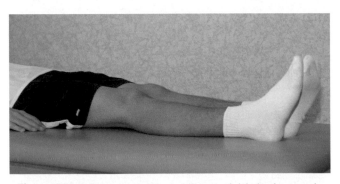

• **Figure 213-1** The reverse pivot shift test of Jakob: the examiner places the patient's affected lower extremity in full extension and neutral rotation.

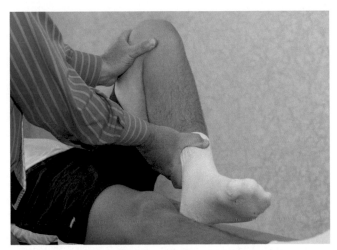

• **Figure 213-2** The reverse pivot shift test of Jakob: the examiner then quickly flexes the patient's affected extremity while placing firm continuous valgus stress and allowing the foot to rotate externally.

To perform the tibial external rotation test for injury to the posterolateral corner, the patient is placed in the prone position with the feet in neutral rotational position and the knees flexed to 30 degrees (Fig. 214-1). The knees are then flexed to 90 degrees with the examiner observing the feet; a decrease in external rotation as the knees are flexed toward 90 degrees is indicative of posterolateral corner injury (Fig. 214-2).

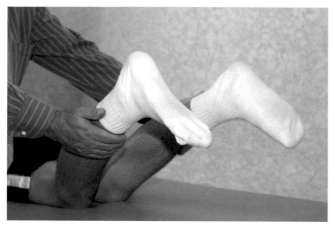

• **Figure 214-1** The tibial external rotation test for injury to the posterolateral corner: the patient is placed in the prone position with the feet in neutral rotational position and the knees flexed to 30 degrees.

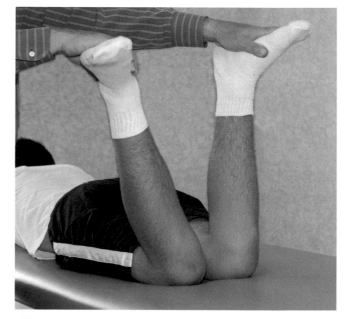

• **Figure 214-2** The tibial external rotation test for injury to the posterolateral corner: the patient's knees are flexed to 90 degrees with the examiner observing the feet; a decrease in external rotation as the knees are flexed toward 90 degrees is indicative of posterorlateral corner injury.

The Perkins test for patellofemoral pain syndrome can provide the clinician with useful information as to whether the patellofemoral joint is responsible for the patient's anterior knee pain. To perform the Perkins test for patellofemoral pain syndrome, the examiner has the patient assume the supine position on the examination table, and the knee is slightly flexed. With the knee relaxed, the examiner moves the patella laterally and medially (Fig. 215-1). The test is considered positive for patellofemoral pain syndrome if the side-to-side movement of the patella reproduces the patient's pain.

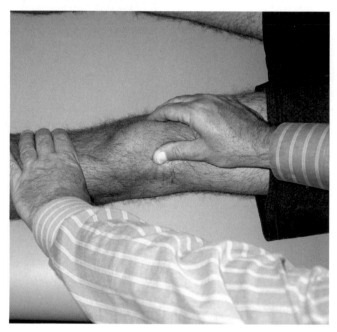

• **Figure 215-1** The Perkins test for patellofemoral pain syndrome.

The patellar grind test is useful in the identification of patellofemoral pathology. To perform the patellar grind test, the patient is placed in the supine position and the examiner applies pressure to the patella and then displaces it medially, laterally, superiorly, and inferiorly (Fig. 216-1). Any complaint of pain or apprehension on the part of the patient with such movement is highly suggestive of patellofemoral pathology, and plain radiographs, ultrasound imaging, and magnetic resonance imaging of the knees should be considered (Fig. 216-2).

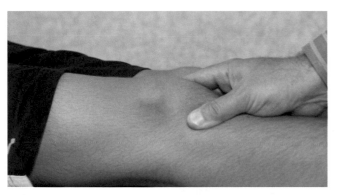

• **Figure 216-1** The patellar grind test for patellofemoral pain syndrome.

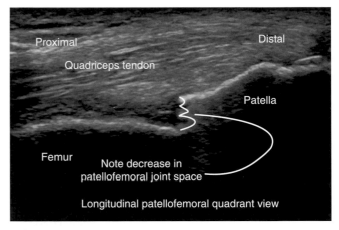

• **Figure 216-2** Longitudinal ultrasound view of the patellar-femoral quadrant.

The Fairbanks apprehension test for lateral patellar subluxation can provide the clinician with useful information as to whether the patellar subluxation is responsible for the patient's anterior knee pain. To perform the Fairbanks apprehension test for lateral patellar subluxation, the examiner has the patient assume the supine position on the examination table, and the knee is flexed 30 degrees. With the knee relaxed, the examiner exerts constant lateral pressure on the medial border of the mid-patella (Fig. 217-1). The test is considered positive for lateral patellar subluxation if the lateral pressure causes the patient apprehension.

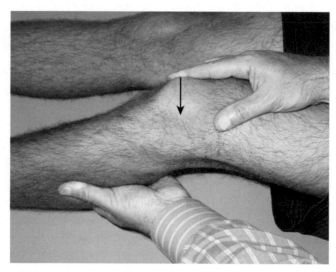

• **Figure 217-1** The Fairbanks apprehension test for lateral patellar subluxation.

The patellar tilt test is useful in the identification of excessive lateral retinacular tightness that may be responsible for patellofemoral pain syndrome. To perform the patellar tilt test for lateral retinacular dysfunction, the patient is placed in the supine position. The examiner places his or her fingers on the medial border of the patella and his or her thumb on the lateral aspect (Fig. 218-1). The examiner then attempts to gently raise the lateral aspect of the patella to the horizontal plane of the affected knee (Fig. 218-2). The inability to raise the lateral aspect of the patella that far indicates excessive lateral retinacular tightness that may be responsible for the patient's anterior knee pain.

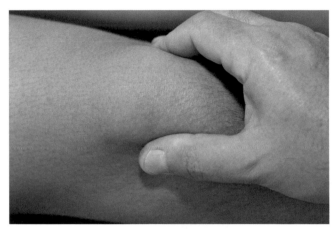

• **Figure 218-1** The patellar tilt test: the examiner places his or her fingers on the medial border of the patella and his or her thumb on the lateral aspect.

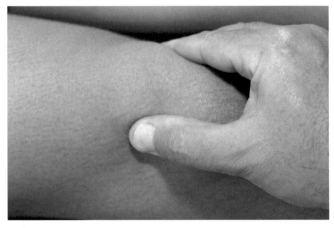

• **Figure 218-2** The patellar tilt test: the examiner then attempts to gently raise the lateral aspect of the patella to the horizontal plane of the affected knee.

The McMurray test for torn meniscus can provide the clinician with useful information as to whether a torn medial or lateral meniscus is responsible for the patient's knee pain. To perform the McMurray test for torn meniscus, the examiner has the patient assume the supine position on the examination table with the knee maximally flexed. With the affected extremity relaxed, the examiner grasps the ankle and palpates the knee while simultaneously rotating the lower leg internally and externally and extending the knee (Fig. 219-1). The test is considered positive for torn meniscus if the examiner appreciates a palpable or auditory click while rotating and extending the knee.

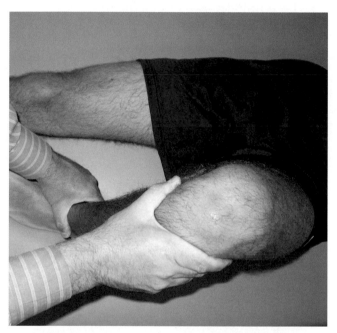

• **Figure 219-1** The McMurray test for torn meniscus.

The Apley grinding test for meniscal tear can provide the clinician with useful information as to whether a torn medial or lateral meniscus is responsible for the patient's knee pain. To perform the Apley test for torn meniscus, the examiner has the patient assume the prone position on the examination table. The examiner has the patient flex his or her knee 90 degrees and relax the entire lower extremity.

The examiner then pushes down on the foot of the affected extremity and internally and externally rotates the lower leg (Fig. 220-1). The Apley grinding test is considered positive if the patient complains of pain, if the examiner appreciates an audible or palpable click, or if there is locking of the knee.

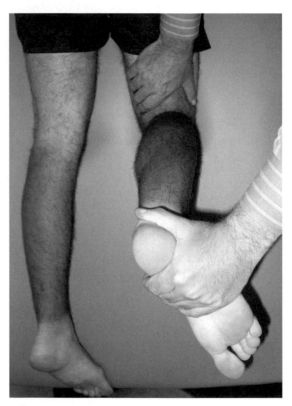

• **Figure 220-1** The Apley grinding test for meniscal tear.

The squat test for meniscal tear is a useful confirmatory test in those patients who have a positive McMurray test or Apley grinding test for torn meniscus (Figs. 221-1 and 221-2; also see Chapters 219 and 220). To perform the squat test for torn meniscus, the patient is asked to perform 2 successive full squats, the first with the feet and legs fully externally rotated (Fig. 221-3) and the second with the feet and legs fully internally rotated (Fig. 221-4). The location of pain is usually the strongest indicator of the location of the torn meniscus, with medial pain highly suggestive of a torn medial meniscus and lateral pain highly suggestive of a lateral torn meniscus. Furthermore, an increase in the intensity of pain with internal rotation of the legs and feet is suggestive of a torn lateral meniscus, and an increase in pain with external rotation of the legs and feet is suggestive of a torn medial meniscus.

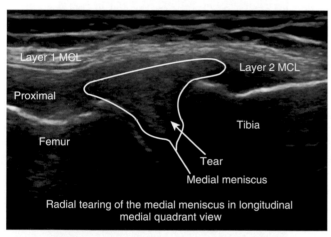

Radial tearing of the medial meniscus in longitudinal medial quadrant view

• **Figure 221-1** Longitudinal ultrasound image of the medial knee demonstrating a radial tear of the medial meniscus. *MCL,* Medial collateral ligament.

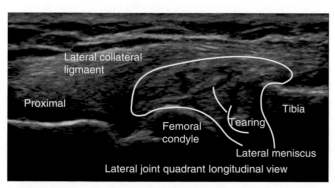

Lateral joint quadrant longitudinal view

• **Figure 221-2** Longitudinal ultrasound image of the lateral knee demonstrating a torn lateral meniscus.

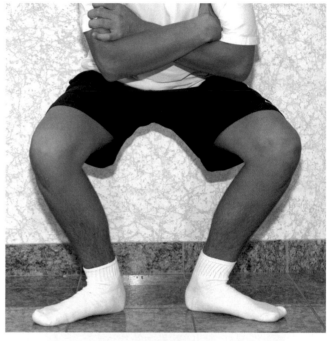

• **Figure 221-3** The squat test for meniscal tear: the patient is asked first to perform a full squat with the feet and legs fully externally rotated.

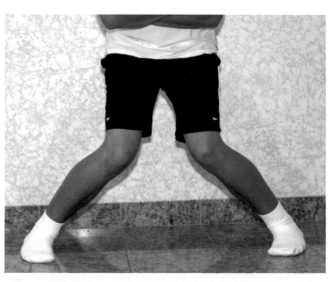

• **Figure 221-4** The squat test for meniscal tear: the patient is then asked to perform a full squat with the feet and legs fully internally rotated.

The premise behind the Thessaly test for meniscal tear is that abnormal loading of the diseased meniscus of the knee is likely to reproduce the knee pain, locking, and clicking that the patient is experiencing. To perform the Thessaly test, the patient is asked to stand with both feet flat on the floor while the examiner helps stabilize the patient by holding both of the patient's hands (Fig. 222-1). The patient is then asked to stand on the nonpainful lower extremity and lift the affected lower extremity off the floor by flexing the nonaffected knee 90 degrees. The patient is then asked to flex the painful knee approximately 5 degrees (Fig. 222-2). The patient then is asked to rotate his or her body and knee externally and internally 3 times with the weight-bearing knee kept at 5 degrees flexion (Fig. 222-3). The test is then repeated with the weight-bearing knee flexed to 20 degrees (Fig. 222-4). The test is now repeated with the painful knee bearing the weight. The test is positive if the patient experiences reproduction and/or exacerbation of the pain, locking, and clicking in the painful knee.

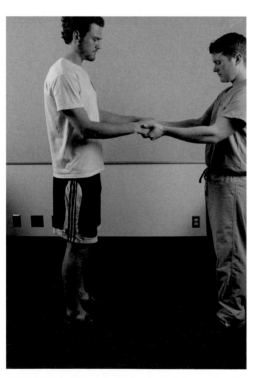

• **Figure 222-1** To perform the Thessaly test, the patient is asked to stand with both feet flat on the floor while the examiner helps stabilize the patient by holding both of the patient's hands.

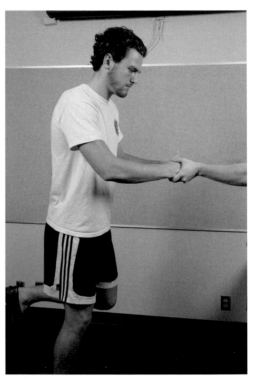

• **Figure 222-2** The patient is then asked to stand on the nonpainful lower extremity and lift the affected lower extremity off the floor by flexing the nonaffected knee 90 degrees. The patient is then asked to flex the painful knee approximately 5 degrees.

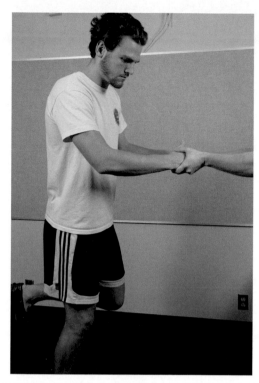

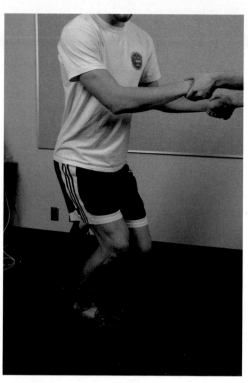

• **Figure 222-3** The patient then is asked to rotate his or her body and knee externally and internally 3 times with the weight-bearing knee kept at 5 degrees flexion.

• **Figure 222-4** The same procedure is then repeated with the weight-bearing knee flexed to 20 degrees.

Semimembranosus insertion syndrome is a constellation of symptoms including a localized tenderness over the posterior aspect of the medial knee joint with severe pain being elicited on palpation of the attachment of the semimembranosus muscle at the posterior medial condyle of the tibia (Fig. 223-1). Semimembranosus insertion syndrome occurs most commonly following overuse or misuse of the knee, often after overaggressive exercise regimens. Direct trauma to the posterior knee by kicks or tackles during football also can result in the development of semimembranosus insertion syndrome. Coexisting inflammation of the semimembranosus bursa that lies between the medial head of the gastrocnemius muscle, the medial femoral epicondyle, and the semimembranosus tendon can exacerbate the pain of semimembranosus insertion syndrome.

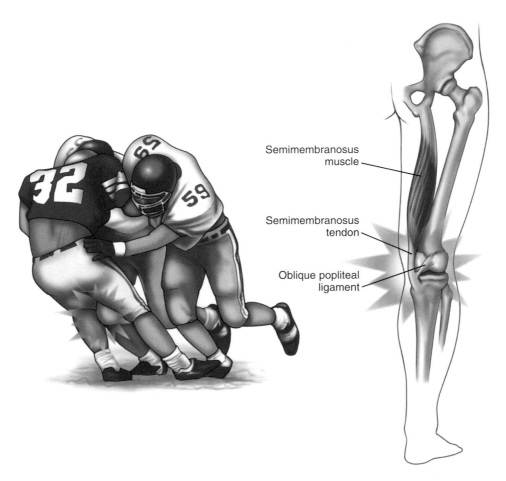

Semimembranosus muscle

Semimembranosus tendon

Oblique popliteal ligament

• **Figure 223-1** Semimembranosus insertion syndrome. (From Waldman SD: *Atlas of uncommon pain syndromes*, Philadelphia, 2003, Saunders, p 213.)

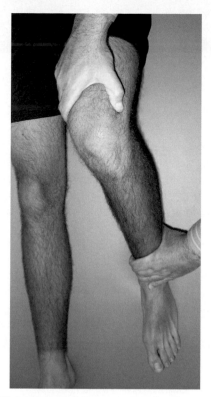

• **Figure 223-2** The twist test for semimembranosus insertion syndrome. The patient is supine.

To perform the twist test for semimembranosus insertion syndrome, the patient is placed in the supine position on the examination table with the ankle and foot of the patient's affected leg held firmly under the examiner's axilla. The patient's knee is placed in 20 degrees of flexion, and the tibia is rotated internally and externally while the examiner applies pressure with his or her thumb over the point of attachment of the semimembranosus muscle on the posterior lateral tibial condyle of the affected leg (Fig. 223-2). The test is considered positive for semimembranosus insertion syndrome if the patient experiences point tenderness beneath the examiner's thumb during rotation.

The quadriceps tendon is made up of fibers from the 4 muscles that make up the quadriceps muscle: the vastus lateralis, the vastus intermedius, the vastus medialis, and the rectus femoris. These muscles are the primary extensors of the lower extremity at the knee. The tendons of these muscles converge and unite to form a single, exceedingly strong tendon. The patella functions as a sesamoid bone within the quadriceps tendon, with fibers of the tendon expanding around the patella and forming the medial and lateral patella retinacula, which help strengthen the knee joint (Fig. 224-1). These fibers are called the quadriceps or patellar expansions and are subject to strain; the

tendon proper is subject to the development of tendinitis (Fig. 224-2). The quadriceps tendon also is subject to acute calcific tendinitis, which can coexist with acute strain injuries. Calcific tendinitis of the quadriceps has a characteristic radiographic appearance of whiskers on the antero-superior patella.

The quadriceps expansion syndrome is characterized by pain at the superior pole of the patella. It is usually the result of overuse or misuse of the knee joint, such as running marathons, or direct trauma to the quadriceps tendon, such as that from kicks or head butts during football. Patients with quadriceps expansion syndrome present with pain over

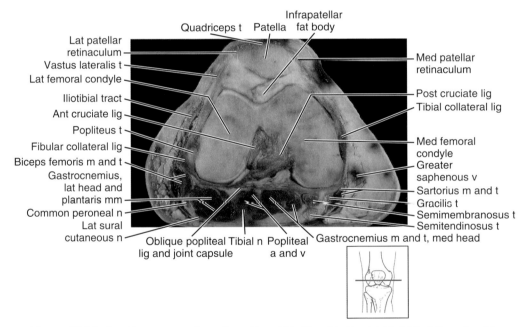

• **Figure 224-1** Quadriceps expansions. (From Kang HS, Ahn JM, Resnick D: *MRI of the extremities*, Philadelphia, 2002, Saunders, p 319.)

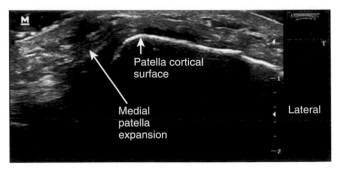

• **Figure 224-2** Ultrasound image demonstrating the medial patellar (quadriceps) expansion.

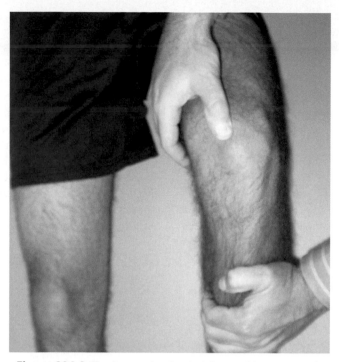

• **Figure 224-3** The knee extension test for quadriceps expansion syndrome.

the superior pole of the sesamoid, more commonly on the medial side. The patient notes increased pain on walking down slopes or stairs. Activity that uses the knee makes the pain worse, with rest and heat providing some relief. The pain is constant and is characterized as aching in nature. The pain may interfere with sleep.

On physical examination, there is tenderness under the superior edge of the patella, more commonly on the medial side. Patients with quadriceps expansion syndrome also exhibit a positive knee extension test. To perform the knee extension test for quadriceps expansion syndrome, the patient is placed in the supine position on the examination table and is then asked to maximally flex his or her affected knee. The examiner places his or her thumb on the superior medial pole of the patella of the affected leg and then has the patient extend the leg against active resistance (Fig. 224-3). The knee extension test for quadriceps expansion syndrome is considered positive if the patient experiences sharp pain at the superior medial pole of the patella as the affected leg extends.

Because of the complex nature of the knee's range of motion and the tremendous and varied physical stresses that are placed on the knee, it is not surprising that the knee is one of the most common anatomic sites for the occurrence of bursitis. Bursae are formed from synovial sacs whose purpose is to allow easy sliding of muscles and tendons across one another at areas of repeated movement. These synovial sacs are lined with a synovial membrane that is invested with a network of blood vessels that secrete synovial fluid. Inflammation of the bursa results in an increase in the production of synovial fluid with swelling of the bursal sac. With overuse or misuse, the bursa may become inflamed, enlarged, and, on rare occasions, infected. Although there is significant intrapatient variability as to the number, size, and location of bursae, anatomists have identified a number of clinically relevant bursae, including the suprapatellar, prepatellar, superficial and deep infrapatellar, and pes anserine bursae, that are commonly the cause of a painful knee. It is important for the clinician to remember, when considering the diagnosis of bursitis of the knee, that bursitis frequently coexists with other pathologic processes and might not be the sole source of the patient's pain and joint dysfunction. This chapter discusses some of the more common types of knee bursitis encountered in clinical practice.

SUPRAPATELLAR BURSITIS

The suprapatellar bursa extends superiorly from beneath the patella under the quadriceps femoris muscle and its tendon (Fig. 225-1). The bursa is held in place by a small portion

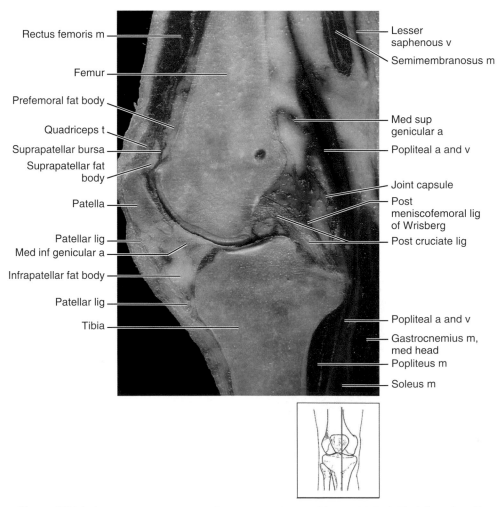

• **Figure 225-1** Sagittal view of the knee. (From Kang HS, Ahn JM, Resnick D: *MRI of the extremities*, Philadelphia, 2002, Saunders, p 337.)

of the vastus intermedius muscle, called the articularis genus muscle. This bursa may exist as a single bursal sac or, in some patients, as a multisegmented series of sacs that may be loculated in nature. The suprapatellar bursa is vulnerable to injury from both acute trauma and repeated microtrauma (Fig. 225-2). Acute injuries frequently take the form of direct trauma to the bursa via falls directly onto the knee or from patellar fractures, as well as from overuse injuries, including running on soft or uneven surfaces, or from jobs that require crawling on the knees, such as carpet laying. If the inflammation of the suprapatellar bursa becomes chronic, calcification of the bursa may occur.

The patient who suffers from suprapatellar bursitis will frequently complain of pain in the anterior knee above the patella that can radiate superiorly into the distal anterior thigh. Often the patient is unable to kneel or walk down stairs. The patient also might complain of a sharp "catching" sensation with range of motion of the knee, especially on first rising. Suprapatellar bursitis often coexists with arthritis and tendinitis of the quadriceps tendon, and these other pathologic processes can confuse the clinical picture.

Physical examination may reveal point tenderness in the anterior knee just above the patella. Passive flexion and active resisted extension of the knee reproduce the pain. Sudden release of resistance during this maneuver markedly increases the pain. There may be swelling in the suprapatellar region with a "boggy" feeling to palpation. Occasionally the suprapatellar bursa may become infected, with systemic symptoms, including fever and malaise, as well as local symptoms, including rubor, color, and dolor being present.

PREPATELLAR BURSITIS

The prepatellar bursa lies between the subcutaneous tissues and the patella (Fig. 225-3). This bursa may exist as a single bursal sac or, in some patients, as a multisegmented series of sacs that may be loculated in nature.

The prepatellar bursa is vulnerable to injury from both acute trauma and repeated microtrauma. Acute injuries frequently take the form of direct trauma to the bursa via falls

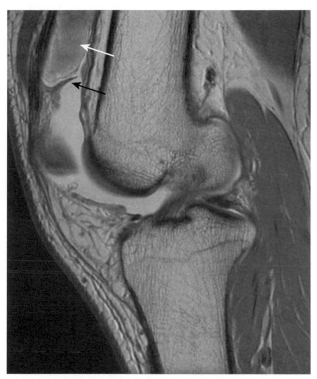

•**Figure 225-2** Sagittal T2W magnetic resonance (MR) image of an imperforate plica *(black arrow)* in a patient with a loculated hematoma in the suprapatellar bursa *(white arrow)* following an acute injury. (From Waldman SD, Campbell, RSD: *Imaging of pain,* Philadelphia, 2010, Saunders/Elsevier, p 402, fig 156-2.)

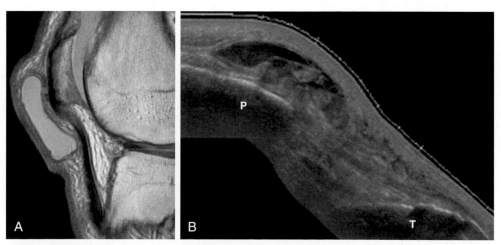

• **Figure 225-3 A,** Sagittal T2W magnetic resonance (MR) image showing prominent high signal intensity (SI) fluid within the prepatellar bursa. There is also an advanced osteoarthritic change in the patellofemoral joint. **B,** The corresponding longitudinal ultrasound image shows the extensive low-echo fluid collection. *P,* Patella; *T,* tibia. (From Waldman SD, Campbell, RSD: *Imaging of pain,* Philadelphia, 2010, Saunders/Elsevier, p 407, fig 157-3.)

directly onto the knee or from patellar fractures, as well as from overuse injuries, including running on soft or uneven surfaces. Prepatellar bursitis also may result from jobs that require crawling or kneeling, such as carpet laying or scrubbing floors; the other name for prepatellar bursitis is housemaid's knee (Fig. 225-4). If the inflammation of the prepatellar bursa becomes chronic, calcification of the bursa can occur.

The patient who suffers from prepatellar bursitis frequently complains of pain and swelling in the anterior knee over the patella that can radiate superiorly and inferiorly into the area surrounding the knee. Often the patient is

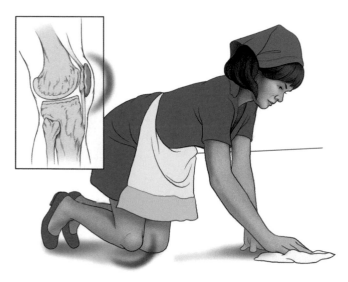

• **Figure 225-4** Prepatellar bursitis is also known as housemaid's knee because of its prevalence in people whose work requires prolonged crawling or kneeling. (From Waldman SD: *Atlas of common pain syndromes,* Philadelphia, 2002, Saunders, p 259.)

unable to kneel or walk down stairs. The patient also may complain of a sharp, "catching" sensation with range of motion of the knee, especially on first rising. Prepatellar bursitis often coexists with arthritis and tendinitis of the knee joint, and these other pathologic processes can confuse the clinical picture.

Physical examination may reveal point tenderness in the anterior knee just above the patella. Swelling and fluid accumulation surrounding the patella are often present. Passive flexion and active resisted extension of the knee reproduce the pain. Sudden release of resistance during this maneuver markedly increases the pain. The prepatellar bursa can become infected, with systemic symptoms, including fever and malaise, as well as local symptoms, including rubor, color, and dolor, also present.

SUPERFICIAL AND DEEP INFRAPATELLAR BURSITIS

The superficial infrapatellar bursa lies between the subcutaneous tissues and the upper part of the ligamentum patellae (Fig. 225-5). The deep infrapatellar bursa lies between the ligamentum patellae and the tibia (Fig. 225-6). These bursae may exist as single bursal sacs or, in some patients, as a multisegmented series of sacs that may be loculated in nature.

Both infrapatellar bursae are vulnerable to injury from both acute trauma and repeated microtrauma. Acute injuries frequently take the form of direct trauma to the bursae via falls directly onto the knee or from patellar fractures, as well as from overuse injuries, including long-distance running. Infrapatellar bursitis also can result from jobs that require crawling or kneeling, such as carpet laying or

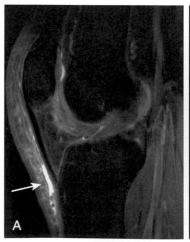
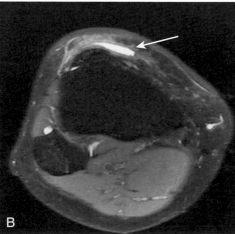
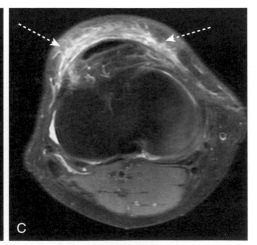

• **Figure 225-5 A,** Sagittal T2-weighted with fat suppression (FST2W) magnetic resonance (MR) image demonstrating a small area of high signal intensity (SI) fluid superficial to the distal patellar tendon and tibial tuberosity *(arrow).* **B,** This area of fluid *(arrow)* is also evident on the axial FST2W MR image. A small amount of fluid may be a normal finding. **C,** In this case, however, more extensive diffuse high-SI edema *(broken arrows)* is demonstrated in the adjacent soft tissues on the proximal axial FST2W MR image, representing a diffuse advential bursitis. (From Waldman SD, Campbell, RSD: *Imaging of pain,* Philadelphia, 2010, Saunders/Elsevier, p 406, fig 158-1.)

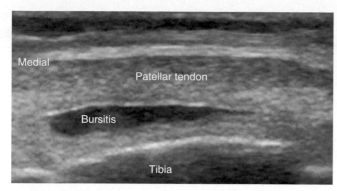

• **Figure 225-6** Longitudinal ultrasound image demonstrating deep infrapatellar bursitis.

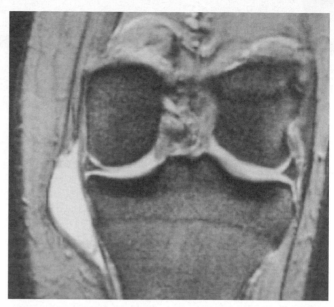

• **Figure 225-7** Pes anserine bursitis. This coronal gradient echo image shows a fluid collection medially, just inferior to the joint line. (From Kaplan PA, Helms CA, Dussault R, et al: *Musculoskeletal MRI*, Philadelphia, 2001, Saunders, p 385.)

scrubbing floors. If the inflammation of the infrapatellar bursae becomes chronic, calcification of the bursae can occur.

The patient who suffers from infrapatellar bursitis frequently complains of pain and swelling in the anterior knee below the patella that can radiate inferiorly into the area surrounding the knee. Often the patient is unable to kneel or walk down stairs. The patient also may complain of a sharp, "catching" sensation with range of motion of the knee, especially on first rising. Infrapatellar bursitis often coexists with arthritis and tendinitis of the knee joint, and these other pathologic processes can confuse the clinical picture.

Physical examination may reveal point tenderness in the anterior knee just below the patella. Swelling and fluid accumulation that surround the lower patella are often present. Passive flexion and active resisted extension of the knee reproduce the pain. Sudden release of resistance during this maneuver markedly increases the pain. The superficial infrapatellar bursa can become infected, with systemic symptoms, including fever and malaise, as well as local symptoms, including rubor, color, and dolor, also present.

PES ANSERINE BURSITIS

The pes anserine bursa lies beneath the pes anserine tendon, which is the insertional tendon of the sartorius, gracilis, and semitendinous muscle to the medial side of the tibia (Fig. 225-7). This bursa may exist as a single bursal sac or, in some patients, as a multisegmented series of sacs that may be loculated in nature.

Patients with pes anserine bursitis present with pain over the medial knee joint and increased pain on passive valgus and external rotation of the knee. Activity, especially that involving flexion and external rotation of the knee, makes the pain worse. Rest and heat provide some relief. Often the patient is unable to kneel or walk down stairs. The pain is constant and characterized as aching in nature. The pain may interfere with sleep. Coexistent bursitis, tendinitis, arthritis, or internal derangement of the knee can confuse the clinical picture after trauma to the knee joint. Frequently the medial collateral ligament also is involved if the patient has sustained trauma to the medial knee joint. If the inflammation of the pes anserine bursa becomes chronic, calcification of the bursa can occur.

Physical examination may reveal point tenderness in the anterior knee just below the medial knee joint at the tendinous insertion of the pes anserine tendon. Swelling and fluid accumulation that surrounds the bursa are often present. Active resisted flexion of the knee reproduces the pain. Sudden release of resistance during this maneuver markedly increases the pain. Rarely the pes anserine bursa becomes infected in a manner analogous to infection of the prepatellar bursa.

Plain radiographs of the knee are indicated for all patients who suffer from bursitis. These may reveal calcification of the bursa and associated structures, including ligaments and tendons, indicating inflammation. Magnetic resonance imaging is indicated if internal derangement, occult mass, or tumor of the knee is suspected. Electromyography helps to distinguish bursitis from neuropathy, lumbar radiculopathy, and plexopathy.

The musculotendinous insertion of the hamstring group of muscles is susceptible to the development of tendinitis for 2 reasons. First, the knee joint is subjected to significant repetitive motion under weight-bearing conditions. Second, the blood supply to the musculotendinous unit is poor, making healing of microtrauma difficult (Fig. 226-1). Calcium deposition around the tendon can occur if the inflammation continues, thereby complicating subsequent treatment. If the inflammation of the tendinous insertions of these muscles becomes chronic, they may rupture if subjected to sudden trauma during exercise or injection. Tendinitis of the musculotendinous insertion of the hamstring frequently coexists with bursitis of the associated bursae of the knee joint, creating additional pain and functional disability.

The onset of hamstring tendinitis is usually acute, occurring after overuse or misuse of the muscle group. Inciting factors may include long-distance running, dancing injuries, or the vigorous use of exercise equipment for lower extremity strengthening. The pain is constant and severe, with sleep disturbance often reported. The patient may attempt to splint the inflamed tendon by holding the knee in a slightly flexed position and assuming a lurch-type antalgic gait. Patients with hamstring tendinitis exhibit severe pain to palpation over the tendinous insertion, the medial portion of the tendon being affected more commonly than the lateral portion.

Patients who suffer from hamstring tendinitis will exhibit a positive creaking tendon sign. To elicit a creaking tendon sign for hamstring tendinitis, the patient is placed prone on the examination table with the knee of the affected leg extended. The examiner palpates the tendinous insertion of the hamstrings and then has the patient flex his or her knee (Fig. 226-2). The creaking tendon sign for hamstring tendinitis is positive if the examiner appreciates a creaking sensation over the tendon while the patient flexes the affected knee.

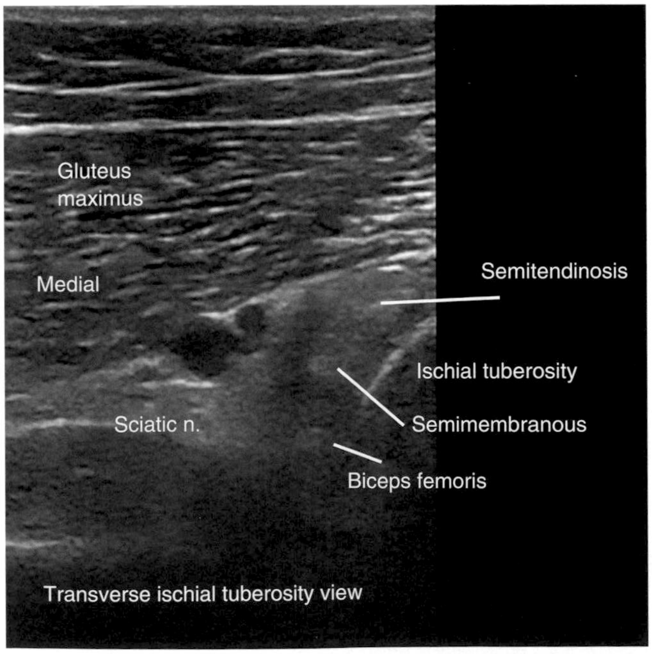

Gluteus maximus

Medial

Semitendinosis

Ischial tuberosity

Sciatic n.

Semimembranous

Biceps femoris

Transverse ischial tuberosity view

• **Figure 226-1** Ultrasound image demonstrating the insertion of the muscles that comprise the hamstring.

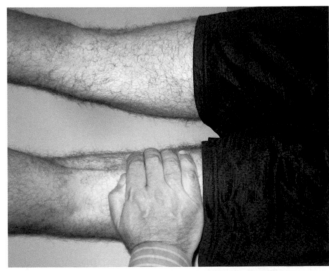

• **Figure 226-2** Eliciting the creaking tendon sign for hamstring tendinitis.

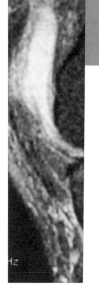

The Nobel compression test is a useful indicator of iliotibial band syndrome. To perform the Nobel compression test for iliotibial band syndrome, the patient is placed in the supine position on the examination table and is asked to flex the affected knee to 90 degrees. The examiner then applies firm pressure with his or her thumb to the lateral femoral condyle (Fig. 227-1). The patient's knee is then passively extended (Fig. 227-2). At approximately 30 degrees of extension, the examiner will feel the iliotibial band translate anteriorly over the lateral femoral epicondyle. A snapping or popping sensation may be appreciated by both the patient and the examiner. The test is positive if the pain is reproduced as the iliotibial band pops anteriorly over the lateral femoral condyle. Ultrasound and magnetic resonance imaging may help identify pathology of the iliotibial band responsible for the patient's pain (Fig. 227-3).

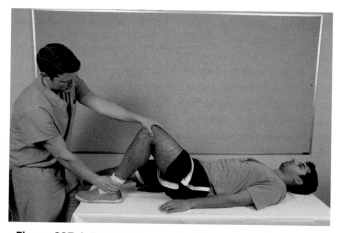

• **Figure 227-1** The examiner applies firm pressure with his or her thumb to the lateral femoral condyle.

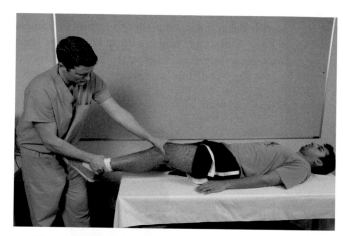

• **Figure 227-2** The patient's knee is then passively extended.

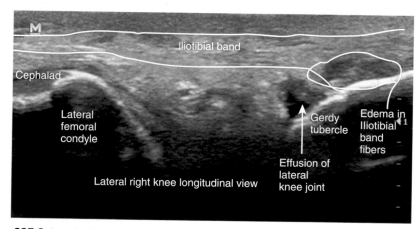

• **Figure 227-3** Longitudinal ultrasound image demonstrating edema and loss of normal echotexture of the iliotibial band. Note the effusion in the lateral knee joint.

231 Palpation of the Ankle and Foot

Palpation of the ankle joint can provide the examiner with much information as to the cause of ankle and foot pain. To adequately palpate the ankle and foot, the patient should be seated comfortably on the edge of the examination table with the shoes and socks removed. The affected ankle is allowed to assume its natural slightly plantar-flexed position, and the examiner gently palpates the anterior aspect of the joint with his or her thumbs while gently supporting the joint with the other fingers (Fig. 231-1). The examiner should be readily able to identify synovial thickening or joint effusion. Tenosynovitis will be palpated as a tender, linear swelling that extends across the joint. Bursitis of the medial and lateral malleolar bursae or last bursae will be easily palpated as painful areas over the medial or lateral malleoli.

The Achilles tendon should be palpated for nodules or insertional tendinitis. Retrocalcaneal bursitis will present as a swelling to palpation overlying the distal Achilles tendon. The plantar surface of the foot should be palpated for localized heel pain caused by subcalcaneal bursitis or calcaneal spur. The plantar surface should be palpated for painful sesamoid bones, plantar warts, cysts, plantar fasciitis, and plantar nodular fibromatosis, which is the foot's analog of a Dupuytren contracture in the hand (Figs. 231-2 and 231-3).

The midtarsal joints are then palpated by supporting the foot with the fingers and using the thumb of the examining hand to palpate the dorsal surface. Careful palpation of this area should readily reveal any bony abnormality and synovial thickening (Fig. 231-4).

The metatarsophalangeal and interphalangeal joints are then each individually palpated to identify obvious bony abnormality, pain, or synovial thickening (Fig. 231-5). Palpation of the metatarsophalangeal and interphalangeal joints is best carried out by using the thumbs of both hands (Fig. 231-6).

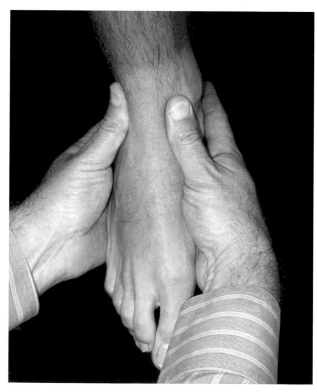

• **Figure 231-1** Palpation of the ankle.

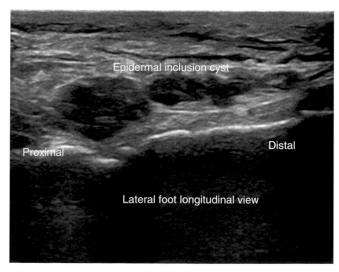

• **Figure 231-2** Longitudinal ultrasound image of the plantar surface of the foot demonstrating large epidermoid cysts.

• **Figure
complain
Waldman
Saunders

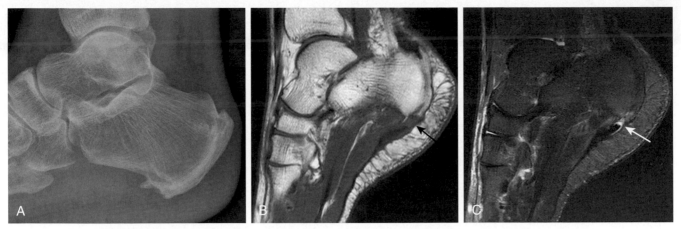

• **Figure 231-3 A,** Lateral radiograph of a plantar spur on the calcaneus. **B,** The sagittal T1W magnetic resonance (MR) image demonstrates thickening and increased signal intensity (SI) within the plantar fascia origin *(black arrow).* There is high-SI fatty marrow within the bony spur. **C,** High-SI fluid *(white arrow)* is seen within the plantar fascia origin on the sagittal FST2W MR image. The appearances are consistent with plantar fasciitis and partial tearing of the origin of the fascia. (From Waldman SD, Campbell, RSD: *Imaging of pain,* Philadelphia, 2010, Saunders/Elsevier, p 458, fig 178-1.)

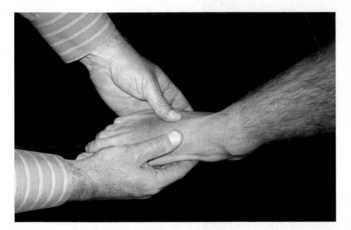

• **Figure 231-4** Palpation of the midtarsal joints.

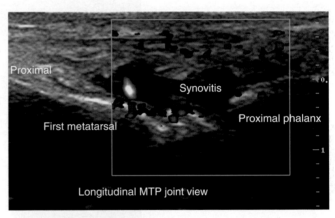

• **Figure 231-5** Longitudinal ultrasound image of the first metatarsophalangeal joint demonstrating active synovitis in a patient with rheumatoid arthritis. *MTP,* Metatarsophalangeal.

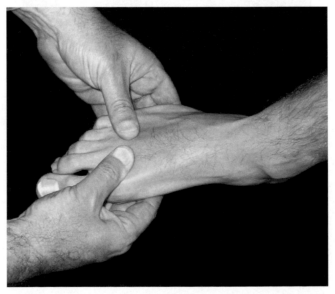

• **Figure 231-6** Palpation of the metatarsophalangeal and interphalangeal joints.

Effusions of the ankle joint are commonly seen in patients who suffer from rheumatoid arthritis and other collagen vascular diseases. Although small effusions of the ankle joint can be missed owing to the strong overlying ligaments and multiple tendons, larger effusions can be identified with the wave test.

To perform the wave test for ankle joint effusion, the patient should be seated comfortably on the edge of the examination table with the shoes and socks removed. The affected ankle is allowed to assume its natural slightly plantar-flexed position. The examiner places pressure on the anterolateral ankle while palpating the opposite side of the ankle joint for a transmission of excess fluid (Fig. 232-1).

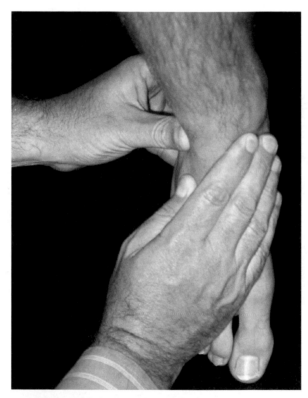

• **Figure 232-1** The wave test for ankle joint effusion.

The anterior drawer test for insufficiency of the talofibular ligament is performed by having the patient sit comfortably on the edge of the examination table with the shoes and socks removed. The affected ankle is allowed to assume its natural slightly plantar-flexed position, and the distal tibia and fibula are stabilized by being grasped. The examiner then cups the calcaneus and talus of the patient's affected ankle in his or her other hand and firmly draws these bones forward (Fig. 233-1). Movement of greater than 5 mm is considered positive and highly suspect for insufficiency of the talofibular ligament. Magnetic resonance and ultrasound imaging can quantify the extent of talofibular ligament damage and also help to identify other ankle pathology (Figs. 233-2 and 233-3).

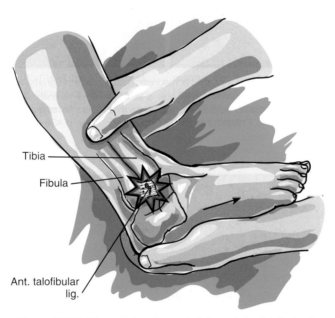

Tibia

Fibula

Ant. talofibular lig.

• **Figure 233-1** The anterior drawer test for anterior talofibular ligament insufficiency.

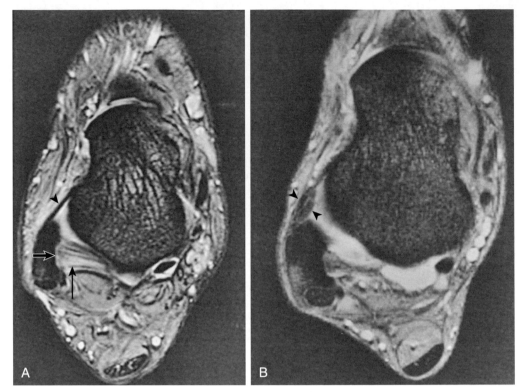

• **Figure 234-2** T2* axial images, ankle. **A,** The anterior talofibular ligament *(arrowhead)* and striated posterior talofibular ligament *(arrows)* are well seen on the level of the malleolar fossa. **B,** In a different patient, the lateral aspect of the anterior talofibular ligament is markedly thickened *(arrowheads)* and has low signal. This indicates previous rupture with scarring and fibrosis that mimics an intact ligament. (From Kaplan PA, Helms CA, Dussault R, et al: *Musculoskeletal MRI*, Philadelphia, 2001, Saunders, pp 408–409.)

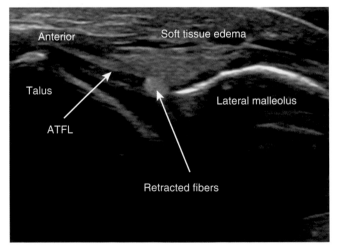

• **Figure 234-3** Ultrasound image demonstrating a high grade tear of the anterior talofibular ligament (ATFL) in a patient who suffered an acute inversion injury to the ankle when stepping in a gopher hole.

The deltoid ligament is susceptible to strain from acute injury from sudden overpronation of the ankle or from repetitive microtrauma to the ligament from overuse or misuse, such as long-distance running on soft or uneven surfaces. The deltoid ligament has 2 layers. Both attach above to the medial malleolus (Fig. 235-1). A deep layer attaches below to the medial body of the talus, with the superficial fibers attaching to the medial talus, the sustentaculum tali of the calcaneus, and the navicular tuberosity. Patients with strain of the deltoid ligament complain of pain just below the medial malleolus. Activities that require plantar flexion and eversion of the ankle joint exacerbate the pain.

On physical examination, patients who are suffering from insufficiency of the deltoid ligament will exhibit point tenderness over the medial malleolus. With acute trauma, ecchymosis over the ligament may be noted. Patients who are suffering from insufficiency of the deltoid ligament will also exhibit a positive ankle eversion test.

The ankle eversion test is performed by having the patient sit comfortably on the edge of the examination table with the shoes and socks removed. The affected ankle is allowed to assume its natural slightly plantar-flexed position, and the distal tibia and fibula are stabilized by being grasped. The examiner then cups the calcaneus and talus of the patient's affected ankle in his or her other hand and firmly everts the ankle joint (Fig. 235-2). The ankle eversion test is considered positive if the patient experiences localized pain over the medial malleolus. To confirm the diagnosis of deltoid ligament insufficiency and to rule out coexistent fracture or bursitis, plain radiographs and sonographic and magnetic resonance images of the ankle should be obtained (Figs. 235-3 and 235-4).

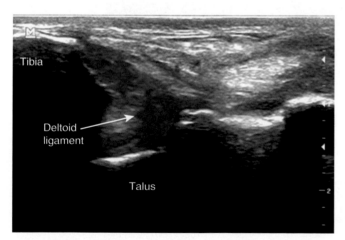

• **Figure 235-1** Longitudinal ultrasound image of the deltoid ligament. Note the proximal attachment to the medial malleolus of the tibia.

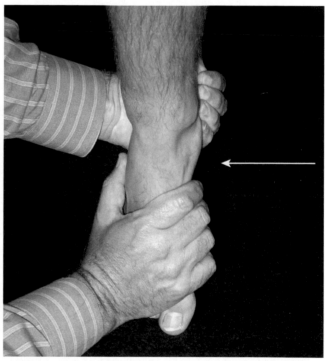

• **Figure 235-2** The eversion test for deltoid ligament insufficiency. Push in the direction of the arrow.

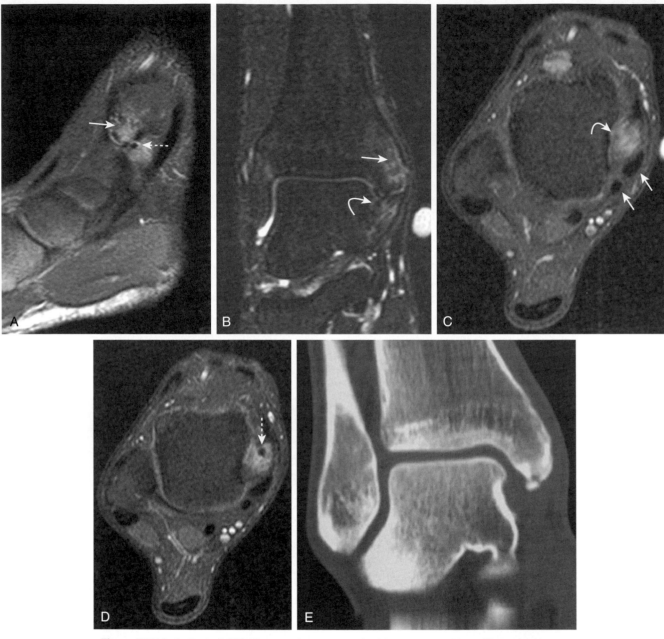

• **Figure 235-3 A,** Sagittal FST2W magnetic resonance (MR) image of an athlete with a subacute eversion ankle sprain. There is marrow edema in the tip of the medial malleolus *(arrow)* and a possible small bony avulsion injury *(broken arrow)*. **B,** The coronal FST2W MR image also shows the marrow edema *(arrow),* and there is high signal intensity (SI) within the deltoid ligament edema *(curved arrow)* as a result of partial tearing. **C** and **D,** Consecutive axial FST2W MR images more clearly demonstrate the deltoid ligament edema *(curved arrow)* anterior to the flexor tendons *(arrows).* The bony avulsion fragment is demonstrated as a small round area of low SI *(broken arrow).* **E,** The coronal computed tomographic image confirms the presence of an avulsion fracture of the tip of the medial malleolus. (From Waldman SD, Campbell, RSD: *Imaging of pain,* Philadelphia, 2010, Saunders/Elsevier, p 441, fig 171-2.)

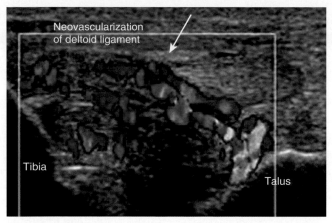

• **Figure 235-4** Color Doppler image of a severe sprain of the deltoid ligament in a patient who sustained an acute eversion injury to the ankle when a step was missed. Note the significant neovascularization of the ligament.

Rupture of the ligaments that hold the distal tibia and fibula is usually associated with trauma severe enough to cause fractures of the medial and lateral malleolus, although occasionally isolated disruption in the absence of fractures can occur, and the only other finding is concurrent rupture of the deltoid ligament. With disruption of the tibiofibular ligaments, with or without fractures of the distal tibia and fibula, widening of the ankle mortise occurs with significant pain and dysfunction (Fig. 236-1). In the absence of fractures, the patient's pain may seem out of proportion to the demonstrable injury on x-ray; the squeeze test may help identify damage to the tibiofibular ligaments.

To perform the squeeze test for syndesmosis ankle strain, the patient is placed in the sitting position and the calf of the affected extremity is squeezed by the examiner (Fig. 236-2). Distal pain and spreading of the tibia and fibula is strongly suggestive of significant ankle strain including disruption of the tibiofibular ligaments.

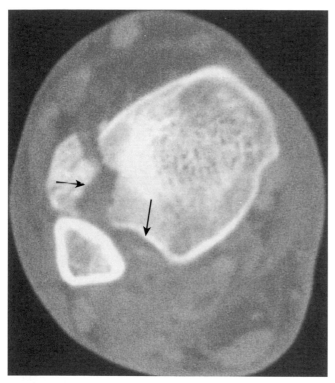

• **Figure 236-1** Axial computed tomographic image of the lower leg demonstrates disruption of the distal tibia and fibular articulation, with the fibula subluxated anteriorly out of its sulcus *(long arrow)*. A large avulsion fragment is seen at the tibial insertion of the anterior tibiofibular ligament *(short arrow)*. This avulsion represents an adult Tillaux fracture. (From Haaga J, Lanzieri C, Gilkeson R, editors: *CT and MR imaging of the whole body,* vol 2, ed 4, Philadelphia, 2002, Mosby, p 1857.)

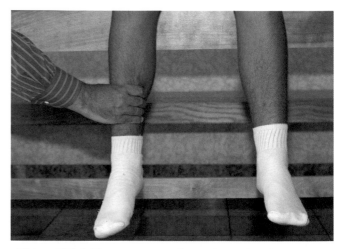

• **Figure 236-2** The squeeze test for syndesmosis ankle strain: the patient is placed in the sitting position and the calf of the affected extremity is squeezed by the examiner.

Rupture of the ligaments that hold the distal tibia and fibula is usually associated with trauma severe enough to cause fractures of the medial and lateral malleolus, although occasionally isolated disruption in the absence of fractures can occur, and the only other finding is concurrent rupture of the deltoid ligament. With disruption of the tibiofibular ligaments, with or without fractures of the distal tibia and fibula, widening of the ankle mortise occurs with significant pain and dysfunction (see Fig. 236-1). In the absence of fractures, the patient's pain may seem out of proportion to the demonstrable injury on x-ray; the external rotation test may help identify damage to the tibiofibular ligaments.

To perform the external rotation test for syndesmosis ankle strain, the patient is placed in the sitting position and the knee of the affected extremity is grasped to stabilize the knee in 90 degrees of flexion while the examiner gently externally rotates the foot and ankle (Fig. 237-1). Pain on external rotation over the anterior or posterior tibiofibular ligaments is strongly suggestive of significant ankle strain including disruption of the tibiofibular ligaments.

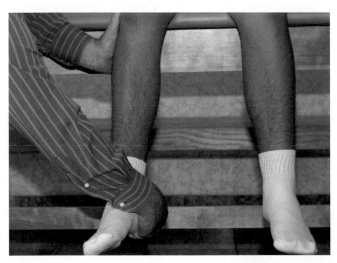

• **Figure 237-1** The external rotation test for syndesmosis ankle strain.

Anterior tarsal tunnel syndrome is caused by compression of the deep peroneal nerve as it passes beneath the superficial fascia of the ankle (Fig. 238-1). The most common cause of compression of the deep peroneal nerve at this anatomic location is trauma to the dorsum of the foot. Severe, acute plantar flexion of the foot has been implicated in anterior tarsal tunnel syndrome, as has the wearing of overly tight shoes or squatting and bending forward, as when planting flowers. Anterior tarsal tunnel syndrome is much less common than posterior tarsal tunnel syndrome.

This entrapment neuropathy presents primarily as pain, numbness, and paresthesias of the dorsum of the foot that radiates into the first dorsal web space. These symptoms also may radiate proximal to the entrapment into the anterior ankle. There is no motor involvement unless the distal lateral division of the deep peroneal nerve is involved. Nighttime foot pain analogous to the nocturnal pain of carpal tunnel syndrome often is present. The patient may report that holding the foot in the everted position decreases the pain and paresthesias of anterior tarsal tunnel syndrome.

Physical findings include tenderness over the deep peroneal nerve at the dorsum of the foot. A positive Tinel sign just medial to the dorsalis pedis pulse over the deep peroneal nerve as it passes beneath the fascia usually is present (Fig. 238-2). Active plantar flexion often reproduces the symptoms of anterior tarsal tunnel syndrome. Weakness of the extensor digitorum brevis muscle may be present if the lateral branch of the deep peroneal nerve is affected.

Anterior tarsal tunnel syndrome is often misdiagnosed as arthritis of the ankle joint, lumbar radiculopathy, or diabetic polyneuropathy. Patients with arthritis of the ankle joint have radiographic evidence of arthritis. Most patients who suffer from a lumbar radiculopathy have reflex, motor, and sensory changes associated with back pain, whereas patients with anterior tarsal tunnel syndrome have no reflex changes, and motor and sensory changes are limited to the distal deep peroneal nerve. Diabetic polyneuropathy generally presents as symmetric sensory deficit involving the entire foot, rather than being limited to the distribution of the deep peroneal nerve. It should be remembered that lumbar radiculopathy and deep peroneal nerve entrapment

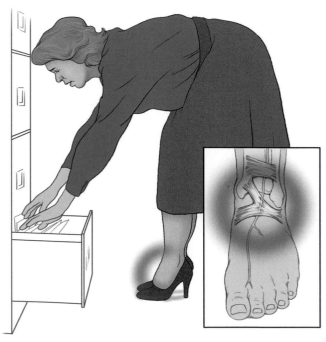

• **Figure 238-1** Anterior tarsal tunnel syndrome will present as deep, aching pain in the dorsum of the foot, weakness of the extensor digitorum brevis, and numbness in the distribution of the deep peroneal nerve. (From Waldman SD: *Atlas of common pain syndromes*, Philadelphia, 2002, Saunders, p 287.)

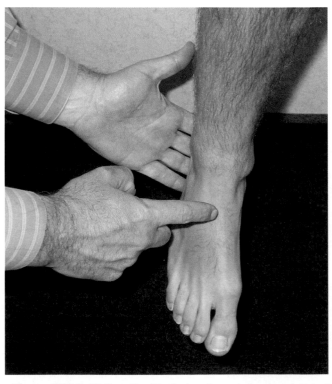

• **Figure 238-2** Eliciting the Tinel sign for anterior tarsal tunnel syndrome.

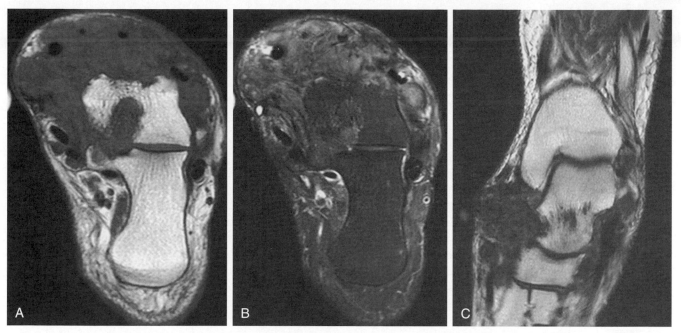

• **Figure 238-3** Axial T1W **(A)** and FST2W **(B)** magnetic resonance (MR) images of a patient with ankle pain and paresthesia over the dorsal aspect of the foot. A mass of synovitis arising from the ankle joint surrounds the extensor tendons and the anterior neurovascular bundle. The synovium has intermediate signal intensity on both images and also on the coronal T2W MR image **(C).** There is also bony erosion. These appearances are typical pigmented villondular synovitis.

may coexist as the so-called double crush syndrome. Furthermore, because anterior tarsal tunnel syndrome is seen in patients with diabetes, it is not surprising that diabetic polyneuropathy is usually present in diabetic patients with anterior tarsal tunnel syndrome.

Electromyography helps to distinguish lumbar radiculopathy and diabetic polyneuropathy from anterior tarsal tunnel syndrome. Plain radiographs are indicated for all patients who present with anterior tarsal syndrome to rule out occult bony pathology. On the basis of the patient's clinical presentation, additional testing may be indicated, including complete blood count, uric acid, sedimentation rate, and antinuclear antibody testing. Magnetic resonance and ultrasound imaging of the ankle and foot is indicated if joint instability or a space-occupying lesion is suspected (Fig. 238-3).

Posterior tarsal tunnel syndrome is caused by compression of the posterior tibial nerve as it passes through the posterior tarsal tunnel. The posterior tarsal tunnel is made up of the flexor retinaculum, the bones of the ankle, and the lacunate ligament. In addition to the posterior tibial nerve, the tunnel contains the posterior tibial artery and a number of flexor tendons, which are subject to tenosynovitis (Fig. 239-1). The most common cause of compression of the posterior tibial nerve at this anatomic location is trauma to the ankle, including fracture, dislocation, and crush injuries. Thrombophlebitis involving the posterior tibial artery also has been implicated in the evolution of posterior tarsal tunnel syndrome. Patients with rheumatoid arthritis have a

higher incidence of posterior tarsal tunnel syndrome than does the general population. Posterior tarsal tunnel syndrome is much more common than anterior tarsal tunnel syndrome.

Posterior tarsal tunnel syndrome presents in a manner analogous to carpal tunnel syndrome. The patient complains of pain, numbness, and paresthesias of the sole of the foot. These symptoms also may radiate proximally to the entrapment into the medial ankle. The medial and lateral plantar divisions of the posterior tibial nerve provide motor innervation to the intrinsic muscles of the foot. The patient might note weakness of the toe flexors and instability of the foot caused by weakness of the lumbrical muscles.

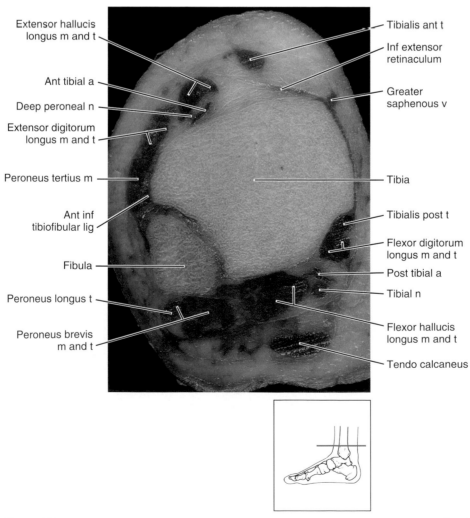

• **Figure 239-1** The structure of the posterior tarsal tunnel. (From Kang HS, Ahn JM, Resnick D: *MRI of the extremities*, Philadelphia, 2003, Saunders, p 411.)

Nighttime foot pain analogous to the nocturnal pain of carpal tunnel syndrome is often present.

Physical findings include tenderness over the posterior tibial nerve at the medial malleolus. A positive Tinel sign just below and behind the medial malleolus over the posterior tibial nerve is usually present (Fig. 239-2). Active inversion of the ankle often reproduces the symptoms of the posterior tarsal tunnel syndrome. Weakness of the flexor digitorum brevis and the lumbrical muscles may be present if the medial and lateral branches of the posterior tibial nerve are affected.

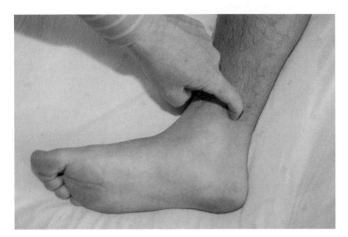

• **Figure 239-2** Eliciting the Tinel sign for posterior tarsal tunnel syndrome.

Posterior tarsal tunnel syndrome is often misdiagnosed as arthritis of the ankle joint, lumbar radiculopathy, or diabetic polyneuropathy. Patients with arthritis of the ankle joint have radiographic evidence of arthritis. Most patients who suffer from a lumbar radiculopathy have reflex, motor, and sensory changes associated with back pain, whereas patients with posterior tarsal tunnel syndrome have no reflex changes, and motor and sensory changes are limited to the distal posterior tibial nerve. Diabetic polyneuropathy generally presents as a symmetric sensory deficit involving the entire foot, rather than being limited to the distribution of the posterior tibial nerve. It should be remembered that lumbar radiculopathy and posterior tibial nerve entrapment may coexist as the so-called double crush syndrome. Furthermore, because posterior tarsal tunnel syndrome is seen in patients with diabetes, it is not surprising that diabetic polyneuropathy is usually present in diabetic patients with posterior tarsal tunnel syndrome.

Electromyography helps to distinguish lumbar radiculopathy and diabetic polyneuropathy from posterior tarsal tunnel syndrome. Plain radiographs are indicated for all patients who present with posterior tarsal tunnel syndrome to rule out occult bony pathology. On the basis of the patient's clinical presentation, additional testing may be indicated, including complete blood count, uric acid, sedimentation rate, and antinuclear antibody testing. Magnetic resonance and ultrasound imaging of the ankle and foot is indicated if joint instability or a space-occupying lesion is suspected (Figs. 239-3 and 239-4).

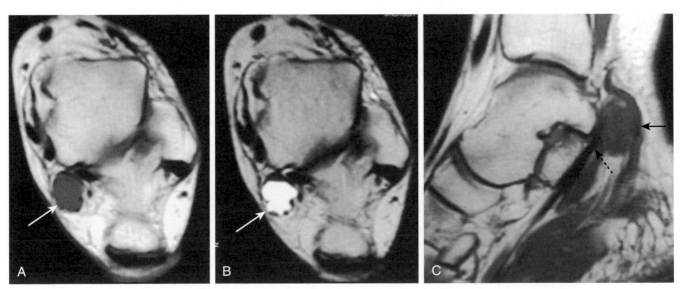

• **Figure 239-3** Axial proton density (PD) **(A)** and T2-weighted (T2W) **(B)** magnetic resonance (MR) images of the ankle in a patient with medial foot pain. There is a discrete rounded lesion *(white arrow)* within the tarsal tunnel. It has intermediate signal intensity (SI) on the PD MR images and high SI on the T2W MR images consistent with a fluid-filled ganglion cyst. **(C)** The sagittal T1W MR image demonstrates the mass posterior to the talus and the flexor hallucis longus tendon *(broken arrow)*, and one of the posterior tibial vessels runs over the superficial surface of the mass *(black arrow)*. The cyst is causing mass effect within the tarsal tunnel, compressing the posterior tibial nerve and producing symptoms of posterior tarsal tunnel syndrome. (Reproduced with permission from Spratt JD et al: The role of diagnostic radiology in compressive and entrapment neuropathies, *European Radiology* 12:2352–2364, 2002.)

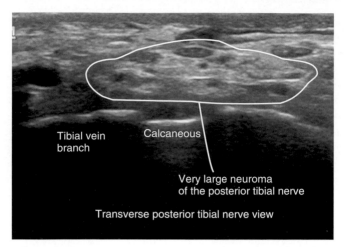

Tibial vein
branch

Calcaneous

Very large neuroma
of the posterior tibial nerve

Transverse posterior tibial nerve view

• **Figure 239-4** Transverse ultrasound image of the ankle demonstrating a large posttraumatic neuroma of the posterior tibial nerve in a patient presenting with symptoms of posterior tarsal tunnel syndrome.

The Achilles tendon is susceptible to the development of tendinitis both at its insertion on the calcaneus and at its narrowest part, at a point approximately 5 cm above its insertion. The Achilles tendon is subject to repetitive motion, which can result in microtrauma that heals poorly because of the tendon's avascular nature. Running is often implicated as the inciting factor of acute Achilles tendinitis (Fig. 240-1). Tendinitis of the Achilles tendon frequently coexists with bursitis of the associated bursae of the tendon and ankle joint, creating additional pain and functional disability. Calcium deposition around the tendon can occur if the inflammation continues, making subsequent treatment more difficult. Continued trauma to the inflamed tendon ultimately might result in tendon rupture.

The onset of Achilles tendinitis usually is acute, occurring after overuse or misuse of the ankle joint. Inciting factors may include activities such as running and sudden stopping and starting, as occurs when playing tennis. Improper stretching of the gastrocnemius and Achilles tendon prior to exercise also has been implicated in the development of Achilles tendinitis, as well as contributing to acute tendon rupture. The pain of Achilles tendinitis is constant and severe and is localized in the posterior ankle. Significant sleep disturbance is often reported. The patient might attempt to splint the inflamed Achilles tendon by adopting a flat-footed gait to avoid plantar-flexing the affected tendon. Patients with Achilles tendinitis exhibit pain with resisted plantar flexion of the foot as well as a positive creak sign. To elicit the creak sign for Achilles tendinitis, the patient is asked to sit on the side of the examination table with his or her legs hanging over the side of the table. The examiner then palpates the area overlying the Achilles tendon and with the other hand passively plantar-flexes and dorsi-flexes the foot (Fig. 240-2). The creak sign is considered positive if the examiner can appreciate a creaking or grating sensation with these movements.

Plain radiographs are indicated for all patients who present with posterior ankle pain. On the basis of the patient's clinical presentation, additional testing may be indicated, including complete blood count, sedimentation rate, and antinuclear antibody testing. Magnetic resonance and ultrasound imaging of the ankle will help to confirm the extent of damage to the Achilles tendon and to identify Achilles bursitis or bone spurs or xanthomas that might be causing repetitive trauma to the tendon (Figs. 240-3 and 240-4).

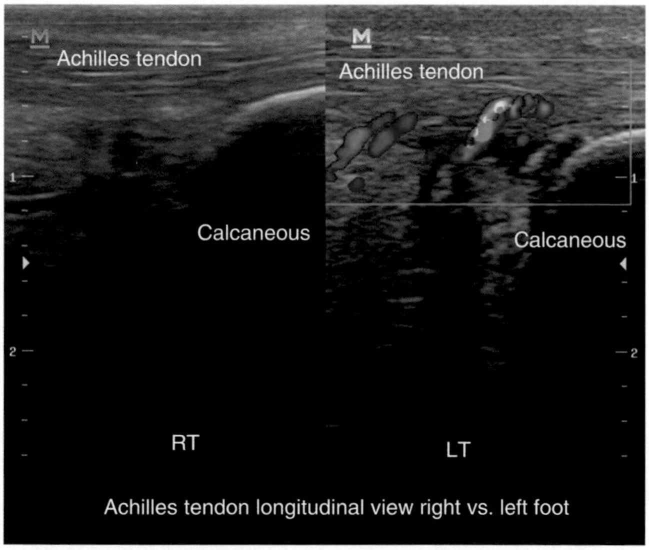

• **Figure 240-1** Longitudinal color Doppler images of the left and right ankles in the same patient demonstrating Achilles tendinitis. Note the neovascularization of the tendon on the *left*.

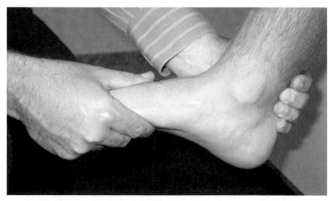

• **Figure 240-2** Eliciting the creak sign for Achilles tendinitis.

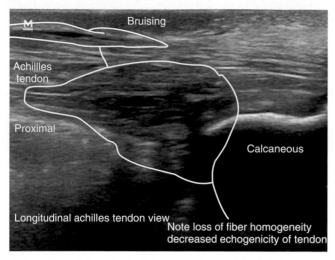

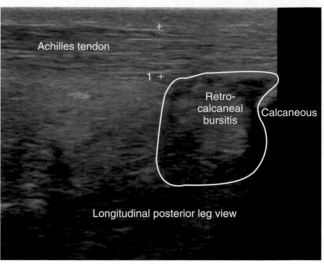

• **Figure 240-3** Longitudinal ultrasound image of the Achilles tendon in a patient with an acute ankle injury demonstrating significant tendinopathy of the Achilles tendon. Note the subcutaneous bruising and the loss of the normal echotexture of the tendon.

• **Figure 240-4** Longitudinal ultrasound image demonstrating retrocalcaneal bursitis in a long-distance runner.

The Achilles tendon is susceptible to rupture following either direct trauma to the tendon or sudden forced dorsiflexion of the ankle or plantar-flexed foot. Push-off injuries to the tendon occur when sudden stress is placed on the weight-bearing forefoot. The toe raise test is useful in the identification of rupture of the Achilles tendon. To perform the toe raise test for Achilles tendon rupture, the patient is asked to stand in a comfortable position and then to raise himself or herself up on tiptoes (Fig. 241-1). An inability to perform a toe raise on the affected side provides a presumptive diagnosis of rupture of the Achilles tendon, and magnetic resonance and/or ultrasound imaging of the tendon is indicated (Figs. 241-2 and 241-3).

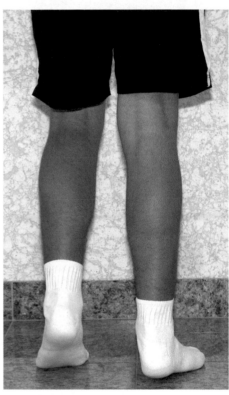

• **Figure 241-1** To perform the toe raise test for Achilles tendon rupture, the patient is asked to stand in a comfortable position and then to raise himself or herself up on tiptoes.

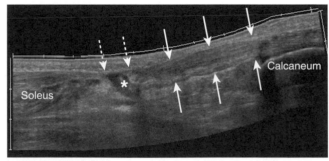

• **Figure 241-2** Longitudinal ultrasound image of an acute mid-Achilles tendon rupture. The distal tendon *(arrows)* appears relatively normal, although there is some low-reflective fluid within the deep portion of the paratenon. The torn ends of the tendon are visualized *(broken arrows),* and there is a low-reflective hematoma in the tendon gap *(asterisk).* (From Waldman SD, Campbell, RSD: *Imaging of pain,* Philadelphia, 2010, Saunders/Elsevier, p 432, fig 167-1.)

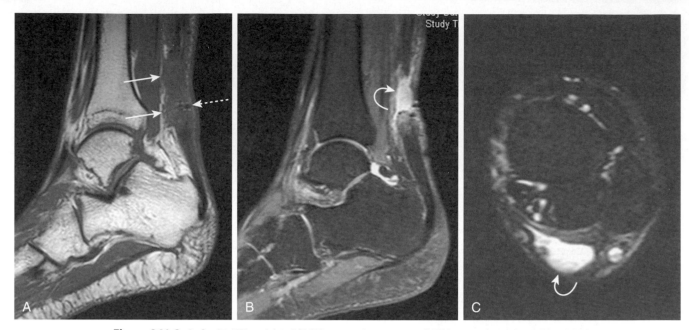

• **Figure 241-3 A,** Sagittal T1-weighted (T1W) magnetic resonance (MR) image of a patient with a failed Achilles tendon repair. The midportion of the tendon is thickened, irregular, and of intermediate signal intensity (SI) *(arrows)*. There are some areas of susceptibility artifact due to the previous tendon repair *(broken arrow)*. The sagittal **(B)** and axial **(C)** T2W with fat suppression (FST2W) MR images demonstrate the tendon gap filled by high-SI hematoma *(curved arrows)*.

The Achilles tendon is susceptible to rupture following either direct trauma to the tendon or sudden forced dorsiflexion of the ankle or plantar-flexed foot. Push-off injuries to the tendon occur when sudden stress is placed on the weight-bearing forefoot. The Thompson squeeze test is useful in the identification of rupture of the Achilles tendon. To perform the Thompson squeeze test for Achilles tendon rupture, the patient is asked to assume the sitting position with his or her feet hanging off the examination table. The examiner then grasps the calf on the patient's affected side just below the point of the calf's maximum girth and firmly squeezes the calf (Fig. 242-1). The absence of plantar flexion on the affected side provides a presumptive diagnosis of rupture of the Achilles tendon, and magnetic resonance imaging of the tendon is indicated (see Figs. 241-2 and 241-3).

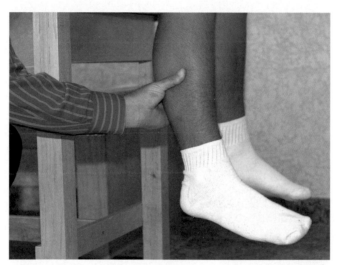

• **Figure 242-1** To perform the Thompson squeeze test for Achilles tendon rupture, the examiner grasps the calf on the patient's affected side just below the point of the calf's maximum girth and firmly squeezes the calf. Absence of plantar flexion on the affected side provides a presumptive diagnosis of rupture of the Achilles tendon.

The Achilles tendon is susceptible to rupture following either direct trauma to the tendon or sudden forced dorsiflexion of the ankle or plantar-flexed foot. Push-off injuries to the tendon occur when sudden stress is placed on the weight-bearing forefoot. The Matles test is useful in the identification of rupture of the Achilles tendon. To perform the Matles test for Achilles tendon rupture, the patient is asked to assume the prone position with his or her feet hanging off the examination table. The examiner then passively flexes the patient's knees to 90 degrees while both of the patient's feet are in neutral position. If the Achilles tendon is ruptured, there will be no plantar flexion of the affected foot (Fig. 243-1).

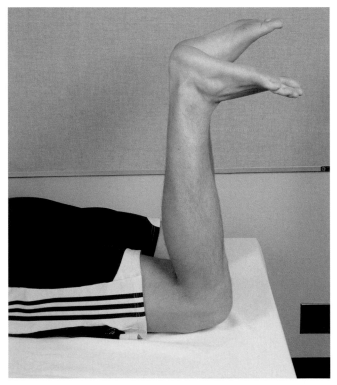

• **Figure 243-1** To perform the Matles test for Achilles tendon rupture, the patient is placed in the prone position and the examiner passively flexes the patient's knees to 90 degrees while both of the patient's feet are in neutral position. If the Achilles tendon is ruptured, there will be no plantar flexion of the affected foot.

Plantar fasciitis is characterized by pain and tenderness over the plantar surface of the calcaneus. Occurring twice as often in women as in men, plantar fasciitis is thought to be caused by an inflammation of the plantar fascia. This inflammation can occur alone or as part of a systemic inflammatory condition, such as rheumatoid arthritis, Reiter syndrome, or gout. Obesity also seems to predispose one to the development of plantar fasciitis, as does going barefoot or wearing house slippers for prolonged periods. High-impact aerobic exercise has also been implicated. The pain of plantar fasciitis is most severe on first walking after not bearing weight and is made worse by prolonged standing or walking.

On physical examination, the patient who suffers from plantar fasciitis will exhibit a positive calcaneal jump sign. To elicit the calcaneal jump sign, the patient is placed in a prone position on the examination table. The examiner uses his or her index finger to firmly press on the skin overlying the plantar medial calcaneal tuberosity (Fig. 244-1). The calcaneal jump sign is considered positive if this maneuver reproduces the patient's pain and causes the patient to jump or withdraw from the sudden onset of pain. The patient with plantar fasciitis also may have tenderness along the plantar fascia as it moves anteriorly. Pain is increased by dorsiflexing the toes, which pulls the plantar fascia taut, and then palpating along the fascia from the heel to the forefoot.

Plain radiographs are indicated for all patients who present with pain that is thought to emanate from plantar fasciitis to rule out occult bony pathology and tumor. On the basis of the patient's clinical presentation, additional testing including complete blood count, prostate-specific antigen, sedimentation rate, and antinuclear antibody testing might be indicated. Magnetic resonance and ultrasound imaging of the plantar surface of the foot can help to confirm the clinical diagnosis of plantar fasciitis and to rule out occult mass, fracture, or tumor (Figs. 244-2 and 244-3).

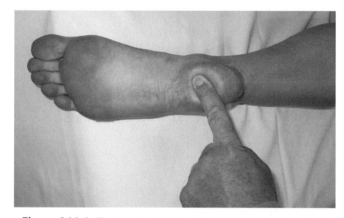

• **Figure 244-1** Eliciting the calcaneal jump sign for plantar fasciitis.

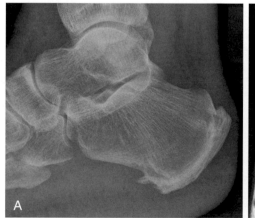
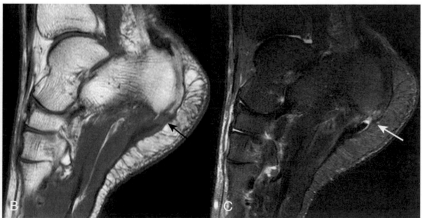

• **Figure 244-2 A,** Lateral radiograph of a plantar spur on the calcaneus. **B,** The sagittal T1W magnetic resonance (MR) image demonstrates thickening and increased signal intensity (SI) within the plantar fascia origin *(black arrow)*. There is high-SI fatty marrow within the bony spur. **C,** High-SI fluid *(white arrow)* is seen within the plantar fascia origin on the sagittal FST2W MR image. The appearances are consistent with plantar fasciitis and partial tearing of the origin of the fascia.

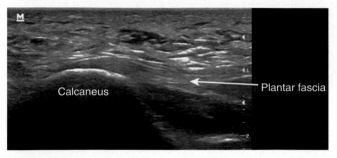

• **Figure 244-3** Longitudinal ultrasound image demonstrating the insertion of the plantar fascia on the calcaneus.

The plantar fascia plays an important role in stabilizing the calcaneus and the metatarsal heads when walking and running during the terminal stance when the heel is off the ground and the toes are in dorsiflexion. This is because dorsiflexion of the toes tightens the plantar fascia around the convex surface of the metatarsal heads, producing the windlass effect (Fig. 245-1). To perform the windlass test for plantar fasciitis, the patient is placed in the supine position with the knee flexed to 90 degrees and the affected foot in neutral position. The examiner then stabilizes the head of the first metatarsal and dorsiflexes the great toe (Fig. 245-2). The test is positive if it reproduces or exacerbates the patient's pain.

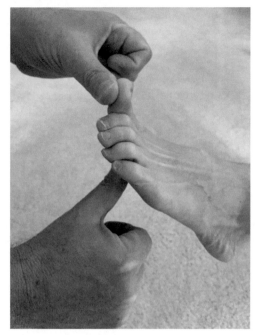

• **Figure 245-2** To perform the windlass test for plantar fasciitis, the patient is placed in the supine position and the examiner then stabilizes the head of the first metatarsal and dorsiflexes the great toe. The test is positive if it reproduces or exacerbates the patient's pain.

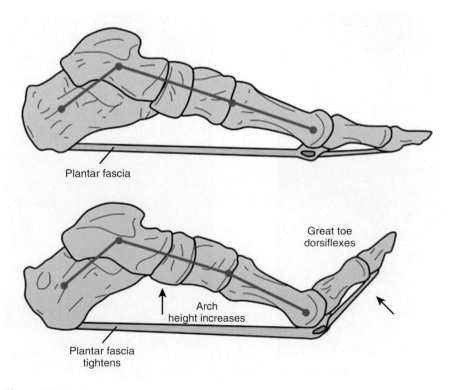

Plantar fascia

Great toe dorsiflexes

Arch height increases

Plantar fascia tightens

• **Figure 245-1** The windlass effect. Note how dorsiflexion of the toes tightens the plantar fascia.

Morton neuroma is one of the most common pain syndromes that affects the forefoot. Morton neuroma is characterized by tenderness and burning pain in the plantar surface of the forefoot, with associated painful paresthesias into the affected 2 toes. This pain syndrome is thought to be caused by perineural fibrosis of the interdigital nerves. Although the nerves between the third and fourth toes are most commonly affected, the second and third toes and, rarely, the fourth and fifth toes can be affected. The patient often feels that he or she is walking with a stone in his or her shoe. The pain of Morton neuroma worsens with prolonged standing or walking for long distances and is exacerbated by improperly fitted or padded shoes. As with bunion, bunionette, and hammer toe deformities, Morton neuroma is most often associated with the wearing of tight, narrow-toed shoes.

On physical examination, patients who suffer from Morton neuroma will exhibit a positive Mulder sign. To elicit the Mulder sign, the examiner has the patient assume the supine position on the examination table. The pain of Morton neuroma can be reproduced by firmly squeezing the 2 metatarsal heads together with 1 hand while placing firm pressure on the interdigital space with the other hand (Fig. 246-1). In contradistinction to metatarsalgia, in which the tender area remains over the metatarsal heads, with Morton neuroma the tender area is localized to only the plantar surface of the affected interspace, with paresthesias radiating into the 2 affected toes. The patient with Morton neuroma often exhibits an antalgic gait in an effort to reduce weight bearing during walking.

Plain radiographs are indicated in all patients who present with Morton neuroma to rule out stress fractures and to identify sesamoid bones that might have become inflamed. On the basis of the patient's clinical presentation, additional testing might be indicated, including complete blood count, sedimentation rate, and antinuclear antibody testing. Magnetic resonance and ultrasound imaging of the foot with contrast enhancement will readily identify Morton neuroma and is also useful if joint instability, occult mass, or tumor is suspected (Figs. 246-2 and 246-3). Radionucleotide bone scanning may be useful in identifying subtle stress fractures of the metatarsal bones or fractures of the sesamoid bones that might be missed on plain radiographs of the foot.

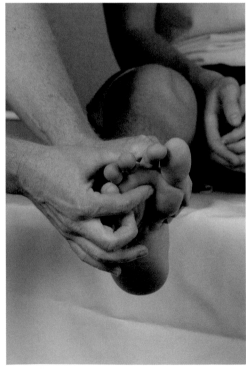

• **Figure 246-1** Mulder's maneuver is accomplished by firmly squeezing the 2 metatarsal heads together with 1 hand while placing firm pressure on the interdigital space with the other hand.

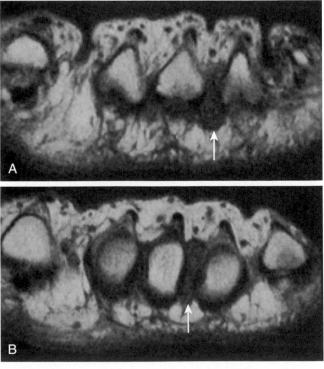

• **Figure 246-2** **A** and **B,** Consecutive coronal T1W magnetic resonance images of a low signal intensity Morton neuroma *(arrows)* arising between the third and fourth metatarsal heads. (From Waldman SD, Campbell, RSD: *Imaging of pain,* Philadelphia, 2010, Saunders/Elsevier, p 460, fig 179-2.)

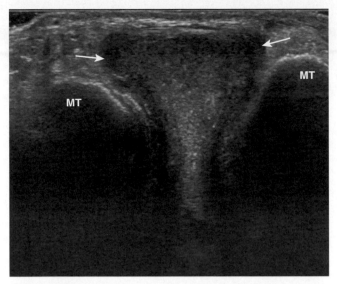

• **Figure 246-3** Transverse ultrasound image of an echogenic inter-metatarsal bursa *(arrows)* arising between the metatarsal necks (MT). The mass was easily compressible with sonopalpitation. (From Waldman SD, Campbell, RSD: *Imaging of pain,* Philadelphia, 2010, Saunders/Elsevier, p 460, fig 179-3.)

Index

Pages followed by *b, t,* or *f* refer to boxes, tables, or figures, respectively.